D1476209

ESTHETIC DENTISTRY IN CLINICAL PRACTICE

ESTHETIC DENTISTRY IN CLINICAL PRACTICE

Editor

Marc Geissberger, DDS, MA, BS, CPT
Chair, Department of Restorative Dentistry
Arthur A. Dugoni School of Dentistry
University of the Pacific
San Francisco, CA

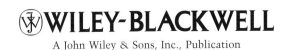
A John Wiley & Sons, Inc., Publication

Edition first published 2010
© 2010 Blackwell Publishing

Blackwell Publishing was acquired by John Wiley & Sons in February 2007. Blackwell's publishing program has been merged with Wiley's global Scientific, Technical, and Medical business to form Wiley-Blackwell.

Editorial Office
2121 State Avenue, Ames, Iowa 50014-8300, USA

For details of our global editorial offices, for customer services, and for information about how to apply for permission to reuse the copyright material in this book, please see our website at www.wiley.com/wiley-blackwell.

Authorization to photocopy items for internal or personal use, or the internal or personal use of specific clients, is granted by Blackwell Publishing, provided that the base fee is paid directly to the Copyright Clearance Center, 222 Rosewood Drive, Danvers, MA 01923. For those organizations that have been granted a photocopy license by CCC, a separate system of payments has been arranged. The fee codes for users of the Transactional Reporting Service are ISBN-13: 978-0-8138-2825-1/2010.

Designations used by companies to distinguish their products are often claimed as trademarks. All brand names and product names used in this book are trade names, service marks, trademarks or registered trademarks of their respective owners. The publisher is not associated with any product or vendor mentioned in this book. This publication is designed to provide accurate and authoritative information in regard to the subject matter covered. It is sold on the understanding that the publisher is not engaged in rendering professional services. If professional advice or other expert assistance is required, the services of a competent professional should be sought.

Disclaimer
The contents of this work are intended to further general scientific research, understanding, and discussion only and are not intended and should not be relied upon as recommending or promoting a specific method, diagnosis, or treatment by practitioners for any particular patient. The publisher and the author make no representations or warranties with respect to the accuracy or completeness of the contents of this work and specifically disclaim all warranties, including without limitation any implied warranties of fitness for a particular purpose. In view of ongoing research, equipment modifications, changes in governmental regulations, and the constant flow of information relating to the use of medicines, equipment, and devices, the reader is urged to review and evaluate the information provided in the package insert or instructions for each medicine, equipment, or device for, among other things, any changes in the instructions or indication of usage and for added warnings and precautions. Readers should consult with a specialist where appropriate. The fact that an organization or Website is referred to in this work as a citation and/or a potential source of further information does not mean that the author or the publisher endorses the information the organization or Website may provide or recommendations it may make. Further, readers should be aware that Internet Websites listed in this work may have changed or disappeared between when this work was written and when it is read. No warranty may be created or extended by any promotional statements for this work. Neither the publisher nor the author shall be liable for any damages arising herefrom.

Companies and the products and instruments cited in this book are solely to assist clinicians. The authors have no financial arrangements and derive no benefits from any of these companies.

Library of Congress Cataloging-in-Publication Data

Geissberger, Marc.
   Esthetic dentistry in clinical practice / Marc Geissberger. – 1st ed.
      p. ; cm.
   Includes bibliographical references and index.
   ISBN 978-0-8138-2825-1 (hardback : alk. paper)
1. Dentistry–Aesthetic aspects.   I. Title.
   [DNLM: 1. Esthetics, Dental. WU 100 G313e 2010]
   RK54.G45 2010
   617.6–dc22
                                              2009041422

A catalog record for this book is available from the U.S. Library of Congress.

Set in 9.5 on 12 pt Palatino by Toppan Best-set Premedia Limited
Printed in Singapore

1   2010

This text is dedicated to our colleague,
Dudley Cheu, DDS, MBA, BS
Assistant Professor
University of the Pacific
School of Dentistry

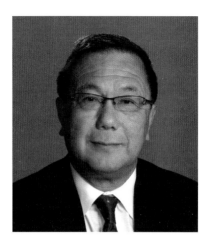

March 25, 1941–July 3, 2009

Dudley completed his undergraduate work in sociology and biology at Pacific Union College, University of California–Berkeley, and University of Southern California; he received his DDS from Northwestern University in 1970. He earned his MBA from University of the Pacific in 1999. After leading a successful private dental practice for over twenty-five years, Dudley taught dentistry at University of the Pacific for fifteen years. During his term at the dental school, he was recognized several times by faculty and students in recognition of teaching excellence. He was an active member of the ADA and CDA, volunteering at countless events and programs, serving on many committees, and helping with local arrangements at scientific sessions. His contribution to University of the Pacific and to dental societies, and even his recent trip to Cambodia teaching local dental students were fine examples of his life work and interest. His contributions to this text are greatly appreciated. He will be missed but never forgotten.

Contents

Contributors

Editor

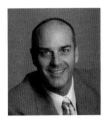

Marc Geissberger DDS, MA, BS, CPT

Marc Geissberger is an associate professor and chair of the Department of Restorative Dentistry at the University of the Pacific, Arthur A. Dugoni School of Dentistry. He has eighteen years of experience in dental education. Additionally, he mentors many students and young dentists in the arena of esthetic dentistry and serves as the university representative to the American Academy of Cosmetic Dentistry's University Council.

Contributing Authors

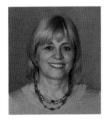

Gabriela Pitigoi-Aron DDS

Gabriela Pitigoi-Aron is an assistant professor and course director within the Department of Restorative Dentistry at the University of the Pacific, Arthur A. Dugoni School of Dentistry. She is a graduate of the Institute of Medicine and Pharmacy, School of Dentistry, in Bucharest, Romania, where she further completed the Advanced General Dentistry Program.

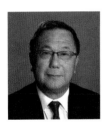

Dudley Cheu DDS, MBA

Dudley Cheu received his DDS from Northwestern University School of Dentistry and an MBA from the University of the Pacific Eberhardt School of Business. Dr. Cheu is an assistant professor and codirector of the International Dental Studies Curriculum in the Restorative Department at the University of the Pacific.

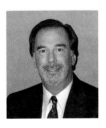

Daniel Castagna DDS

Dan Castagna received his Doctor of Dental Surgery from the University of the Pacific School of Dentistry in 1981. From graduation to 1989, he participated in full-time private practice in South San Francisco and was part-time faculty at Pacific. In 1990 he transitioned to full-time dental education, acquiring the rank of assistant clinical professor in fixed prosthodontics and removable prosthodontics.

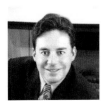

Foroud Hakim DDS, MBA, BS

Foroud Hakim earned his DDS from the University of the Pacific in 1991. In addition to his private practice in general and esthetic dentistry, he currently holds a full-time position at Pacific as assistant professor and curriculum director for the Department of Restorative Dentistry.

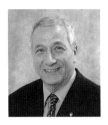

Robert Hepps DDS, BS

Robert Hepps is an assistant professor in the Department of Restorative Dentistry at the University of the Pacific. He is a 1971 graduate of the Ohio State University School of Dentistry and has lectured and directed programs on esthetics, practice growth, and development of the comprehensive practice in New York, Florida, and California. He is founder and director of the California Academy of Aesthetic Dentistry and maintains a private practice in San Francisco.

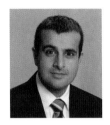

Parag R. Kachalia DDS, BS

Parag Kachalia is an assistant professor in the Department of Restorative Dentistry and codirector of the Pre-doctoral Fixed Prosthodontics Program at the University of the Pacific. He also maintains a private practice in San Ramon, California, with a focus on restorative and cosmetic dentistry.

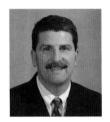

Brian J. Kenyon DMD, BA

Brian Kenyon completed his undergraduate studies at Brown University and graduated from Tufts University School of Dental Medicine in 1982. He was in private practice in Smithfield, Rhode Island, for seventeen years prior to accepting a full-time faculty position at the University of the Pacific. Dr. Kenyon is currently an associate professor in the Department of Restorative Dentistry and maintains a private practice in San Francisco, California.

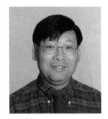

Kenneth G. Louie DDS, MA, BA

Kenneth Louie completed his undergraduate studies at the University of California–Berkeley and graduated from the University of the Pacific in 1988. Dr. Louie is the codirector of Pre-clinical Operative and teaches in the senior clinic generalist model. He maintains a private practice in San Francisco, California, in restorative and esthetic dentistry.

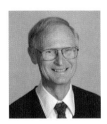

Richard G. Lubman DDS

Richard Lubman is a graduate of the Loyola University School of Dentistry in Chicago, Illinois, and has practiced esthetic and restorative dentistry for over thirty years in California. Following retirement from private practice, he joined the faculty as an assistant professor of restorative dentistry at the University of the Pacific.

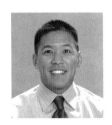

Mark Macaoay DDS, BS

Mark Macaoay graduated from the University of the Pacific, Arthur A. Dugoni School of Dentistry, and completed an Advanced Education in General Dentistry residency at the Naval Dental Center in San Diego, California. He currently is an assistant professor in the Department of Restorative Dentistry at the University of the Pacific and maintains a private practice in the San Francisco Bay Area.

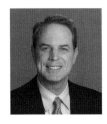

James Milani DDS, BA

Jim Milani received a DDS degree from the University of the Pacific in 1982. He is an assistant professor in the Department of Restorative Dentistry and maintains a private practice in Lakeport, California.

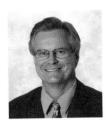

Jeffrey P. Miles DDS

Jeff Miles graduated from the University of California–San Francisco in 1980. Following twenty-one years of private practice in the San Francisco Bay Area, he joined the faculty at the University of the Pacific, Arthur A. Dugoni School of Dentistry.

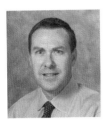

James B. Morris DDS, BS

Brad Morris graduated from the University of the Pacific with a degree in dentistry in 1991. He continued his education at Columbia University and graduated in 1995 with a certificate in the specialty of prosthodontics. Dr. Morris currently has a practice in Mill Valley, California, and is an assistant professor in the Department of Restorative Dentistry at the University of the Pacific.

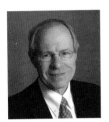

Warden Noble DDS, MS, BS

Ward Noble graduated from the University of California at San Francisco with a degree in Dentistry in 1965, and he obtained a master's in education in 1968 as well as a master's in restorative dentistry in 1970. Dr. Noble is a certified prosthodontist and has worked in private practice for more than thirty years. He is currently a professor in the Department of Restorative Dentistry at the University of the Pacific.

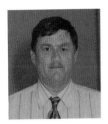

Donnie G. Poe, CDT

Donnie Poe has been a certified dental technician since 1974. He has served the dental laboratory profession since 1981 at the local, state, and national levels. Since 1987 Mr. Poe has given clinics and lectured nationally on waxing, casting, and use of the stereo microscope in dental technology, and he is now on staff at the University of the Pacific.

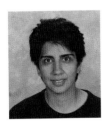

Gitta Radjaeipour DDS, EdD

Gitta Radjaeipour is an assistant professor of restorative dentistry at the University of the Pacific and has practiced esthetic and restorative dentistry for seventeen years in Northern California. She graduated from Pacific's dental school in 1992 and has been on faculty continuously since her graduation.

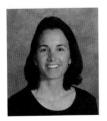

Laura Reid DDS, BS

Laura Reid is an assistant professor in the Department of Restorative Dentistry at the University of the Pacific. She has taught dental anatomy and fixed prosthodontics for the past eight years and practices in Santa Rosa, California.

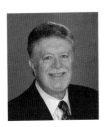

Eugene Santucci DDS, MA, BS

Eugene Santucci is full-time faculty in the Department of Restorative Dentistry and director of the second-year restorative curriculum. He is a frequent lecturer in the Predoctoral Occlusion course and directs the Occlusion Plus postgraduate program. He maintains a private practice with his wife in Atherton, California.

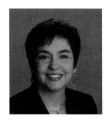

Noelle Santucci DDS, MA, BS

Noelle Santucci is an assistant professor in the Department of Restorative Dentistry at the University of the Pacific, Arthur A. Dugoni School of Dentistry. She maintains a private practice with her husband in Atherton, California.

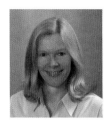

Karen A. Schulze DDS, PhD

Karen Schulze graduated in 1992 from the dental program and in 1998 from the PhD program at the University of Leipzig, School of Dentistry in Germany. She is currently an assistant professor and director of the Restorative Research Division in the Department of Restorative Dentistry at the University of the Pacific and maintains a private practice in San Francisco, California.

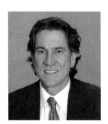

Ai B. Streacker DDS, BS

Ai Streacker graduated from the University of the Pacific School of Dentistry in 1979, and in 2002 retired from a successful two-decade-plus private practice in San Francisco specializing in esthetic and reconstructive dentistry. He is now an assistant professor in the Department of Restorative Dentistry at the University of the Pacific School of Dentistry. He is the recipient of the Mark Hagge award and the Lucien Schmyd memorial award for excellence in teaching.

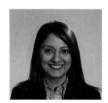

Bina Surti DDS

Bina Surti graduated from the University of Detroit Mercy School of Dentistry and completed a residency in Advanced Education in General Dentistry and a fellowship in Implant Restoration at Case Western Reserve University School of Dentistry. She is currently an assistant professor at University of the Pacific in the Department of Restorative Dentistry.

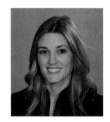

Jessie Vallee DDS, BS

Jessie Vallee is an assistant professor in the Department of Restorative Dentistry at the University of the Pacific. She is a 2004 graduate of Pacific who served three years in the United States Naval Dental Corps upon graduation. She is currently an instructor of Occlusion, Pre-Clinical Fixed Prosthodontics, Integrated Clinical Sciences and maintains a part-time private practice in San Francisco, California.

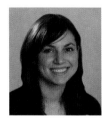

Marina Wasche DDS, BS

Marina Wasche graduated with honors from the University of California–Davis where she received her Bachelor of Science in biological sciences. She received her Doctor of Dental Surgery with honors from the University of the Pacific and has since become full-time faculty at the Arthur A. Dugoni School of Dentistry. She was recently appointed the director of New Technologies for the Department of Restorative Dentistry.

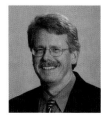

Richard H. White DDS, BA

Richard White is an assistant professor in the Department of Restorative Dentistry at the University of the Pacific. He has a BA from Albion College and is a graduate of the University of Michigan School of Dentistry. He completed a Dental General Practice residency with the United States Public Health Service, where he continued for a twenty-seven-year career and achieved the rank of dental director. He currently lectures in the occlusion course and restorative dentistry courses at the University of the Pacific.

ESTHETIC DENTISTRY IN CLINICAL PRACTICE

Chapter 1
Introduction to Concepts in Esthetic Dentistry

Marc Geissberger DDS, MA, BS, CPT

General Principles of Esthetics

Esthetics (also spelled aesthetics) is a subdiscipline of value theory or axiology, which is a branch of philosophy that studies sensory values, sometimes called judgments of sentiment or taste. Esthetics is closely associated with the philosophy of High Art. Esthetics includes art as well as the very purpose behind it. Esthetics as a branch of philosophy studies art, the methods of evaluating art, and judgments of art. Art has existed through all recorded human history. Art is unique to human beings because of our innate ability to abstract. Esthetics is important because it examines the reasons why art has always existed and attempts to bring clarity to a vastly complex intellectual human need (Manns 1997).

The term *aesthetics* is derived from the Greek $a\ \sigma\theta\eta\tau\iota\kappa\acute{\eta}$ "aisthetike" and was coined by the philosopher Alexander Gottlieb Baumgarten in 1735 to mean "the science of how things are known via the senses." The term was used in German, shortly after Baumgarten introduced its Latin form (*Aesthetica*), but it did not come into popular use in English until the beginning of the nineteenth century (Kivy 1998). However, much the same study was called studying the "standards of taste" or "judgments of taste" in English, following the vocabulary set by David Hume prior to the introduction of the term *aesthetics* (Hume 1987).

It has been said that "beauty is in the eye of the beholder." This very concept suggests that there may not be universal agreement on what constitutes art or beauty. Look at the two images that follow (figs.1-1 and 1-2). Both are paintings, one abstract and one realistic. Do both appeal to you as a viewer? If so, why? If not, why not? By nature, all esthetic undertakings will elicit an emotional response from its creator, the receipient of the esthetic work, and the larger viewing audience. Successful art must not only appeal to its creator but to the recipient and larger viewing audience as well. Additionally, what one group or society may deem esthetic, another may dismiss as overtly unappealing. Esthetics and art do not necessarily cross cultural, political, generational, or societal boundaries. This being said, can there be a set of guidelines that increase the likelihood of art being deemed esthetic?

Although esthetics studies the broader context of art and may be difficult to fully conceptualize, principles do exist within the field of art that can dramatically enhance the aesthetic appeal of any piece of artwork. This textbook will provide dental practitioners with several tools designed to enhance the beauty of the dental restorations they create. Throughout this text, practitioners will be introduced to several guiding principles, techniques, and methods that, when followed, can dramatically increase the esthetic appeal of their efforts. The goal of this text is to organize and define concepts of esthetics into tangible, meaningful tools that can be applied to the practice of esthetic dentistry.

Esthetic (Cosmetic) Dentistry

For years, the focus of the practice of dentistry was primarily the prevention and treatment of dental disease. This has been loosely described as "need"-based dentistry (Christensen 2000). In the mid to late twentieth century, dentistry evolved as a highly organized profession with advanced treatment methodologies and protocols enabling dentists to successfully treat dental disease. As tooth-colored restorative materials were developed, both dentists and the public began to recognize the esthetic improvements that could be obtained with these advances. During the later part of the twentieth century, practitioners began to see a shift in the type of dentistry the public was seeking. The public was no longer forced to select between metallic restorative materials that restored function but presented esthetic compromises. With the rapid improvements in tooth-colored restorative materials, the discovery of tooth-whitening agents, and the American preoccupation with appearance, patients were suddenly seeking selective procedures that focused on the esthetic improvement of

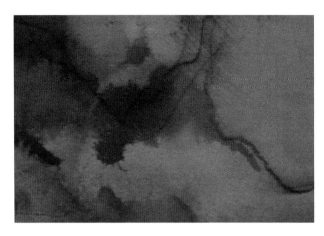

Figure 1-1. Abstract artwork, watercolor on paper, artist unknown.

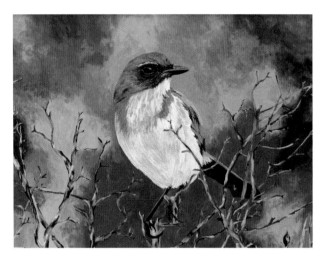

Figure 1-2. Scrub jay, guache on paper. Artist: Marc Geissberger.

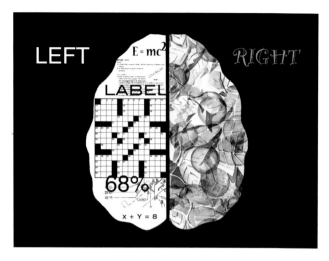

Figure 1-3. Schematic representation of the left and right hemispheres of the brain.

To be successful, the practitioner must be able to put aside personal bias and allow the patient to guide esthetic decisions. Once this occurs, the likelihood of esthetic success dramtically increases. If the dentist is too controlling of the process, superimposing his or her esthetic preconceptions over those of the patient, chances of success will decrease.

Why Is Esthetic Dentistry Stimulating?

Roger W. Sperry PhD, a professor of psychobiology, won a Nobel Peace Prize for Physiology or Medicine in 1981 for his discoveries concerning the functional specialization of the cerebral hemispheres, namely, defining the different function of the left and right hemispheres of the brain. His work led to the belief that the left brain is associated with verbal, logical, and analytical thinking. It excels in naming and categorizing things, symbolic abstraction, speech, reading, writing, and arithmetic. The right brain, on the other hand, functions in a nonverbal manner and excels in visual, spatial, perceptual, and intuitive information (Sperry 1973; fig. 1-3). Dentistry, as a profession, is a relatively left-brain activity where facts rule, strategies are formed, and detail-oriented behavior is commonplace. A well-constructed, logical plan and implementation of any surgical procedure or treatment is essential for clinical success. Esthetics and art are largely right-brain functions, where imagination is prevalent, spatial perception abounds, and possibilities are explored. Success in this area requires imagination, vision, and flexibility.

The successful practice of esthetic dentistry capitalizes on a combination of left-and right-brain behavior. The

their dentitions. The age of "want"-based dentistry was born (Christensen 2000).

Esthetic (cosmetic) dentistry is a discipline within dentistry in which the primary focus is the modification or alteration of appearance of a patient's oral structures, in conjunction with the treatment and prevention of structural, functional, or organic oral disease. Through cosmetic dentistry, the appearance of the mouth is altered to more closely match the patient's subjective concept of what is visually pleasing. Under this definition, successful cosmetic dentistry adheres to the principal that "beauty is in the eye of the beholder." Furthermore, it requires the practitioner, as the artist, to recognize the subjective nature of all esthetic undertakings.

Under this principle, the dentist is the artist and the patient is the recipient of the artwork. Both individuals have an emotional investment in the process and results.

left-brain behavior allows practitioners to develop sound, logical, and predictable treatment plans. Additionally, they can accomplish the detail work that is required for successful clinical outcomes. The artistic mindset required for esthetic dentistry allows practitioners to engage the right brain in visual, spatial, and intuitive behavior. This total brain engagement may help explain why esthetic dentistry is so appealing and professionally rewarding for dental professionals. Esthetic dentistry can provide a highly stimulating body of work, requiring the practitioner to balance logic, facts, and the known with feeling, perception, and the unknown.

A Brief History of Esthetic Dentistry

Ancient Esthetics

Examples of prehistoric art exist, but they are rare, and the context of their production and use is not very clear, so we can little more than guess at the esthetic culture that guided their production and interpretation. Ancient art was largely, but not entirely, based on the six great ancient civilizations: Egypt, Mesopotamia, Greece, Rome, India, and China. Each of these centers of early civilization developed a unique and characteristic style in its art. Greece had the most influence on the development of esthetics in the West. The period dominated by Greek art saw a veneration of the human physical form and the development of corresponding skills to show musculature, poise, beauty, and anatomically correct proportions.

Greek philosophers initially felt that esthetically appealing objects were beautiful in and of themselves. Plato felt that beautiful objects incorporated proportion, harmony, and unity among their parts. Similarly, in the *Metaphysics*, Aristotle found that the universal elements of beauty were order, symmetry, and definiteness (Ahmad 2005). These "mathematical" theories of esthetics have been used to establish many of today's concepts in esthetic dentistry. It must be noted that although several mathematical principles can be applied to beauty and esthetics, they are merely tools and do not constitute absolutes; they will be discussed in greater detail in later chapters.

In twenty-first century United States, dental esthetics may be simplified to include a full dentition consisting of straight, white teeth. The so-called "Hollywood" smile, popularized by American cinema and television, can be recognized worldwide. History shows us that throughout the world, this may not have always been the case. There are several examples of tooth modification for esthetic reasons that do not adhere to the standard of the "Hollywood" smile. Recognizing that there have been and still remain many different concepts of esthetic dentistry helps illustrate that dental beauty is truly in the eye of the beholder. Furthermore, what is appealing to one group may be unappealing to another.

So Much for White Teeth: The Japanese Tradition of Tooth Blackening

An examination of skeletal remains and art from the Asuka to the Edo period (from the seventh to the nineteenth century) reveals a tradition of intentional tooth blackening as a practice among both women and men. The custom, an esthetic symbol from ancient times in Japan called *ohaguro*, became popular among married women as a way of distinguishing themselves from unmarried women and providing contrast to their white painted faces. The artwork pictured here depicts women from this era with intentionally blackened teeth (fig. 1-4). The black dye was an oxidized mixture of iron shavings melted in vinegar and powdered gallnuts. The tradition of ohaguro became popular among males, especially court nobles and commanders. Among samurais, the custom of ohaguro was a symbol of loyalty to one master within a lifetime. In the case of men, the custom is said to have ended around the Muromati Era (1558–1572) and was far less popular and short-lived compared with the female tradition (Hara 2001). With its origin in Japan, this tradition spread throughout Asia.

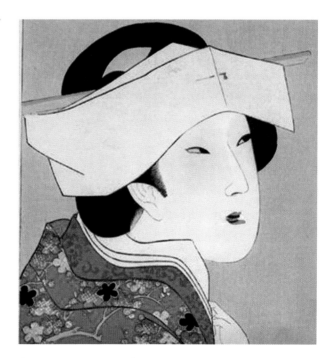

Figure 1-4. Japanese art depicting a woman with blackened teeth, circa sixteenth century.

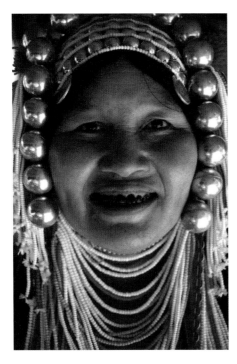

Figure 1-5. Modern version of *ohaguro* depicting Asian female with ceremonially blackened teeth.

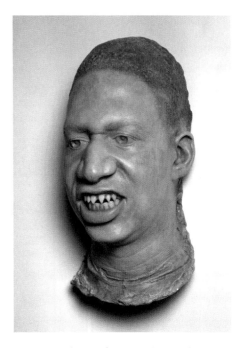

Figure 1-6. Cast reproduction of a Bantu tribesman depicting typical tooth modification. Courtesy Dr. Scott Swank, curator, the Dr. Samuel D. Harris National Museum of Dentistry.

The tradition of blackening of teeth can still be seen in small pockets of Asian culture today (fig. 1-5).

African Tooth Modification

The Bantu people of Africa have a myth that holds that death enters the human body through the teeth. Due to this longstanding belief, the Bantu file teeth into points in an attempt to create a portal trough which death may exit the body (Favazza 1996). Figure 1-6 is a photograph of cast reproduction of a Bantu tribesman depicting typical tooth modification associated with these people. Although this tooth modification process has its roots in ancient tribal mythology, over time, this custom became the esthetic norm for many Bantu adults. This created a cultural shift in what constituted a beautiful smile for the Bantu people. Although some may find these tooth modifications to be utterly unaesthetic, the Bantu accept them as beautiful.

Esthetics during the Roman Empire

Roman citizens were acutely aware of tooth-related esthetics. Some practices of the Romans may provide the first real evidence of a cultural bias for whiter teeth. First-century Roman physicians advocated brushing teeth with Portuguese urine to achieve a whiter appearance.

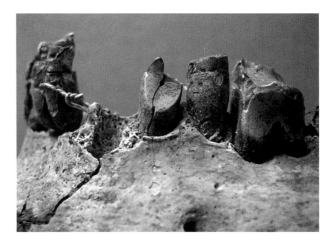

Figure 1-7. First- to second-century attempt at a fixed partial denture involving the lower anterior teeth of a female Roman citizen.

The appearance of missing teeth had a significant social impact in Roman culture. Teeth were crudely replaced for both functional and esthetic purposes. One of the earliest known dental prostheses can be traced to the early Roman Empire. The prosthetic devise utilized multi-karat gold wire to string together "artificial teeth." The teeth, pictured here, date from the first to the second century AD. They were found in the mouth of an unidentified woman who was buried in an elaborate mausoleum within a Roman necropolis (fig. 1-7).

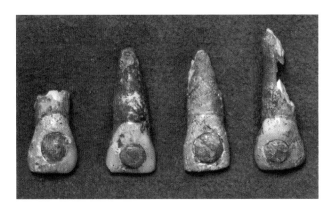

Figure 1-8. Mayan jadeite inlays. Courtesy Dr. Scott Swank, curator, the Dr. Samuel D. Harris National Museum of Dentistry.

Central American Esthetic Dentistry

Little is known about the Mayan empire because early settlers from Europe destroyed most of its written history. Despite the lack of recorded history, a fair amount has been discovered from Mayan archeological findings. Human remains discovered in Mayan burial sites display two types of esthetic tooth modification. The first is tooth filing, which created a step appearance in the incisors. The second is a sophisticated technique of inlaying various semiprecious stones on the facial aspect of anterior teeth and some first premolars (Ring 1985). This technique utilized round inlay preparations placed in the enamel with corresponding round inlays of jadeite, turquoise, hematite, or other locally available minerals (fig. 1-8).

Victorian Era Esthetics

The Victorian age saw many advances in technological breakthroughs and science. With the advent of marketing and direct sales, the public was inundated with new products touting many great benefits in the marketplace. Many examples of esthetic treatment offerings emerged in the form of trade cards. These advertising trade cards often made several exaggerated claims regarding the benefits of the products or services being sold, although the public largely accepted their claims with little hesitation or skepticism (Croll and Swanson 2006).

Current State of Esthetic Dentistry in the United States

The previous sections have illustrated many different types of nontherapeutic tooth modifications centered on esthetic enhancement of the dentition and smile. In 2000

at its annual convention, the American Dental Association asked its member dentists which services were most requested by their forty- to sixty-year-old patients. More than 66% of the dentists surveyed reported that tooth whitening was the first request among that age group. Furthermore, 65% of dentists reported other cosmetic procedures such as crowns and bonding as the second most sought after treatment (McCann 2001). In a 2005 survey of 9,000 American dentists, the American Academy of Cosmetic Dentistry (AACD) found that dentists experienced a 12.5% increase in the number of esthetic procedures done in their offices over a five-year period. The dentists reported that tooth whitening was the number-one requested esthetic procedure (29%; Levin 2005).

Since its creation, the AACD has surveyed American patients regarding esthetic dentistry and their personal preferences. The findings have remained quite consistent over the last two decades. Ninety-two percent of Americans report that an attractive smile is an important social asset. Only 50% of Americans report being happy with their smile. In 2004, the AACD asked Americans, "What is the first thing you notice in a person's smile?" The most common responses were

1. Straightness
2. Whiteness and color of teeth
3. Cleanliness of teeth
4. Sincerity of smile
5. Any missing teeth?
6. Sparkle of smile

When the same group of Americans was asked, "What types of things do you consider make a smile unattractive?" the most common responses were

1. Discolored, yellow, or stained teeth
2. Missing teeth
3. Crooked teeth
4. Decaying teeth and cavities
5. Gaps and spaces in teeth
6. Dirty teeth

And finally, when respondents were asked, "What would you most like to improve about your smile?" the most common response was they wished they had whiter and brighter teeth (AACD 2004).

A Broader View of Esthetics

Although the overwhelming American concept of what constitutes a beautiful smile and teeth may be somewhat uniform, it must be noted that there still remains some variation on just what constitutes a beautiful smile. The concept that big, straight, white teeth with full lips and

Table 1-1.   Organizations dedicated to esthetic dentistry.

Academy Name	Year Established	Web Address
American Academy of Esthetic Dentistry	1975	www.estheticacademy.org
American Academy of Cosmetic Dentistry	1984	www.aacd.com
European Academy of Esthetic Dentistry	1986	www.eaed.org
Japanese Academy of Esthetic Dentistry	1990	www.jdshinbi.net
Indian Academy of Aesthetic & Cosmetic Dentistry	1991	www.iaacd.org
Brazilian Society of Aesthetic Dentistry	1994	www.sboe.com.br
British Academy of Aesthetic Dentistry	1995	www.baad.org.uk
Scandinavian Academy of Esthetic Dentistry	1996	www.saed.nu
European Society of Esthetic Dentistry	2003	www.esed-online.com
Canadian Academy for Esthetic Dentistry	2004	www.caed.ca
Australian Academy of Cosmetic Dentistry	2005	www.aacd.com.au

minimal gingival display represent a beautiful smile is a relatively narrow perspective. If one accepts the notion advanced by the early Greek philosophers that beauty and esthetics is a harmonious blend of symmetry and proportion, one could argue that unaesthetic or unattractive things may, by default, lack symmetry and have poor proportion. When this concept is applied to the smile, we could hypothesize that a beautiful smile would be harmonious, symmetrical, and well proportioned. The human eye may be predisposed to identify objects as symmetrical and well proportioned. The further an object is from this predisposition, the less likely that object would be perceived as beautiful.

Professional Organizations that Promote Esthetic Dentistry

With the increased awareness of esthetic dentistry throughout the world, it became increasingly important for dental professionals to have focused resources where they could grow their knowledge base, share information with colleagues, and meet formally at annual sessions. This led to the formation of numerous professional organizations with esthetic dentistry as their main focus. Above is a table containing several leading organizations in chronological order from their founding year (table 1-1).

Works Cited

AACD. 2004. *Survey of American Public.* American Academy of Cosmetic Dentistry.

Ahmad I. 2005. Anterior dental aesthetics: Historical perspective. *British Dental Journal* 198:737–72.

Christensen GJ. 2000. Elective vs. mandatory dentistry. *J Am Dent Assoc* 131(10):1496–8.

Croll TP, Swanson BZ. 2006. Victorian era esthetic and restorative dentistry: An advertising trade card gallery. *J Esthet Restor Dent* 18(5):235–54.

Favazza AR. 1996. *Bodies Under Siege, Self-mutilation and Body Modification in Culture and Psychiatry,* JHU Press.

Hara Y. 2001. *Green Tea: Health Benefits and Applications,* CRC Press.

Hume D. 1987. *Essays, Moral, Political, and Literary,* Liberty Fund, Inc.

Kivy P. 1998. *The Blackwell Guide to Aesthetics.* Oxford, England: Blackwell.

Levin RP. 2005. *North American Survey: The State of Cosmetic Dentistry.* Levin Group Study Commissioned by the American Academy of Cosmetic Dentistry. Madison, Wisconsin.

Manns JW. 1997. *Explorations in Philosophy: Aesthetics.* M E Sharpe.

McCann D. 2001. Who needs Geritol? Give us brighter smiles! *Dental Practice Report,* pp. 24–6.

Ring ME. 1985. *Dentistry, an Illustrated History.* New York: Harry N. Abrams & Mosby-Year Book.

Sperry RW. 1973. *Hemispheric Specialization of Mental Faculties in the Brain of Man.* New York: Random House.

Chapter 2
Guiding Principles of Esthetic Dentistry

Marina Wasche DDS, BS

Robert Hepps DDS, BS

Marc Geissberger DDS, MA, BS, CPT

Esthetic dentistry—complicated, multifaceted, and emotionally charged—can be quite intimidating for the new practitioner. Many general principles of esthetic dentistry must be considered for successful esthetic treatment. Although esthetic dentistry is as much an art form as a science, there are several guiding principles that can dramatically improve the success of esthetic treatment. These principles or guidelines should govern the decision-making process of the esthetic dentist. The purpose of this chapter is to outline the basic guidelines of esthetic dentistry by discussing the following core concepts in detail:

Ethical principles
Frame of reference—macroesthetics
Lip assessment
Smile pattern
Gingival tissue assessment
Phonetics
Extent of treatment and material selection
Microesthetics

Ethical Principles

The American Dental Association has outlined several ethical principles that define the ethical practice of dentistry of its members. As with all aspects of dentistry, ethical principles must be maintained throughout esthetic treatment. Patient autonomy or self-governance refers to the quality or state of being independent, free, and self-directing (Oxford University Press 2005). This principle is paramount in the practice of esthetic dentistry and must never be marginalized. The patient must be intimately involved in the esthetic decision-making process. Although dentists should never perform any treatment to which they are opposed, they must take the patient's wishes into consideration.

Nonmalfeasance is the ethical principle of doing no harm, based on the Hippocratic maxim, *primum non nocere*, "first do no harm" (Oxford University Press 2005). Treatment rendered by the esthetic dentist should

never bring harm to the patient. Esthetic treatment should not be undertaken if there is a reasonable chance the patient will end up in worse shape than they were prior to treatment. Close attention to detail during treatment planning and case design can greatly decrease the chance of this occurring.

Beneficence and justice refer to the dentist's duty to demonstrate kindness and fairness throughout treatment. Esthetic treatment, in various forms, should be available to all, regardless of race or socioeconomic condition. The esthetic dentist should always practice to the highest standard of care possible, staying current on methods and materials in order to provide their patient with quality treatment.

Being honest and having integrity demonstrate the ethical principle of veracity, which is also expected of all dental practitioners. An esthetic dentist should always practice within the scope of his or her ability, never misleading the patient, and making sure that the patient's periodontal health, occlusal stability, proper phonetics, and masticatory function are maintained in the course of all comprehensive oral healthcare. Esthetic treatment must follow this same principle.

Macroesthetics

Traditional dental training in most universities tends to focus on microesthetics. Students are taught line angles, point angles, and heights of contour, and they focus on the minutia of dental morphology. This intense focus can often create an unfortunate perspective where practitioners are able to recognize the "tree but not the forest." One of the most critical features of esthetic success has far less to do with microesthetics and far more to do with macroesthetics. Taking into account the relationship of the teeth to each other and surrounding anatomic features trumps all concepts of microesthetics.

Regardless of how attractive or natural teeth appear individually, the overall impression will not be esthetic if they do not blend harmoniously with the rest of the facial structures. Macroesthetics guides the creation of tooth arrangement in harmony with the gingiva, lips, and face of the patient (Morley 2001). Combinations of tooth forms, when positioned together, have the potential to create an effect that is greater than, equal to, or less than the sum of the parts (Golub-Evans 1994). Taking into account macroesthetic elements such as midline location, intertooth relationships, lip assessment, and gingival architecture when designing an esthetic case is essential for achieving superior results.

Dental Midline

The dentist must make several observations about the individual facial features of each patient in order to determine the correct placement of the dental midline. The first observation should be an assessment of the symmetry of the patient's face. It is not uncommon to encounter patients that possess some form of facial asymmetry. The dental midline should coincide with the facial midline whenever possible. However, as long as the dental midline is within 4 mm of the facial midline and is parallel to the long axis of the face, the public generally does not perceive it as unaesthetic (figs. 2-1 and 2-2; Kokich, Kiyak, and Shapiro 1999). There are several principles that must be considered when addressing the maxillary dental midline. They are listed in order of importance:

1. The maxillary dental midline should always be positioned parallel to the facial midline.
2. The maxillary dental midline should be centered as close to the facial midline as possible.
3. The incisal edge of the maxillary incisors should be set perpendicular to the dental midline of the maxillary incisors.

4. The incisal edge of the maxillary incisors should parallel the interpupillary line in individuals with eyes positioned symmetrically.
5. The dental midlines of both arches should correspond with each other whenever possible.

In order to make an appropriate assessment of these landmarks and achieve as much symmetry as possible for a patient, dentists should obtain photographs and a facial landmark registration, commonly referred to as a "T-reference" or "stick bite." This procedure uses bite registration material and micro-brushes positioned facial to and over the mandibular central incisors to record the facial midline and interpupillary line. Common landmarks to gauge the proper facial midline are the nasion and the philtrum (fig. 2-3). These may not be accurate in all patients. In most cases it may be better to use the midline of the face from upper bridge of the nose to the chin as the reference for this record. A hori-

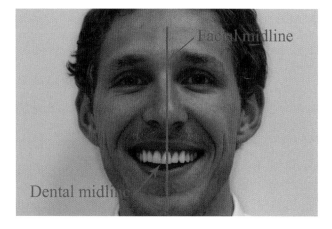

Figure 2-2.   Example of deviated midline with labels.

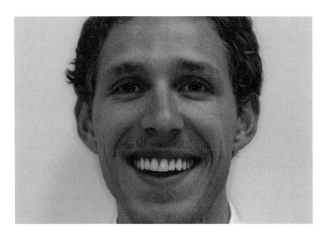

Figure 2-1.   Example of deviated midline.

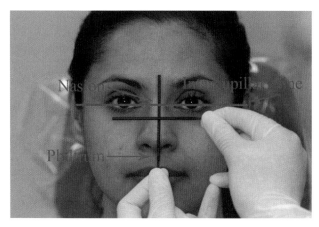

Figure 2-3.   Picture of stick bite with nasion, philtrum, and interpupillary line marked.

zontal reference can be taken from the interpupillary line when symmetry is observed.

If facial asymmetries make the interpupillary line unreliable, a horizontal reference can be simply made perpendicular to the facial midline or parallel to the floor when the patient's head is held in a vertical position (figs. 2-4 and 2-5; Morley 2001). Once the appropriate horizontal and vertical references have been selected, the dentist should position the microbrushes along these planes and secure the proper positions with bite registration material (figs. 2-6, 2-7, and 2-8). Some material should flow between the anterior teeth while the patient is in centric occlusion so the reference can be easily transferred to study models for later use in case design (fig. 2-9). It is important to hold the microbrushes steady until the registration material is completely set to avoid distorting the record. The stick bite not only helps to establish an ideal dental midline, but it also prevents canting, or tilting, of new restorations and consequent asymmetry.

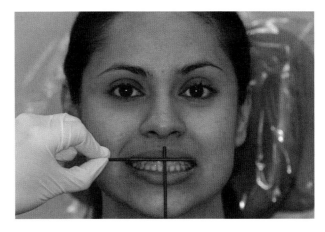

Figure 2-6. Aligning microbrushes to match patient's facial midline and interpupillary line for stick bite.

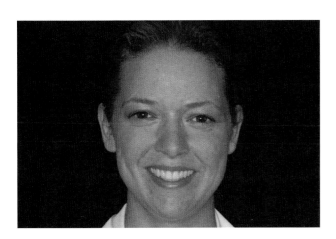

Figure 2-4. Example of facial asymmetry.

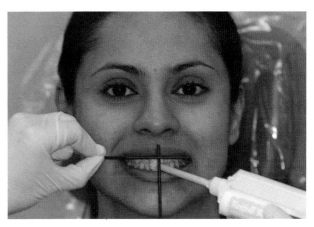

Figure 2-7. Applying bite registration material to secure position of microbrushes for stick bite.

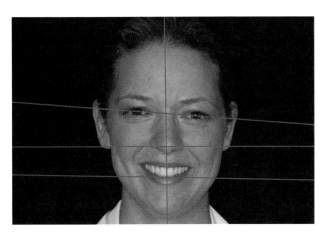

Figure 2-5. Example of facial asymmetry with lines.

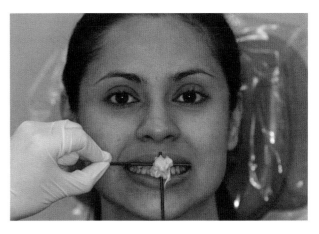

Figure 2-8. Final adjustment before set of registration material for stick bite.

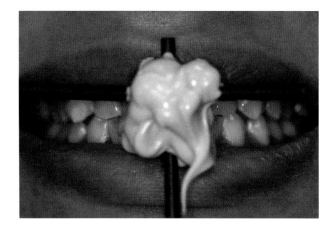

Figure 2-9. Close-up view of stick bite.

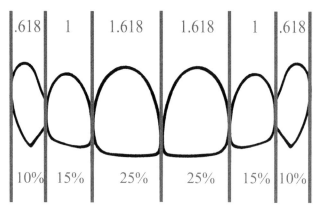

Figure 2-10. Diagram of Golden Proportion and Golden Percentage.

Intertooth Relationships

After establishing an appropriate size for the central incisors, the dentist can use various tooth-to-tooth ratios to help create a symmetrical and harmonious smile. The Golden Proportion has been used for centuries to study proportionality in art and nature. This reference must be viewed as a guideline rather than an absolute rule. While this proportion is well established in nature, subtle deviations decrease the tendency to establish a monotonous smile.

Relating this proportion to teeth, the ratio from central to lateral to canine should follow 1.618:1:0.618, the golden proportion. Reducing case design to a simple mathematic equation can potentially remove the artistic component of esthetic treatment. Practitioners must utilize these proportions to enhance the esthetic quality of their efforts.

For some, the use of mathematical equations to establish a harmonious smile may be a daunting task. For these individuals, a potentially more user-friendly derivative of the Golden Proportion should be employed. The Golden Percentage is a simplified version of the Golden Proportion. This concept, described by Snow, suggests that each maxillary anterior tooth should occupy a certain percentage of the anterior segment from a straight facial view. Ideally, each central should occupy 25% of this space, each lateral should occupy 15% of this space, and each canine should occupy 10% of this space (fig. 2-10). The advantages of using the Golden Percentage include the ability to evaluate the width of each tooth for its contribution to symmetry, dominance, and proportion of the anterior segment. Teeth with identical widths generate identical percentages; asymmetry becomes clearly identifiable and quantifiable, and rough percentages can be easily determined

clinically (Snow 1999). Although it is not always possible to design each case according to the Golden Proportion or the Golden Percentage standards, both methods serve as useful guides and starting points.

The symmetry of the maxillary central incisors and maxillary cuspids is well established. Lateral incisors, on the other hand, tend to have far greater individual variations. Because of this phenomenon, the viewing public is far more accustomed to and tolerant of a smile with symmetrical central incisors and cuspids. Additionally, they are accustomed to seeing lateral incisors with subtle or significant deviations. When perfect symmetry is not achievable, discrepancies in Golden Proportion or Percentage should be placed with the maxillary lateral incisors. Every effort should be made to create symmetrical maxillary central incisors and canines.

Subtle changes occur from anterior teeth to posterior teeth. The changes should be incorporated during the esthetic case design. The contact areas will move apically as the incisal embrasures increase in size, and there should be a subtly increasing axial inclination toward the midline. If the incline is too severe, the smile will appear overly narrow; conversely, if the teeth are too labial, they overfill the buccal corridor. In both cases, the natural anterior/posterior progression is disrupted (Moskowitz and Nayyar 1995).

Perspective can have a significant effect on esthetics as demonstrated by the principle of gradation. When viewing teeth from the frontal perspective, there is an apparent decrease of tooth size and structure moving posteriorly (fig. 2-11). Minor changes made to cusp

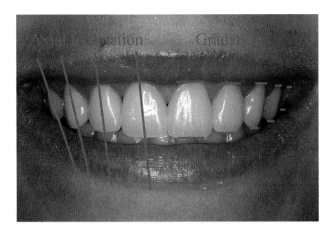

Figure 2-11. Example of axial inclination and gradation with labels.

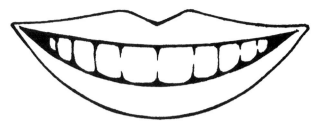

Figure 2-12. Drawing of commissure smile type.

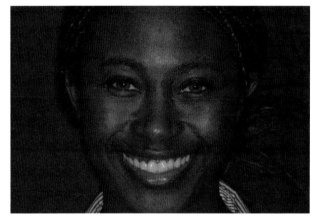

Figure 2-13. Example of commissure smile type.

lengths can actually enhance or detract from this phenomenon and cause an arch to appear wider or narrower due to this effect.

Smile Pattern

The lips must be viewed as the picture frame of all esthetic dentistry. A smile pattern is composed of a combination of a patient's smile style, smile stage, and smile type (Philips 1999). Recognizing the patient's most common smile pattern may help the esthetic dentist determine the complexity of the case.

Smile Style

Three main smile styles were determined by a physician attempting to improve the success of surgical restoration following facial paralysis. A random sample was analyzed, and 67% of people had a "Mona Lisa" or "commissure" smile, where the corners of the mouth are pulled up and outward followed by the upper lip contracting to show the upper teeth. (figs. 2-12 and 2-13) Thirty-one percent of the sample was found to have a "canine" or "cuspid" smile, where the levator labii superioris is dominant, exposing the canines first, followed by the corners of the mouth. (figs. 2-14 and 2-15) The third type, the "full denture" or "complex" smile, was found in only 2% of the sample; it involves simultaneously exposing all of the upper and lower teeth (Rubin 1974; Philips 1999). (figs. 2-16 and 2-17) Celebrities with commissure smiles are Jennifer Aniston and Jerry Seinfeld; recognizable cuspid smiles are found on Drew Barrymore and Tom Cruise; Julia Roberts and Will Smith both have identifiable complex smiles.

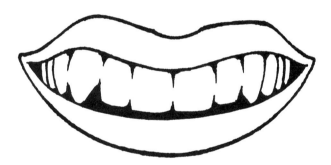

Figure 2-14. Drawing of cuspid smile type.

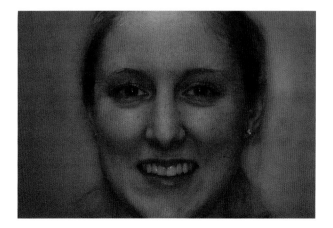

Figure 2-15. Example of cuspid smile type.

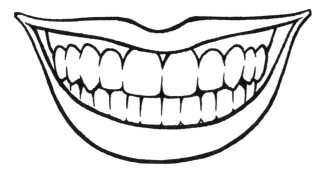

Figure 2-16.   Drawing of complex smile type.

Table 2-1.   Smile types.

Smile Type	Maxillary Anterior Tooth Display	Mandibular Anterior Tooth Display	Amount of Maxillary Gingiva Display
Type I	Yes	No	Up to 3 mm
Type II	Yes	No	Over 3 mm
Type III	No	Yes	None
Type IV	Yes	Yes	None
Type V	No	No	None

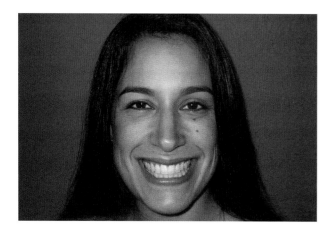

Figure 2-17.   Example of complex smile type.

Smile Stages

There are four stages in a smile cycle, progressing from closed lips (stage I) to resting display (stage II) to natural smile (stage III) to the expanded smile (stage IV). (Philips 1999) It is important to determine the difference between a patient's stage III and stage IV smile. If there is a significant difference between these stages, then esthetic treatment may need to be expanded to include additional teeth exposed during the expanded smile. Generally speaking, patients who are displeased with their smile are far less likely to routinely employ a stage IV smiling pattern than patients who are content with their smile. A guarded smile may be the routine smile stage employed by dissatisfied patients. When attempting to assess the potential smile pattern of these patients, it is essential to encourage them to exaggerate their smile.

Smile Types

There are five possible types of smiles based on which teeth and how much gingiva are exposed during the smile (table 2-1). Type I displays maxillary teeth only,

type II displays maxillary teeth and more than 3 mm of gingiva, type III displays mandibular teeth only, type IV displays both maxillary and mandibular teeth, and type V does not display teeth during the smile (Philips 1999). Obviously, it would be more challenging to restore a type II patient compared with a type V patient. As with smiles stages, patients with esthetic concerns will often present with a guarded smile type, hiding features with which they are dissatisfied. It is important to assess the full degree of smile extension in order to observe the true borders and critical landmarks necessary in designing the esthetic case (Moskowitz and Nayyar 1995).

Esthetic practitioners must get in the habit of classifying each patient's smile. First they should classify the smile style: commissure, canine, or complex. Next, the practitioner should classify the stage generally employed by the patient when smiling: stage I—closed lips, stage II—resting display, stage III—natural smile, or stage IV—expanded smile. Finally, the practitioner should classify the smile type: type I—maxillary teeth displayed with up to 3 mm of gingiva visible, type II—maxillary teeth displayed with over 3 mm of gingiva visible, type III—only mandibular teeth displayed, type IV—both maxillary and mandibular teeth displayed, or type V—no teeth displayed.

Combining these three components will help the esthetic dentist classify the patient's prominent smile pattern. The most common smile pattern is a commissure stage III type I. A patient with a complex stage IV type IV smile may be a more challenging case. The main purpose of recognizing a patient's smile pattern is to help determine the potential complexity of the case and the extent of necessary treatment.

Lip Assessment

The amount of tooth structure that is revealed when a patient is at rest, speaking, smiling, or laughing has a significant effect on the esthetic treatment plan. According to literature, 2–4 mm of tooth structure exposed at rest is esthetically desirable (Morley 2001; McLaren and Rifkin 2002). However, the dentist must consider that as people age, they naturally show less maxillary tooth structure at rest due to incisal wear in the absence of compensatory eruption and loss of elasticity in the upper lip over time. Vig and Brundo (1978) found that the average incisor exposure at rest at age 30 years was 3–3.5 mm, at age 50 years it was 1.0–1.5 mm, and by 70 years of age it was 0–0.5 mm. To help determine the amount of resting tooth reveal, the patient should repeat the letter "M" and allow their lips to part naturally. If little to no tooth structure is exposed in this resting position, the dentist may consider lengthening the teeth, but not at the expense of the function or the width-to-length ratio.

The most esthetically pleasing smiles have the edges of the maxillary teeth follow the curvature of the lower lip. Some patients have what is known as a reverse smile line, where the edges of the premolars and canines are longer than the centrals, creating uneven approximation of the lower lip. Disharmony between the maxillary incisal edges and the lower lip can be esthetically displeasing. Another element for consideration in smile design when evaluating a patient's smile is the amount of negative space created bilaterally between the maxillary teeth and the corners of the lips. Patients with narrow arches and wide smiles have more negative space, whereas patients with wider arches and narrower smiles have less (fig. 2-18). Studies have actually shown that negative space does not significantly affect the overall esthetic evaluation of a smile, so decisions to fill the buccal corridor by increasing the contours of maxillary posterior restorations should be made on a case-by-case basis (Ritter et al. 2006).

Gingival Tissue Assessment

When patients exhibit a high degree of lip mobility or simply display an excessive amount of gingival tissue when smiling, it can cause an unbalanced smile. In extreme cases, involved treatment, such as orthognathic surgery, may need to be considered. Otherwise, the most important factor in establishing harmony between the gingiva and the rest of the smile is symmetry. The gingival height of the maxillary laterals should fall approximately 0.5–1 mm incisal to the similar central and canine heights. The gingival zenith refers to the most apical point of the gingival tissue, and it should be located slightly distal to the long axis of the centrals and canines and coincide with the long axis of the laterals. The gingival scalloping and papilla should be well balanced, and like the teeth, should be perpendicular to the facial midline, parallel to the horizon (fig. 2-19). Healthy tissue is the most esthetic, and all periodontal issues should be resolved prior to initiating esthetic treatment.

Phonetics

Phonetics can be a useful tool in determining if teeth have been positioned correctly to support proper speech patterns and sounds. When the patient makes an "F" or "V" sound, there should be light contact between the central incisors and the "wet-dry" line of the lower lip (Spear 1999). To determine the maximum tooth exposure, presumably what would show during laughing, the patient should be instructed to say an exaggerated letter *E*. If the patient has a high smile line, lengthening the teeth apically may be considered, but extra care must

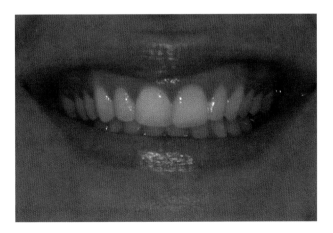

Figure 2-18. Example of buccal corridor with negative space.

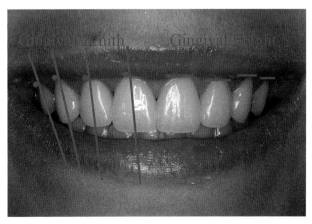

Figure 2-19. Example of gingival landmarks with labels.

be taken with the gingival tissues in this esthetic zone. A general rule suggested by Spear (1999) is the more mobile the lip, the less incisal edge can be shown at rest; the less mobile the lip, the more incisal edge should be shown at rest to achieve a pleasing full smile.

Extent of Treatment and Material Selection

After the dentist has determined the patient's smile pattern and made a sufficient lip and gingival assessment, a decision should be made as to the extent of treatment necessary to achieve the desired result. While some patients will present with their chief concern about a single tooth, others will be dissatisfied with many aspects of their smile. Some patient's concerns can be resolved with extremely conservative treatment such as bleaching, whereas others require extensive maxillary and/or mandibular restoration to achieve the desired result.

Microesthetics

Microesthetics guide the creation of teeth with pleasing intrinsic proportions and appropriate positions with respect to each another. Aspects of the teeth such as width-to-length ratio, shape, characterization, and shade are important microesthetic elements. As Jeff Morley (2001) describes, microesthetics include "the elements that make teeth actually look like teeth." Most authors agree that the maxillary central incisors are key to assessing anterior esthetics (Chiche and Pinault 1994; Goldstein 1997; Lombardi 1973; Rosenstiel, Ward, and Rashid 2000). It is therefore essential to establish proper width-to-length ratios for the central incisors, which according to research, should be between 75% and 80% (Wolfart 2005). The Tooth Indicator, from Dentsply International, is a simple instrument that can also help determine a patient's ideal central incisor size (fig. 2-20). If a patient's teeth deviate significantly from the optimal size, the dentist should consider making the appropriate modifications during case design. Other aspects of microesthetics such as tooth shape, characterization, and shade are largely dependant on patient preferences or, in the case of single-tooth restoration, matching contralateral teeth.

A common microesthetic complaint of patients is undesirable tooth shade caused by endodontic pathology, tetracycline stain, or fluorosis. The dentist, having determined which microesthetic changes are necessary for the case, must establish good communications with a laboratory technician capable of translating them into artistic restorations.

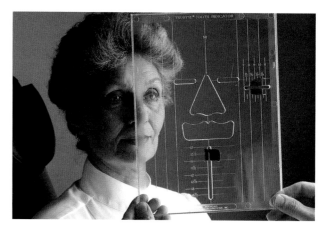

Figure 2-20. Dentsply Tooth Indicator.

Summary

Although there are many things to consider when planning an esthetic case, many principles and guidelines exist that can help direct treatment. It is important to have a good understanding of the overriding ethical principles as well as the elements of microesthetics and macroesthetics prior to performing esthetic dentistry.

A simple rule of thumb is to start with the large features and work toward the smaller features. Look at the face, lips, and gingiva before individual tooth assessments are performed. In other words, look at the forest before you look at the trees. Think of the guiding principles as a dental microscope. When using a microscope, one generally starts at the lowest magnification to establish his or her bearing. The magnification should not be increased until this bearing is established.

Works Cited

Chiche GJ, Pinault A. 1994. *Esthetics of Anterior Fixed Prosthodontics*, 1st ed. Chicago: Quintessence.

Goldstein RE. 1997. *Change Your Smile*, 3rd ed. Chicago: Quintessence.

Golub-Evans J. 1994. Unity and variety: Essential ingredients of a smile design, *Curr Opin Cosmet Dent* 2:1–5.

Kokich VO, Kiyak HA, Shapiro PA. 1999. Comparing the perception of dentists and lay people to altered dental esthetics. *J Esthet Dent* 11:311–24.

Lombardi RE. 1973. The principles of visual perception and their clinical application to denture esthetics. *J Prosthet Dent* 29:358–82.

McLaren EA, Rifkin R. 2002. Macroesthetics: Facial and dentofacial analysis. *J Calif Dent Assoc* 30(11):839–46.

Morley J. 2001. Macroesthetic elements of smile design. *JADA* 132, Jan.

Moskowitz ME, Nayyar A. 1995. Determinants of dental esthetics: A rationale for smile analysis and treatment. *Compendium* 16, no. 12.

Oxford University Press. 2005. *The New Oxford American Dictionary*.

Philips E. 1999. The perfect gap: When are midline diastemas aesthetically acceptable? *Dent Today* 18(5):52–7.

Ritter DE, et al. 2006. Esthetic influence of negative space in the buccal corridor during smiling. *Angle Orthodontist* 76, no. 2.

Rosenstiel SF, Ward DH, Rashid RG. 2000. Dentists' preferences of anterior tooth proportion: A web-based study. *J Prosthodont* 9:123–36.

Rubin LR. 1974. The anatomy of the smile: Its importance in the treatment of facial paralysis. *Plast Reconstr Surg* 53(4):384–7.

Snow S. 1999. Esthetic smile analysis of maxillary anterior tooth width: The golden percentage. *J Esthet Dent* 11:177–84.

Spear F. 1999. The maxillary central incisal edge: A key to esthetic and functional treatment planning. *Compendium* 20, no. 6.

Vig RG, Brundo GC. 1978. The kinetics of anterior tooth display. *J Prosthet Dent* 39(5):502–4.

Wolfart S. 2005. Assessment of dental appearance following changes in incisor proportions. *Eur J Oral Sci* 113:159–65.

Chapter 3
Dental Photography in Esthetic Dental Practice

Parag R. Kachalia DDS, BS

Marc Geissberger DDS, MA, BS, CPT

In this day and age, if a practitioner is going to embark on performing aesthetic dentistry, digital photography must be an integral component of their armamentarium. Digital photography affords the practitioner many benefits such as medico-legal documentation, laboratory and peer communication, patient education, third-party communication, and ease in adaptation to marketing campaigns. However, the single greatest benefit as it relates to aesthetic dentistry is the ability to critically evaluate one's own work. As the general public becomes more dentally educated, one must assume that its expectations of elective treatment outcomes will also rise. In order to meet if not exceed the public's expectations, digital dental photography must be utilized to increase the practitioner's skills in delivering invisible beauty.

Choosing the Correct Equipment

In order to produce high-quality photography that can be used for communication and evaluation, one must consider purchasing the proper equipment that is geared specifically toward the macrophotography of dentistry.

Digital cameras can be broken into two categories: digital viewfinder cameras (DVF) and digital single lens reflex cameras (DSLR). Digital viewfinder cameras offer many advantages in everyday amateur photography. Unfortunately, they have tremendous drawbacks when utilized for dental photography. The primary issue that resides with a DVF camera is that the image visualized through the viewfinder is not the exact image that will be captured by the sensor. The photographer can overcome this drawback by viewing the subject through the LCD screen; however, focusing through the LCD screen can prove somewhat challenging. Generally speaking, dental photography is conducted in a "macro" mode, and DVF cameras are manufactured to take superb casual images of scenery or portrait-type photography; they are not designed for extreme close-up photography. While most DVF cameras on the market today contain macro settings, these settings generally force the

photographer to be incredibly close to the subject being photographed and cause distortion and lighting issues when it comes to intraoral photography. Generally speaking, these cameras should be avoided if the practitioner intends to use the images for any other purpose than basic communication or documentation.

When considering which type of equipment to purchase, the practitioner must consider three major components: the DSLR camera body, the lens, and the type of flash. Selecting each of these components is an essential part of ensuring success. Another drawback of DVF cameras is that these components cannot be selected individually. With DSLR cameras, these components can be selected individually and the practitioner will encounter many different options. This ability to customize the individual camera setup will allow the practitioner far more flexibility and provide a far greater range of capability than a DVF camera will.

Camera Body

High-quality DSLR cameras have been available for a number of years now, and similar to most technological advances, costs have dropped dramatically in this arena. Without question, to repeatedly produce high-quality intraoral images, the dentist should invest in a DSLR camera. The vast majority of DSLR cameras give the dentist the ability to control critical factors such as aperture, shutter speed, and digital film speed. Ultimately, the ability to adjust these factors, along with proper lighting, will help produce high-quality images. When considering a DSLR camera, one must look at the type of sensor in the camera. Digital cameras contain either a charge-coupled device (CCD) sensor or a complementary metal oxide semiconductor (CMOS) sensor. These sensors are analogous to film in a traditional 35-mm camera. The vast majority of DSLR cameras that are commonly used in dentistry have a CMOS sensor. Most DSLR cameras in the marketplace today have a sensor that is smaller than traditional 35-mm film cameras. This is important from the standpoint that standard magnifi-

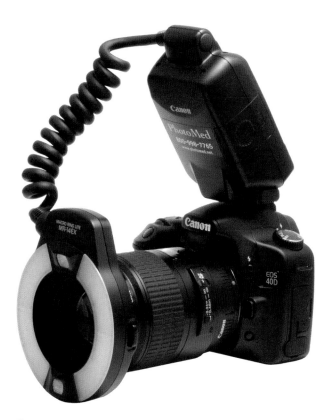

Figure 3-1.   Canon 40D maintains a 1.6 crop factor.

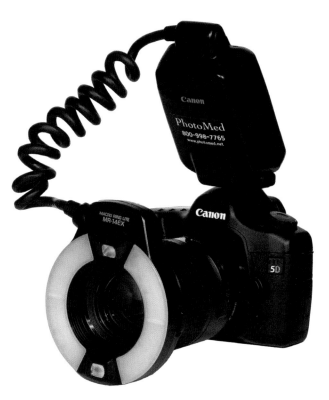

Figure 3-2.   Canon 5D: full-format camera.

cation ratios that may have been used with traditional film photography do not transfer over to the digital world. In traditional film photography, 36 mm would fill a magnification ratio of 1:1, and 72 mm would fill a magnification ratio of 1:2. Conversely, with a camera that has a crop factor of 1.6, the camera lens would have to be zoomed out to accomplish the same 36- and 72-mm width that can be accomplished with a 35-mm camera. In the past few years, manufacturers of DSLR cameras have produced cameras containing full-format sensors that are equivalent in sensor size to 35-mm cameras; however, these cameras tended to be quite expensive. This slight benefit for most dental consumers was not sufficient to offset the tremendous cost differences that came with these cameras, compared with DSLR cameras with different crop ratios. Full-format cameras are currently available in the marketplace at a premium of roughly 50% when compared with DSLR cameras with 1.5 or 1.6 crop factors (figs. 3-1 and 3-2).

Macro Lens

The lens most commonly used in intraoral and limited extraoral dental photography is either a 100-mm or 105-

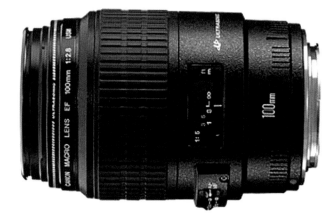

Figure 3-3.   Canon 100 mm macro lens.

mm macro lens (figs. 3-3 and 3-4). These macro lenses allow reproduction ratios of 1:1, whereas most standard everyday photography lenses generally output a maximum reproduction ratio of 1:7. In relation to macro photography, the term *reproduction ratio* is synonymous to the term *magnification ratio*. A reproduction ratio is simply a mathematical equation that relates the image a subject will cast onto traditional film or digital sensor relative to the actual size of the image. When a reproduc-

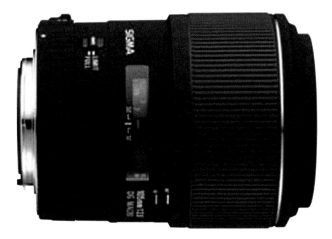

Figure 3-4.   Sigma 105 mm macro lens.

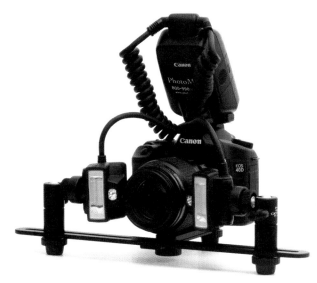

Figure 3-6.   PhotoMed R1 dual point flash bracket with Canon MT-24EX.

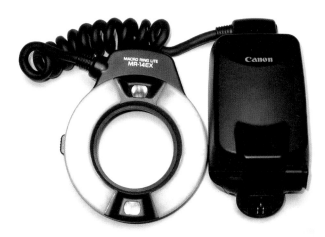

Figure 3-5.   Canon MR-14EX ring flash.

tion ratio of 1:1 is stated, it simply means that the actual size of the subject is displayed on the film or the sensor. Similarly, a reproduction ratio of 1:7 would mean the subject is seven times larger than the image captured on the digital sensor or film.

Flash Systems

The flash systems that should be utilized will fall into two categories: ring system and point system (figs. 3-5 and 3-6). Ring system flashes are placed around the lens in either a sectored format or a more traditional single flash component that surrounds the lens. A sectored format system essentially has multiple flash tubes arranged in a circular format compared with a traditional single flash system that has one tube. Many of the newer sector-based ring flashes can be fired so that all

sectors of the ring flash fire at once or flash power can be varied between sectors. This type of flash offers the advantage of evenly illuminating difficult areas within the oral environment and properly rendering their color. One potential drawback of the ring flash system is that it may light areas up a little too well at times, thus removing all shadows. As shadows dissipate, the photographed object also loses its ability to communicate depth. This drawback is not as evident with intraoral photography because complete illumination of the subject matter is nearly impossible, as the cheeks, lips, and tongue tend to block some light.

Unlike ring systems that distribute light in a circular pattern, point systems are meant to bring light in from the side. In a point system, single or multiple flashes are placed around the lens and the direction and angle of these flashes can be modified. This modification of direction and angle allows the photographer to cast greater shadows onto the subject, allowing greater communication of texture and depth. Many point systems on the market have bilateral flash tubes present and allow the operator to selectively regulate the light output from each of these sources. Properly focused point systems can do a fine job for intraoral photography; however, these systems are more useful in extraoral or portrait photography. With manipulation of the lighting units, point systems allow the benefit of showing more depth in an image with the use of shadows. A system by Lester Dine offers a hybrid system that combines a ring flash with a point flash. This system potentially combines the intraoral photography benefits of the ring flash and an ideal point source for portrait photography.

Photography Accessories

Once the components of the camera have been assembled, the photographer must add a few key components to their armamentarium. These include a compact flash card (to store the images in the short-term), photo mirrors, photographic contrasters, and retractors. Virtually all DSLR cameras accept a compact flash card to store images. Compact flash cards used by DSLR cameras are analogous to film used in standard 35-mm SLR cameras. A compact flash card on the minimum order of 1.0 GB of storage space is sufficient for dental photography.

Many photographic mirrors designed specifically for intraoral photography are available. These mirrors are fabricated with chromium, rhodium, or titanium. Any of the aforementioned mirrors will suffice in capturing quality intraoral images; however titanium-coated mirrors tend to produce slightly brighter images. When selecting intraoral mirrors, one should consider a mirror that can be positioned a sufficient distance from the area that is in focus. Several designs are available that will limit the potential for errors of composition. Mirrors that possess a handle and/or are greater in length decrease the possibility of fingers being captured in the image (fig. 3-7). Once the type of material is selected, it is best to obtain a mirror for buccal images and at least two sizes of occlusal mirrors, so that both large and small mouths can have these mirrors placed comfortably.

In addition to intraoral mirrors, black photographic contrasters should also be utilized in the documentation of aesthetic cases (figs. 3-8 and 3-9). Black photographic contrasters allow the focus to fall on an individual segment of the smile while blocking distracting images of the tongue, lips, or back of the mouth. Contrasters are particularly useful when communicating incisal translucency to your dental laboratory technician.

In order to properly frame images, retractors are a must. The practitioner should consider the purchase of an assortment of retractors, as no single retractor will fit all patients. At a minimum, two sets of retractors in various sizes should be considered. One set should allow the patient or assistant to hold the retractors, and the other set should be auto-expanding (figs. 3-10 and 3-11). Generally speaking, the operator should place the largest retractors feasible into the patient's mouth to provide for maximum retraction.

After the armamentarium of camera body, macro lens, ring flash, mirrors, contrasters, and retractors has been acquired, the equipment is complete and images can be taken. To properly capture digital images, one must

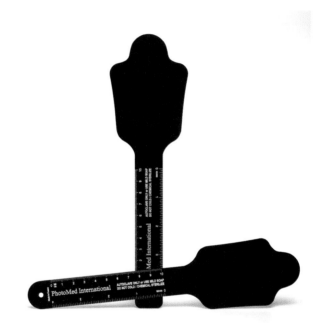

Figure 3-8. Photographic contraster with appropriate contour to allow isolated photo of anterior dentition.

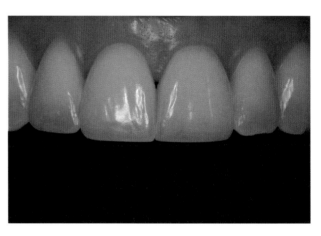

Figure 3-9. Retracted 1:1 image with photo contraster placed.

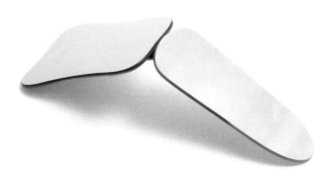

Figure 3-7. PhotoMed Combo Titanium Mirror.

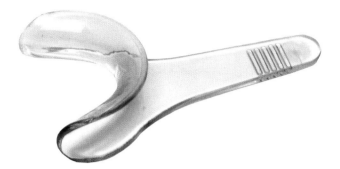

Figure 3-10. Unilateral adult plastic retractor.

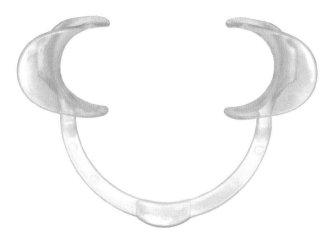

Figure 3-11. Saga adult self-retracting photo retractor.

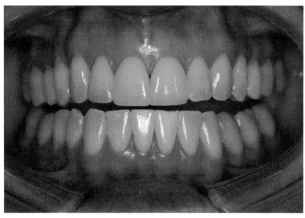

Figure 3-12. 1:2 retracted view with f-stop at f11. Distortion of the posterior dentition is evident.

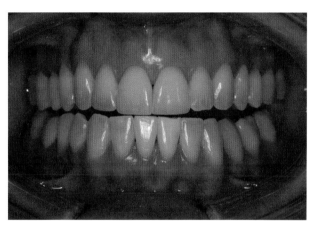

Figure 3-13. 1:2 retracted view with f-stop at f22. Posterior dentition is also in focus.

keep in mind that the quality of the image when using a DSLR camera is dependent on equipment and proper technique. Most DSLR cameras possess the ability to produce very good images in an automatic mode (this mode allows the camera to automatically adjust for lighting and aperture); however, in this mode the camera automatically changes the aperture setting to achieve appropriate lighting of the subject. This often produces an image with poor depth of field. It is the opinion of the authors that far superior images can be produced repeatedly when the camera is set to a manual mode. Utilizing the manual setting of DSLR cameras allows the practitioner to adjust aperture, shutter speed, and reproduction ratios to maximize exposure and depth of field.

Settings

Aperture (also called f-stop) is a feature of the lens that controls how wide the lens is open. On traditional film

cameras this adjustment was made on the lens itself; however, with a DSLR camera the adjustment is made on the camera body. Keep in mind the larger the aperture number, the smaller the opening and vice versa. An aperture of f22 has a smaller diameter opening than an aperture setting of f10; thus, an f22 setting would let in less light than an f10 setting. Depth of field is defined as the distance in front of and beyond the subject that appears to be in focus. Depth of field will automatically improve as the f-stop is increased. This phenomenon occurs primarily because the image is being captured on flattest portion of the lens (figs. 3-12 and 3-13). As the lens is opened to provide more light (lower f-stop), more of the curved surface of the lens is used. The image created will possess far less depth of field. When the f-stop is increased, light is decreased. This will potentially cause an image to be underexposed (dark).

Altering the film speed, shutter speed, or output from the flash can compensate for this loss of light and produce an image that has excellent depth of field and proper exposure. Generally speaking, the aperture setting for intraoral photography will be between f22 and f32. Depth of field becomes less important as the camera moves away from the image. Portrait photography or headshots are taken with an aperture setting of f10 due to the need for greater light.

In addition to aperture, shutter speed is another key component in determining how much light the camera can capture. Shutter speed is defined as how long the shutter is open and thus how long the sensor of the camera is allowed to take in the image. As the amount of time the shutter is open increases, light intake to the sensor also increases. Unfortunately, the longer the shutter is open, the greater the chance that camera movement will produce an image with distortion. Without the use of a tripod or stabilizing device, this phenomenon can occur with shutter speeds of 1/60 of a second or less. Macro dental photography will generally be taken at a shutter speed of 1/100 to 1/200 seconds. Shutter speed settings above 1/200 may produce dark (underexposed) images due to decrease in the amount of time the sensor has to capture light. A shutter speed of 1/200 will help to decrease the yellow hue of light found with operatory lights (Ward 2007).

Reproduction ratios for dental photography can be simplified into three categories: one portrait setting (1:10) and two intraoral settings (1:2 and 1:1). As mentioned earlier, these settings were traditionally based on film photography, and most DSLR sensors tend to be smaller by about 50%. To account for this difference, the photographer would need to be positioned farther away from the subject. Newer cameras with full-size sensors can maintain the standard film ratios. Intraoral images historically fall into two ratios: 1:1 and 1:2. When framing a 1:2 image based on film standards, 72mm should be evident in a horizontal format. In average size arches this image will generally capture at least the mesial buccal line angle from second molar to second molar. DSLR cameras with smaller sensors will need to be set closer to a 1:3 setting to frame a similar image. A more magnified image generally has a reproduction ratio of 1:1. Most of the time these images are taken to display tremendous detail on a small segment of the dental arch. Traditionally speaking, a 1:1 ratio should display 36mm in a horizontal format. When photographing the anterior segment, the 1:1 image should allow display from the center of one canine to the center of the contra lateral canine in the average maxillary dental arch. In a camera with a 1.5 crop factor, this ratio would convert to 1:1.5 to capture a similar image.

Capturing Standard Views

When capturing digital dental images, the order in which images are taken is important. An organized, repeatable order will lead to increased efficiency and minimize the amount of time the patient must tolerate retractors and/or mirrors in their mouth. The photographic series depicted below has been taken in the recommended order. The recommended camera settings for these images are

1. ISO (film speed) set at 100
2. Shutter speed set at 1/200 s.

These two settings will remain constant. Only the aperture (f-stop) and reproduction ratio will be adjusted during the series of images.

Extraoral Images

Portrait View

This image will essentially be the patient's headshot. It is recommended that this image be taken both in a repose and full smile (figs. 3-14 and 3-15). To begin, the patient should be positioned in front of a dark photographic drape to minimize any superfluous distractions. The image should be taken with the midline of the patient's face perpendicular to the floor. The camera is held in a horizontal position with the patient's nose centered in the middle of the frame. Assuming a 100-mm lens is being utilized, the f-stop of the DSLR should be set at f10 and the lens should be set to 1:∞. In addition to the two frontal shots (repose and smiling), a profile image can also be taken with the same settings. This image can be taken both in a repose and natural smile (figs. 3-16 and 3-17).

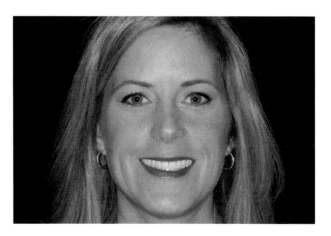

Figure 3-14.   1:10 full headshot with a natural smile depicted.

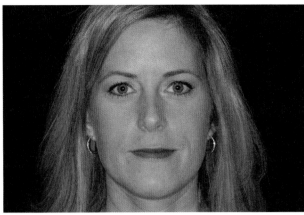

Figure 3-15. 1:10 full headshot with patient in repose.

Close-up

The extraoral close-up view allows the photographer to capture the natural smile as it relates to lips. As discussed in previous chapters, the lips are critically important; they serve as the frame for the teeth and should be captured photographically. Three close-up extraoral smile images are recommended: right and left lateral smile views and a frontal smile view. All of these images should be taken at a reproduction ratio of 1:2 and an aperture setting of f22. Either canine should serve as the focus point for the frontal image. The center of the image should be the interdental papilla between the maxillary central incisors (fig. 3-18). A right and left lateral view should also be taken with the lateral incisors serving as the focus point (figs. 3-19 and 3-20).

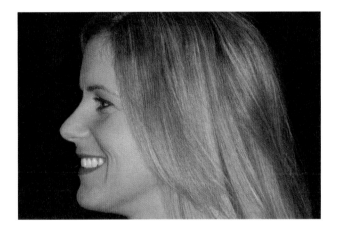

Figure 3-16. 1:10 profile image of patient depicting lateral reveal with natural smile.

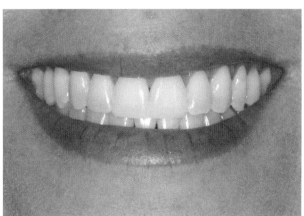

Figure 3-18. 1:2 nonretracted natural smile.

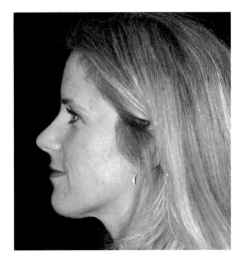

Figure 3-17. 1:10 profile image of patient in repose.

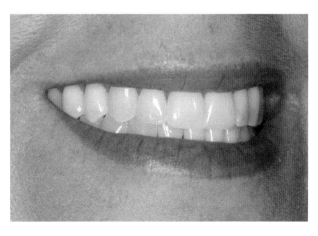

Figure 3-19. 1:2 natural smile with the focal point being on the patient's maxillary right lateral incisor.

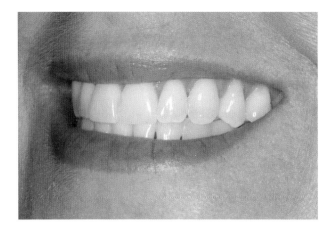

Figure 3-20. 1:2 natural smile with the focal point being on the patient's maxillary left lateral incisor.

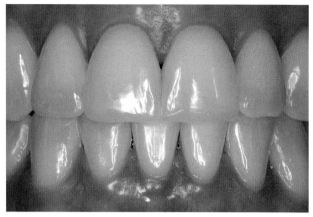

Figure 3-21. 1:1 retracted image of anterior dentition. The maxillary incisal edge serves as the center point of the image.

Intraoral Images

Once the extraoral images have been captured, the intra-oral images should be taken utilizing the selected retractors. All the intraoral images will be taken at a standard ratio of 1:2 with one exception: the magnified anterior image. This image will be captured at 1:1.

Anterior View

Similar to the anterior extraoral images, this image should be taken with the interdental papilla between the maxillary incisors as the center of the image. This photo can either be taken in maximum intercuspation or with the teeth slightly parted to display the incisal edges or cusp tips of both the maxillary and mandibular anterior teeth. To maximize the depth of field, the camera should be focused on a cuspid first at the proper ratio and then the camera should be moved over to the central incisors before the shutter is released. With most DSLR cameras, this technique will allow the cuspid(s) to be the focus point and maximize the quality of the exposure. This image should be taken at a 1:1 ratio first and then 1:2 ratio (figs. 3-21, 3-22, and 3-23).

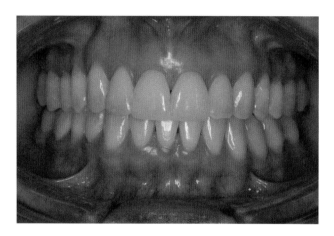

Figure 3-22. 1:2 retracted image. This image is initially focused on the canine to achieve maximum depth of field.

Direct Lateral View

This series of images is designed to visualize the second bicuspid to the midline. The camera should be focused on the first bicuspid before being moved over to the incisal embrasure between the maxillary lateral incisor and the cuspid. Once the camera is at this new position, the photographer should release the shutter and capture the image. To aid with retraction, the retractor closest to the side being photographed should be held taut and the contralateral side loosened (fig. 3-24).

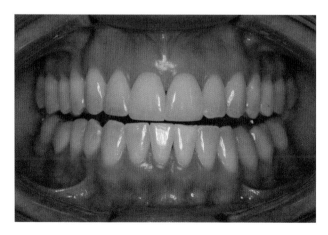

Figure 3-23. 1:2 retracted image taken with anterior dentition slightly separated to convey incisal wear and translucency.

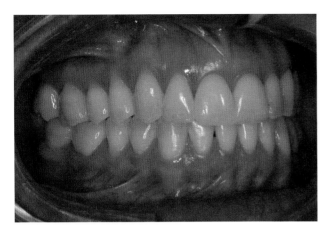

Figure 3-24. 1:2 retracted lateral view with focus occurring directly on the dentition.

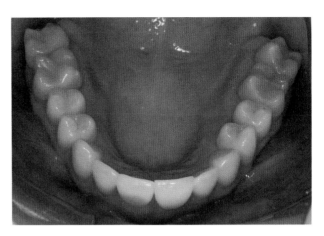

Figure 3-26. 1:2 retracted image of the maxillary arch.

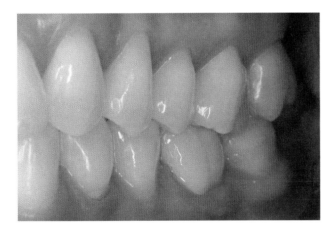

Figure 3-25. 1:2 retracted lateral view with indirect focus through a photographic mirror.

Indirect Lateral View

In order to fully visualize the entire buccal aspect of the posterior dentition, this image must be taken indirectly with the aid of a buccal mirror. The focus point of this image should be the mesial buccal cusp tip of the upper first molar. Ideally, only the side being photographed should be retraced to allow maximum displacement of the patient's cheek. After the retractor is correctly positioned, a lateral view mirror is introduced. The mirror should be pulled laterally to expose the buccal surface of the posterior dentition. When placing the mirror, the operator should pay particular attention to comfort level of the patient and insure that the mirror is not traumatizing the gingiva (fig. 3-25).

Occlusal View

The most challenging photographs in the intraoral series are the maxillary and mandibular occlusal views. To properly capture the entire arch, occlusal mirrors must be utilized. Additionally, retractors should be positioned in a manner that pulls the lip of the arch being captured in an outward and apical direction. Placing the retractors in this position will allow for easy placement of the mirror. The largest end possible should be inserted into the oral cavity with the back edge of the mirror gently resting on the tissue directly distal to the second or third molar region. The front portion of the mirror should come into close contact with the incisal edges of the mandibular incisors. Resting the occusal mirror on the opposing arch of the one being captured is an effective way to ensure proper mirror positioning. The photographer should then focus on the occlusal surface of the molars before centering the image on the midline of the palate and the lingual groove area of the first molars. This image is best captured with the photographer in front of the patient and the patient moderately reclined (fig. 3-26). In addition to the difficulties experienced with the maxillary view, the mandibular image is further complicated with the addition of the tongue. Retractors should be positioned so that they are pulled outward and downward. The widest portion of the mirror that the mouth will accommodate should be utilized. The mirror must extend distal to the second molars and the anterior portion of the mirror should be tilted upward and placed against the incisal edges of the maxillary incisors. The patient should be instructed to lift his or her tongue toward the soft palate, and an assistant should blow a gentle stream of air on to the mirror to keep it from fogging up. Another technique to prevent the mirror from fogging is to presoak the mirror in a bath of warm water. The photographer should center the photo with a horizontal line that bisects the distal lingual aspect of second premolars and a vertical line that bisects the lower central incisors (fig. 3-27).

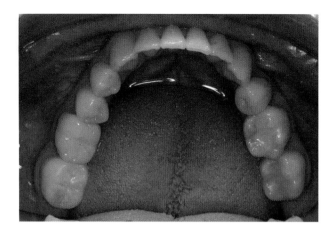

Figure 3-27.   1:2 retracted image of the mandibular arch.

Some Examples of Variations in Photographic Recommendations

There are several variations to the aforementioned photographic series that are utilized throughout our profession. Photographs are standard requirements for Invisalign® treatment and for the accreditation process for the American Academy of Cosmetic Dentistry. Each of these entities has a standard series of photographs that must be submitted for consideration. The American Academy of Cosmetic Dentistry recommends the following before and after photographs for its accreditation process:

1. Full face (1:10 ratio)
2. Full smile (centered 1:2 ratio)
3. Left lateral view of full smile (1:2 ratio)
4. Right lateral view of full smile (1:2 ratio)
5. Retracted view of the dental arches (centered 1:2 ratio)
6. Left lateral view of the retracted dental arches (1:2 ratio)
7. Right lateral view of the retracted dental arches (1:2 ratio)
8. Centered close-up of the teeth (arch) being treated (1:1 ratio)
9. Left lateral view of the teeth (arch) being treated (1:1 ratio)
10. Right lateral view of the teeth (arch) being treated (1:1 ratio)
11. Maxillary occlusal view of the dental arches (1:2 ratio)
12. Mandibular occlusal view of the dental arches (1:2 ratio)

When submitting a case for Invisalign® treatment, the following eight photographs must be submitted in printed or electronic format:

1. Full face with patient smiling (1:10 ratio)
2. Full face with patient repose (1:10 ratio)
3. Profile (1:10 ratio)
4. Retracted view of the dental arches (centered 1:2 ratio)
5. Left lateral view of the retracted dental arches (1:2 ratio)
6. Right lateral view of the retracted dental arches (1:2 ratio)
7. Maxillary occlusal view of the dental arches (1:2 ratio)
8. Mandibular occlusal view of the dental arches (1:2 ratio)

Making Photography a Routine Part of Practice

The idea of incorporating photography into the dental office can seem like a daunting task; however, this task can be managed by establishing a routine. Photographers must take the time to develop a photo sequence that works best for them and seems intuitive. The sequence described above works best for the authors; however, each practitioner should modify the sequence above as they deem appropriate and allow digital dental photography to be a pleasant experience.

Photo credit: Figures 3.1 through 3.8, 3.10, and 3.11 were provided courtesy of Photomed International. Reprinted with permission.

Work Cited

Ward DH. 2007. The vision of digital dental photography. *Dentistry Today* 26(5):100, 102, 104–105.

Suggested Reading

Bengel W. 2006. *Mastering Digital Dental Photography*. New Malden, Surrey, United Kingdom: Quintessence.
Goldstein MB. 2006. Dental digital photo potpourri. *Dentistry Today* 25(5):122–25.
Rinaldi SJ. 2007. The digital age and image of dentistry. *Dentistry Today* 26(6):132, 134.
Snow SR. 2005. Dental photography systems: Required feature for equipment selection. *Compendium Continuing Education in Dentistry* 26(5):309–310, 312–14, 349.

Chapter 4
The Initial Patient Examination

Eugene Santucci DDS, MA, BS

Noelle Santucci DDS, MA, BS

The successful intake of new patients seeking esthetic treatment is of critical importance to a dentist becoming established in this arena. Today's esthetic patient is savvy and will seek out clinicians with the skills, reputation, and rapport necessary to achieve the desired outcomes. To that end, developing an effective intake process can quickly elevate any dental practice. This chapter will outline the general makeup of the intake process, provide detailed information that must be obtained during the process, and provide several useful forms that clinicians may utilize to enhance their current system.

The process of developing esthetic and reconstructive treatment plans cannot be left to chance. To adequately prepare a comprehensive esthetic treatment plan, practitioners must devote an appropriate amount of time and energy to the process. A rushed initial examination may convey the wrong message to patients seeking your expertise. For cases involving several esthetic options it is essential to devote the necessary time to the intake process.

Generally speaking, patients seeking esthetic treatments should be allotted two separate appointments. The first appointment can be described as the information-gathering and assessment appointment. The goals of this appointment are to discuss the patient's desires, obtain all necessary records and information, and discuss some preliminary findings with the patient. The data collected at this appointment will be used to assist the practitioner in developing several different treatment plans. The plans will be discussed in detail at the second appointment, the consultation appointment.

Utilizing an additional appointment affords the clinician adequate time to reflect on the gathered information and develop several treatment approaches. During the consultation appointment, these treatment plans and financial ramifications of each can be discussed in detail. Adequate time must be reserved to answer any questions the patient may have generated between the two appointments or during the consultation appointment itself.

First Impressions

The initial phone call to the dental office is extremely important since this conversation establishes the patient's first impression of the staff. Potential patients will make a judgment concerning the staff's helpfulness. With this in mind, the staff should ensure that new patients feel they have selected the right office for their dental treatment.

During the initial phone call, the receptionist must seamlessly display a genuine message of concern, one that makes potential patients feel as if they have one hundred percent of the receptionist's attention. The receptionist must never display a rushed demeanor. Additionally, it is considered inappropriate to place a potential new patient on hold. The following data are important to obtain from all new potential patients:

1. What type of treatment are they seeking?
2. Are they calling for emergency treatment?
3. Are they seeking a second opinion?
4. Are they calling to establish a routine dental examination appointment?

The receptionist must be in the habit of repeating what the caller is saying. This "active listening" method will ensure that callers feel their needs are being heard and understood. Furthermore, the receptionist must obtain all pertinent information in an exacting but noninvasive fashion. Questions regarding insurance coverage or initial costs are best kept toward the middle of the conversation to give the impression that the office's main concern is patients' oral health, not their financial status.

Another helpful phone skill is to frequently repeat the patient's name during the discussion. The receptionist should advise the patient regarding the length of the initial appointment and clearly set its parameters. Patients must be instructed to bring information regarding their current health, present medications, and any condition that may require premedication for dental procedures. Flexibility is a desirable characteristic. Offer patients the choice of filling out the new patient information at the time of their appointment or receiving the forms via mail to be completed at their leisure, prior to the appointment.

Once an appointment has been established, the receptionist should ask the patient if he or she desires to be called prior to the appointment to reconfirm the time and date. Additionally, the receptionist must ensure that the new patient is given information regarding office location and parking availability. If available, suggest that the patient visit the office Web site. This indicates a sense of pride in the appearance of your office and the services you offer.

In summary, don't cut corners on the patient's first contact with your office; it's time well spent and will create a very positive first impression. Initially, the patient may not be calling for esthetic treatment but rather routine or emergency care. Satisfaction with the initial exposure to the office and staff can open the door to future comprehensive esthetic and reconstructive therapy.

The Initial Visit

At the initial visit, the receptionist should be prepared to greet patients by name as they enter the office. The appearance of the reception area is a strong indicator of the character of your practice. This room should be clean, inviting, and uncluttered. A reception area that possesses a professional environment can establish a strong initial impression on new patients. Staff members should introduce themselves to patients and ask them how they wish to be addressed. The staff should be instructed to offer assistance with any paperwork, answer all insurance-related questions, and make sure all general concerns have been adequately addressed. When escorting patients to the treatment area, allow them to follow closely behind. Never leave patients stranded in the reception area. This is especially critical for the elderly and physically impaired. Remember, it is the little things that can make a lasting impression.

Office space permitting, an introductory meeting between the doctor and patient in a dedicated well-appointed consultation room is advised. This allows both the patient and doctor the opportunity to meet in a safe, private, and nonthreatening environment affording both parties the opportunity to have a free exchange of vital information regarding past dental and medical experiences as well as present dental and medical concerns. Discussing occupational background, common hobbies and interests, or acknowledging the referral source(s) are all effective strategies to quickly establish rapport. During this initial conversation, make sure that the patient is clear on the various components of your examination and the possible need for a follow-up consultation if an extensive treatment plan is anticipated.

Generally speaking, most patients are very impressed with this personal, friendly, and professional preexamination experience.

It must be assumed that the patient has formulated an initial impression of the staff, the facility, and the dentist by the time the initial preexamination conversation is completed. Each step of your intake process is an opportunity to create a positive, long-lasting, professional relationship with every new patient. This is critically important with patients seeking complex esthetic or full-mouth reconstruction therapy.

Dental Examination

Evaluation of the Gnathostomatic System

A comprehensive dental examination must include a thorough assessment of both extraoral and intraoral components. The extraoral examination is an evaluation of the gnathostomatic system with its muscle, nerve, bone, and symmetry components, along with their contribution to the harmonious function or dysfunction of this system. Facial symmetry, interpupillary axis, and lip posture at rest and at full smile may not be major considerations for routine dental procedures but are of major importance for esthetic and reconstructive cases. This information is also critical as we address the fluidity of mandibular movement as well as its range and comfort to the patient during periods of mastication and rest (figs. 4-1, 4-2, and 4-3).

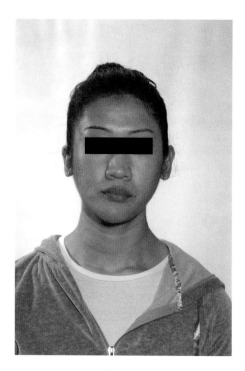

Figure 4-1. Asymmetrical mandible.

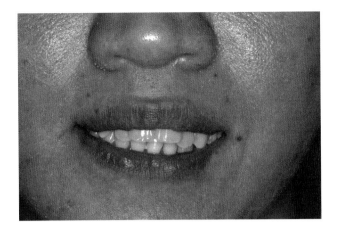

Figure 4-2. Lip sag.

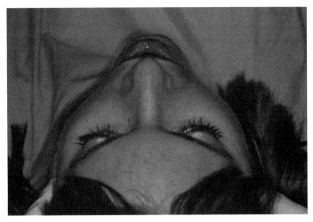

Figure 4-4. View from the twelve o'clock position.

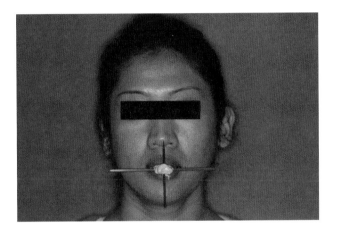

Figure 4-3. Evaluation of vertical and horizontal axis.

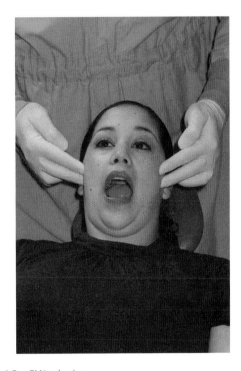

Figure 4-5. TMJ palpation.

When evaluating the path of mandibular motion, the doctor should be positioned behind the patient. The twelve o'clock position allows even the slightest mandibular deviation to be noted throughout the complete opening and closing cycle. Additionally, the twelve o'clock position affords easy access to the external auditory meatus and allows the application of gentle anterior pressure upon the capsule during opening and closing movements to ascertain the presence of joint effusions noted by the patient's increased pain response (figs. 4-4 and 4-5).

Bilateral TMJ evaluation consisting of palpation, auscultation, or synography can also be completed from this twelve o'clock position. When using the stethoscope, it is advised to use the bell-shaped end to minimize false positives frequently encountered with use of the flat end (Wright 2005). The TMJ examination results should not only report if joint sounds are present but also their quality and time of occurrence in the opening and closing cycles. Is the joint sound present early, middle, or late in the opening and in the closing movements? In general, a late opening and early closing joint sound indicates a greater dysfunctional diagnosis than an early opening, late closing joint sound. This information must be considered in the long-term stability of the joint apparatus when extensive reconstructive procedures are anticipated. Sounds can be classified as clicks, pops, or as grating in nature. Clicks and pops are generally attributed to a disc displacement with or without reduction (Yatani et al. 1998). These joint sounds can be very aggravating to the patient and very difficult to eliminate. Physical therapy in conjunction with a dental orthotic can, at best, reduce symptoms in approximately 33% of cases (Okeson and Hayes 1986). The grating or crepitant sound is suggestive of degenerative changes within the articular structure (Schiffman et al. 1989). Dental reconstruction may have a guarded or unfavorable prognosis due to this progressive instability, and such information must be mentioned to the patient as part of the informed consent process.

Thorough evaluation of the TMJ should include questions to the patient regarding spontaneous pain, pain during function, a history of facial trauma, episodes of joint locking in either an open or closed position, and whether self-reduction or emergency treatment was required for these episodes. Does the patient restrict his or her diet to soft foods and consciously limit the range of mandibular opening to avoid such situations? This information has implications on whether extensive dentistry can be performed without initiating or exacerbating these symptoms. If the locking occurs at full opening, the patient may be experiencing episodes of subluxation due to flattening of the crest of the eminence or loss of ligamentous control. If the locking occurs in a restricted opening position, the patient may have an anteriorly displaced disc that is preventing mandibular translation, or they may be experiencing severe spasticity of the opening muscles. In any case, a step-by-step TMD checklist is very helpful in acquiring all the pertinent information and should be considered an invaluable part of the intake treatment record (fig. 4-6).

A thorough examination must also include palpation of the following muscles of mastication:

1. The masseter muscle, deep and superficial bodies
2. The temporalis muscle with its three bodies
3. The anterior and posterior digastric bundle
4. The sternocliedomastoid muscle with its sternal and crevicular heads
5. The medial pterygoid muscle
6. The splenius capitis muscle
7. The insertion of the temporalis tendon

While palpating the masseter and temporalis muscles, you want to look for signs of muscle hypertrophy or symptoms of pain (figs. 4-7 and 4-8). Instruct the patient to clench and relax the jaw and observe any increase in size, bulging, or firmness of those muscles. Direct the patient to place his or her hands on these muscles while clenching to fully experience the increased size and quality of hardness during this activity (fig. 4-9; Schindler et al. 2007). Ask the patient about awareness of any parafunctional activity such as clenching or grinding, early morning muscle fatigue, headaches in the region of the anterior temporalis, or history of migraine headaches (fig. 4-10). If the patient responds positively to any of these inquiries, you must supplement these findings during the intraoral and hard tissue examination. Painful palpation of these muscles may also suggest an etiology for other nondental disease processes such as atypical facial pain (Gotouda et al. 2005), muscle contraction headaches, or misdiagnosed migraine headaches. If there is painful palpation of the posterior bundle of the temporalis muscle, it may suggest that the patient is unconsciously assuming a habitual retruded postural position.

If tenderness is observed while palpating the digastric bundles, first rule out any intraoral contributing factors and attempt to elicit and trace a referred pain pathway (fig. 4-11). In addition, the posterior digastric may be very tender if the patient has a recent restricted opening episode (Wright 2005). This tenderness may be a result of the patient's repeated attempt to open wider during these events. Painful palpation to the sternocleidomastoid muscle may refer pain to the masseter, ear, and TMJ areas (fig. 4-12).

To palpate the splenius capitis, follow the sternocleidomastoid superiorly and posteriorly to its insertion at the base of the skull (fig. 4-13). If one or both of these muscles have a positive response to palpation, with or without referral pain, it may imply a possible cervical component to their pain (Wright 2000). You must consider referring the patient for a full TMD evaluation at a multidisciplinary clinic (Fricton and Dall'Arancio 1994) prior to undertaking any extensive reconstructive procedures (Rosenbaum et al. 1997).

Additionally, an intraoral palpation of the temporalis tendon with its insertion on the neck of the coronoid process should be performed. This procedure is accomplished by palpating distal to the mandibular second molar, up the ascending ramus to the head of the coronoid process (fig. 4-14). Many times, the intraoral palpation of this tendon is painful, while palpation of the external muscle itself may not elicit any discomfort. While in this area, palpate the medial pterygoid muscle. This can be done by palpating in the area of the traditional penetration site for the inferior alveolar nerve block (fig. 4-15). Lastly, palpation of the inferior and superior lateral pterygoid muscles has limited value due to the inability of direct palpation as a result of its anatomical position. To palpate the inferior belly indirectly, press against the deposition site for the posterior superior alveolar injection site. Dysfunction of this muscle can be observed while the patient is opening with a noted deviation of the mandible to the contralateral side. Generally speaking, healthy muscles do not hurt when

Occlusion and TMJ Assessment Form
===

Patient Name:_____   Date: _____

Initial Patient Concerns:

_____

_____

_____

Initial Occlusal & TMJ Findings:

CENTRIC RELATION:
    Location: ☐ easy ☐ difficult ☐ impossible
    TMJ discomfort to pressure: ☐ none ☐ right ☐ left
    Initial tooth contact: _____ vs. _____
CENTRIC RELATION–CENTRIC OCCLUSION DISCREPANCY:
    Vertical slide _____mm Forward slide _____mm
    Lateral slide ☐ right ☐ left _____mm
CENTRIC OCCLUSION:
    Canine classification (I, II, III) right _____ left _____
    Right canine functional vertical overlap _____ mm
    Right canine functional horizontal overlap _____ mm
    Left canine functional vertical overlap _____ mm
    Left canine functional horizontal overlap _____ mm
    Central incisor functional vertical overlap _____ mm
    Central incisor functional horizontal overlap_____mm
    Wear facets ☐ minimal ☐ moderate ☐ severe

CR TO CO INTERFERENCE	1 2 3 4 5 32 31 30 29 28	6 7 8 9 10 11 27 26 25 24 23 22	12 13 14 15 16 21 20 9 18 17
RT. LATERAL	1 2 3 4 5 32 31 30 29 28	6 7 8 9 10 11 27 26 25 24 23 22	12 13 14 15 16 21 20 9 18 17
LT. LATERAL	1 2 3 4 5 32 31 30 29 28	6 7 8 9 10 11 27 26 25 24 23 22	12 13 14 15 16 21 20 9 18 17
PROTRUSIVE	1 2 3 4 5 32 31 30 29 28	6 7 8 9 10 11 27 26 25 24 23 22	12 13 14 15 16 21 20 9 18 17

TEMPOROMANDIBULAR JOINT:
    Maximum opening _____mm
    Joint sounds during opening and closing: ☐ none   ☐ right   ☐ left
Joint sounds during excursions: ☐ none   ☐ right   ☐ left
History of TMJ treatment: ☐ yes   ☐ no
Current joint pain: ☐ none   ☐ right   ☐ left

Supporting Musculature Evaluation   Within Normal Limits
----

1) Palpation of masseter muscle at rest   Yes   No
2) Palpation of anterior temporalis muscle at rest   Yes   No
3) Palpation of masseter muscle while clenching   Yes   No
4) Palpation of anterior temporalis muscle while clenching   Yes   No
5) Palpation of anterior medial pterygoid muscle   Yes   No

Specific Notes or Findings:

_____

_____

_____

Figure 4-6.   TMJ assessment form.

palpated (Okeson 2003). If numerous regions express pain during the examination, extensive dental therapy should be postponed and a complete TMD evaluation should be instituted following the completion of the needed routine dental procedures.

Palpation of the thyroid gland is suggested to rule out thyroiditis (fig. 4-16). Palpation of the carotid arteries is suggested to rule out carotidynia (a painful response locally or to a distant referred site) with a recommend physician referral with either painful response (fig. 4-17;

Wright 2005). Asking the patient to smile, squint their eyes, and wrinkle their brow is a simple way to obtain basic neurological information and assess any potential dysfunction of cranial nerve VII.

Elderly patients require palpation of prominent temporal arteries to rule out temporal arteritis, a potential disastrous condition leading to optic nerve damage and eventual blindness (fig. 4-18). Painful palpation of this region requires referral for a biopsy for definitive diagnosis.

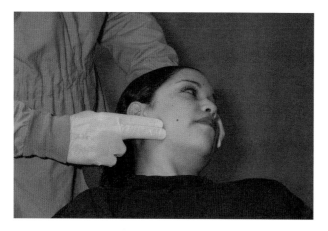

Figure 4-7. Palpation of masseter muscle at rest.

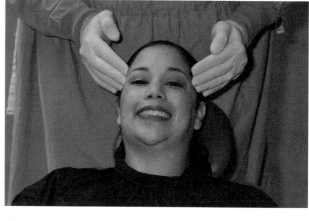

Figure 4-10. Palpation of anterior temporalis muscle while clenching.

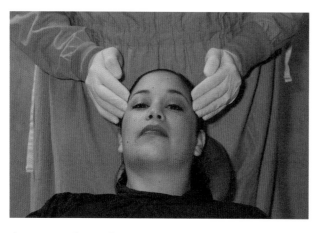

Figure 4-8. Palpation of anterior temporalis muscle at rest.

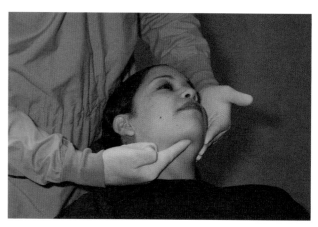

Figure 4-11. Palpation of anterior digastric muscle.

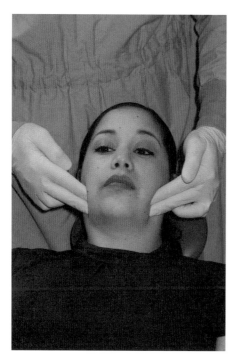

Figure 4-9. Palpation of masseter muscle while clenching.

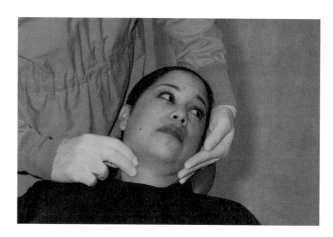

Figure 4-12. Palpation of sternocleidomastoid muscle.

34

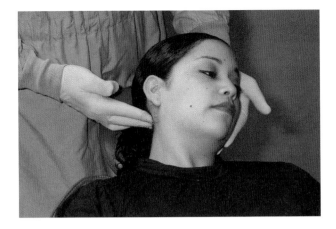

Figure 4-13. Palpation of splenius capitis muscle.

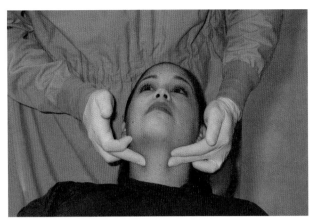

Figure 4-16. Thyroid gland palpation.

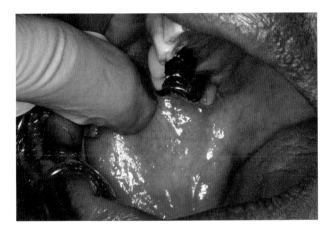

Figure 4-14. Intraoral palpation of temporalis tendon.

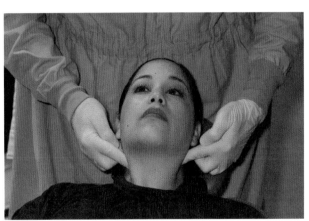

Figure 4-17. Palpation of carotid arteries.

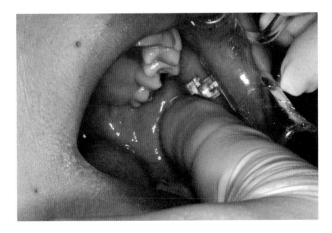

Figure 4-15. Palpation of medial pterygoid muscle.

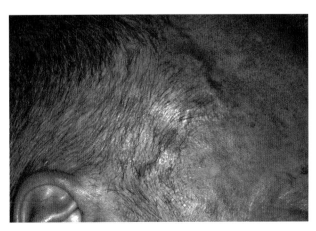

Figure 4-18. Prominent temporal artery.

After the palpation of all aforementioned structures is completed, range of motion values should be obtained. The following ranges should be measured for all patients:

1. Maximum opening
2. Left lateral movement
3. Right lateral movement
4. Protrusive movement

Several devices that can be used to assess the patient's mandibular range of motion include a millimeter ruler, a boley gauge, or a therabite appliance (fig. 4-19). Routinely take these measurements early in the appointment and ask the patient if these movements are within their comfort range.

Maximum mandibular opening is a vertical interincisal measurement recorded by measuring from maxillary incisal edge to mandibular incisal edge at full opening. The millimeters of maxillary/mandibular overbite are added to this measurement since the mandible opened through the overbite several millimeters prior to clearing the incisal edges. However, if an open bite is present, the distance between the incisal edges is subtracted from the measurement of maximum opening to establish a true measurement of vertical interincisal opening (fig. 4-20). The average maximum interincisal opening for men ranges from 45 mm to 55 mm, whereas the average range for women is from 35 mm to 45 mm.

In lateral excursions, the range of movement is from 10 mm to 15 mm and 8 mm to 14 mm on average, in protrusion (figs. 4-21 and 4-22). In addition to these measurements, it is important to note if the patient displays pain during any portion of these excursions. The quality of all movements should also be described as either fluid or guarded throughout its path.

Evaluating tongue function, swallowing patterns, and freeway space adds additional pertinent information and may provide clues to the etiology or presence of any destructive forces at work. The presence of a retained infantile swallowing pattern may be a causative, contributing, or supportive factor when an anterior open bite is

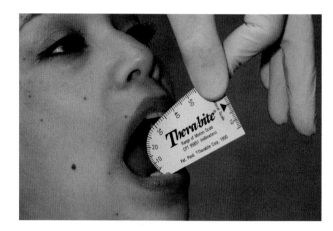

Figure 4-20. Use of Therabite device.

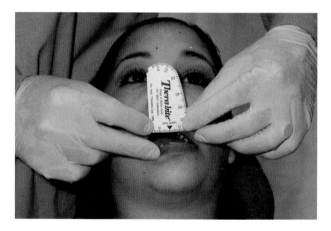

Figure 4-21. Recording lateral excursions.

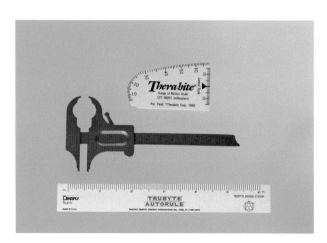

Figure 4-19. Various range of motion devices.

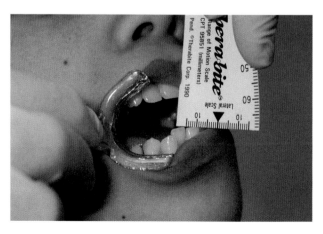

Figure 4-22. Recording protrusive excursion.

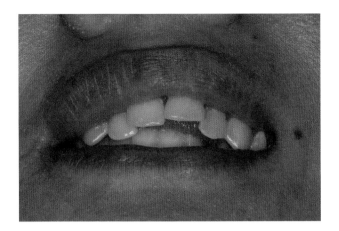

Figure 4-23. Retained anterior swallowing pattern.

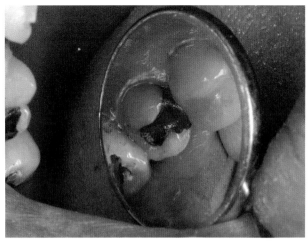

Figure 4-24. Evaluation of restoration, moist.

present (fig. 4-23). A lateral tongue thrust, either unilateral or bilateral, can contribute to a posterior open bite. In such cases a referral to a speech pathologist and orthodontist is the recommended course of pretreatment therapy to help correct this destructive swallowing pattern and increase the stability of the proposed dental reconstruction.

Intraoral Examination

For patients seeking esthetic treatment, the intraoral examination must consist of an objective assessment of the following:

1. Dental disease
   a. Caries assessment
   b. Periodontal assessment
   c. Periapical assessment
2. Supporting soft tissue structures
3. Functional status of the masticatory system
4. Esthetic assessment

Dental Caries

Utilizing a routine system for charting present restorations, caries, and suggested restorations is the simplest way to complete an efficient examination. The doctor and assistant can develop a well-choreographed routine that gathers the necessary information in a timely fashion.

The use of the air/water syringe to remove the excess saliva and debris from the teeth prior to examination with an explorer is recommended when evaluating the dentition for decay and faulty restorations. Additionally, this presents an opportune time to take individual photographs of teeth that will be used in the treatment planning and consultation phases. During this section of the intake process, the practitioner should communicate

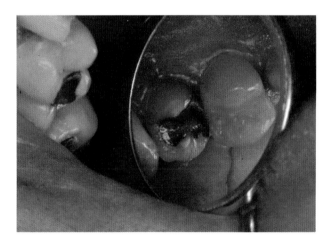

Figure 4-25. Evaluation of restoration, dry.

the potential need for indirect restorations due to new or recurrent decay, fractured cusps, or failing restorations. The use of an intraoral camera is highly recommended to clearly demonstrate these findings for the patient (figs. 4-24 and 4-25).

Periodontal Evaluation

As in charting dental caries, establish a pattern for your periodontal examination that is thorough and time efficient. Along with the straight calibrated probe, include the use of the Nabors probe to evaluate the presence and extent of furcation involvements (fig. 4-26). The probing depths and furcation information results will suggest areas in which thorough radiographic evaluation is essential. In addition to pocket depths, your charting should include tissue quality, bleeding points, attachment loss, detectible plaque and calculus, and

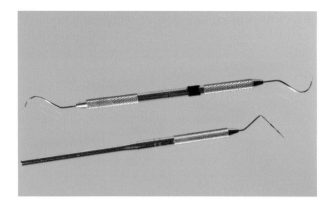

Figure 4-26. Calibrated straight and Nabors probe.

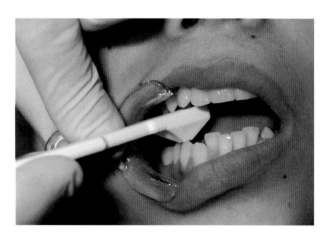

Figure 4-27. Toothsloot assessment.

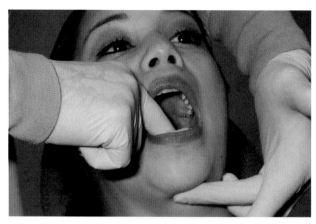

Figure 4-28. Bimanual palpation of floor of the mouth.

areas of recession. It is imperative that all esthetic patients receive a thorough periodontal diagnosis. The diagnosis of the overall periodontal condition will lead to the initial periodontal treatment and help the practitioner to establish a routine supportive periodontal plan that can influence your treatment choices and long-term prognosis.

Periapical Pathology

The intraoral examination must include percussion of all teeth in both axial and nonaxial directions (Okeson 1995). If a patient's history or signs during the examination indicate possible periapical pathology, then thermal testing, transillumination, or tests for fractured cusps must be a part of the protocol (fig. 4-27; Wright and Gullickson 1996, Walton 1986).

If periapical pathology is suspected, supplemental radiographs of suspicious teeth should be added to the customary full mouth series of radiographs.

Supporting Soft Tissue Structures

At this phase of the intraoral examination, it's appropriate to bimanually palpate the floor of the mouth and to complete the oral cancer screening. The use of supportive examination modalities such as dilute acetic acid rinses combined with dark light sources can be very effective in detecting early to late cellular changes. The patient should be advised of the purpose of this procedure and that it is a routine part of the thorough examination (fig. 4-28).

Functional Status of the Masticatory System

On average approximately 90% of our patients will exhibit some form of malocclusion or dysfunction (McNeil 1997). The goal of our initial examination is to capture relevant information that is useful for the case workup and consultation. Since many dental dysfunctional habits are difficult to diagnosis with purely visual examination techniques, properly mounted dental casts should be secured. The use of a semi-adjustable articulator that incorporates a facebow and incisal guide table can properly record the required information. The utilization of centric records will guide the decision whether to design the case in centric relation or centric occlusion. These concepts will be addressed further in chapter 5. Interocclusal records can be attained via manual manipulation or intraoral deprogramming devices (fig. 4-29). Comparison of the initial tooth contacts in centric relation orally with the initial tooth contacts on the mounted casts will verify the exactness of your records. The majority of patients will exhibit a slide from centric relation to centric occlusion. The practitioner must determine whether this slide is detrimental to the dental health of the patient or if the dental structures are adapting to this dysfunction. This determination can affect the final treatment plan. When analyzing the mounted casts, consider the basic type of

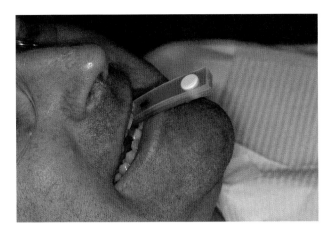

Figure 4-29. Use of an intraoral deprogramming device.

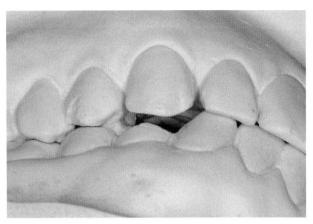

Figure 4-31. Right side cuspid relationship exhibiting excessive functional horizontal overlap.

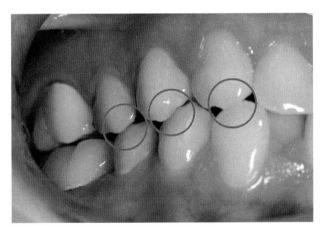

Figure 4-30. Image of working side group function.

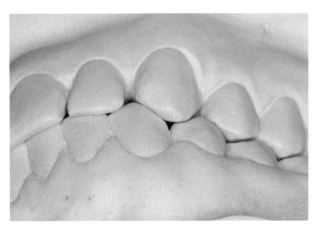

Figure 4-32. Left side cuspid relationship exhibiting minimal functional horizontal overlap.

chewing pattern. Does the patient exhibit a severe bruxing style ("cow clusion") or clenching style ("gator clusion")? Additionally, it is essential that the practitioner ascertain the type of disclusive pattern present on both sides of the dental arches: group function or canine disclusion.

Closer analysis of canine disclusion evaluates the presence of functional horizontal overlap and its influence on the posterior occlusion patterns. If immediate canine disclusion is not present, the mandible travels laterally in group function until canine rise is achieved or the canine participates in the group function through the remainder of the excursion. Be aware that this working group function may also create destructive posterior balancing interferences (fig. 4-30). In these cases, the posterior teeth may exhibit flattened wear patterns and facets. This canine functional horizontal overlap can be corrected to one of immediate canine

disclusion if the patient's dental function is not adapting but rather is exhibiting ongoing signs of dysfunction, excessive wear, symptomatic pain, or lack of effective mastication. If full-mouth reconstruction or anterior rehabilitation is the desired goal, the canine's functional horizontal overlap can be corrected to comply with the patient's habitual chewing pattern (figs. 4-31 and 4-32).

If major treatment is not warranted and the patient's signs and symptoms of dental function are not an issue, the disclusion correction can be optional for the present time, but its importance should be disclosed to the patient.

Recording the range of mandibular disclusion in full right lateral pathways, left lateral pathways, and protrusive excursions is noted not only for their extent but also the quality and fluidity of such movements. For example, a jerky, tentative pattern may indicate the presence of a protective mechanism adopted due to a dental or neuromuscular dysfunction. These issues are covered in greater detail in chapters 5, 7, and 9.

Esthetic Evaluation

The goal of this chapter is not to delve deeply into the fundamentals of esthetic dentistry. This is covered extensively in other chapters of the text. Rather, this chapter outlines the necessary information that must be gathered during the initial examination to develop a comprehensive esthetic treatment plan. The initial esthetic examination must obtain information regarding the patient's needs, desires, and perception of any functional and esthetic reconstructive issues. With this in mind, it becomes imperative to gather all essential information that allows the doctor to develop one or multiple treatment plans that simultaneously treat existing dental defects and achieve the patient's desired esthetic outcomes.

To assist the practitioner in developing a comprehensive esthetic and restorative treatment plan, certain references must be obtained during the initial appointment. These items will be used to assist the practitioner with his or her diagnosis and treatment plan development. During the first appointment, it is essential to gather the following:

1. Quality full-mouth radiographic survey
2. Pretreatment photographs (outlined in chapter 3)
3. Centric relation bite registration
4. Vinyl Polysiloxane impression to yield several sets of high-quality study casts
   a. One unaltered set of the pretreatment condition
   b. One set mounted in centric relation
5. Facial landmark registration (discussed in chapter 2)

Consultation Appointment

Even when the required dental treatment involves basic restorative procedures, a separate consultation visit allows the doctor to discuss various optional esthetic proposals that may be considered by the patient in the future. Extensive esthetic and reconstructive treatment plans are difficult to thoroughly develop during a short, initial patient examination and necessitate a separate consultation visit to provide adequate time for complete diagnosis on the part of the practitioner. Additionally, the time between the two appointments provides the practitioner with an opportunity to develop an esthetic wax-up or computer-generated smile design, both of which are effective communication tools. The diagnostic wax-up also provides the opportunity to establish improved occlusal schemes when necessary. At the consultation appointment, various restorative designs and

options such as direct, indirect, fixed, or removable partial dentures or implants are presented to the patient. For example, are veneers the only option or is whitening and enamel recontouring acceptable?

This appointment with its printed treatment plans, along with financial and treatment time estimates, establishes the record framework and goals agreed to by the patient.

This structured methodology of the initial patient examination encourages the doctor to plan the case, involve the patient in pretreatment decisions, and hopefully eliminate the concept of "prep and pray" dentistry.

Works Cited

Fricton JR, Dall'Arancio D. 1994. Myofascial pain of the head and neck: Controlled outcome study of an interdisciplinary pain program. *J Musculoske Pain* 2(2):81–99.

Gotouda A, Yamaguchi T, Okada K, Matsuki T, Gotouda S, Inoue N. 2005. Influence of playing wind instruments on activity of masticatory muscles. *Clin Anat* 18(5):318–22.

McNeil C. 1997. Management of temporomandibular disorders: Concepts and controversies. *J Pros Dent* 77:510–22.

Okeson JP, Hayes DK. 1986. Long-term results of treatment for temporomandibular disorders: An evaluation by patients. *J Am Dent Assoc* 112(4):473–8.

Okeson JP. 1995. *Bell's Orofacial Pains*, 5th ed. Chicago: Quintessence.

Okeson JP. 2003. *Management of Temporomandibular Disorders and Occlusion*, 5th ed. St. Louis: CV Mosby.

Rosenbaum RS, Gross SG, Pertes RA, Ashman LM, Kreisberg MK. 1997. The scope of TMD/orofacial pain (head and neck pain management) in contemporary dental practice. Dental Practice Act Committee of the American Academy of Orofacial Pain. *J Orofac Pain* 11(1):78–83.

Schiffman E, Anderson G, Fricton J, Burton K, Schellhas K. 1989. Diagnostic criteria for intraarticular T.M. disorders. *Community Dent Oral Epidemiol* 17(5):252–27.

Schindler HJ, Rues S, Turp JC, Schweizerhof K, Lenz J. 2007. Activity patterns of the masticatory muscles during feedback-controlled simulated clenching activities. *Cranio* 25(3):193–9.

Walton RE. 1986. Distribution of solutions with the periodontal ligament injection: Clinical, anatomical and histological evidence. *J Endod* 12:492–500.

Wright EF, Gullickson DC. 1996. Dental pulpalgia contributing to bilateralpreauricular pain and tinnitus. *J Orofac Pain* 10(2):166–8.

Wright EF. 2000. Patterns of referred craniofacial pain in TMD patients. *J Am Dent Assoc* 131(9):1307–15.

Wright EF. 2005. *Manual of Temporomandibular Disorders and Occlusion*, 1st ed. Ames, IA: Blackwell.

Yatani H, Sonoyama W, Kuboki T, Matsuka Y, Orsini MG, Yamashita A. 1998. The validity of clinical examination for diagnosiing anterior disc displacement with reduction. *Oral Surg Oral Med Oral Pathol Oral Radiol Endod* 85:647–53.

Suggested Reading

Austin DG, Pertes RA. 1995. Examination of the TMD patient. In *Clinical Management of Temporomandibular Disorders and Orofacial Pain*, ed. Pertes RA, Gross SG, 148–49. Chicago: Quintessence.

Bell WE. 1989. *Orofacial Pains: Classification, Diagnosis, Management*, 4th ed. Chicago: Yearbook Medical Publishers.

Bush FM, Abbott FM, Butler JH, Harrington WG. 1998. Oral orthotics: Design, indications, efficacy and care. In *Clark's Clinical Dentistry*, vol. 2, ed. Hardin JF, chap. 39. Philadelphia: JB Lippincott.

Dawson PE. 2007. *Functional Occlusion: From TMJ to Smile Design*, St. Louis: Mosby/Elsevier.

Dworkin SF, LeResche L. 1992. Research diagnostic criteria for temporomandibular disorders: Review, criteria, examinations and specifications, critique. *J Craniomandib Disord* 6(4):301–55.

Magnusson T, Egermark I, Carlson GE. 2000. A longitudinal epidemiologic study of signs and symptoms of temporomandibular disorders from 15 to 35 years of age. *J Orofac Pain* 14(4):310–9.

Monaco A, Cattaneo R, Spadaro A, Giannoni M, DiMartino S, Gatto R. 2007. Visual input effect on EMG activity of masticatory and postural muscles in healthy and in myopic children. *J Oral Rehab* 34(9):645–51.

Ribeiro RF, Tallents RH, Katzberg RW, Murphy WC, Moss ME, Magalhaes AC, Tavano O. 1997. The prevalence of disc displacement in symptomatic and asymptomatic volunteers aged 6 to 25 years. *J Orofac Pain* 11(1):37–47.

Simons DG, Travell JG, Simons LS. 1999. *Travell & Simons Myofascial Pain and Dysfunction: The Trigger Point Manual*, vol. 1, 2nd ed. Baltimore: Williams & Wilkins.

Stegenga B. 2001. Osteoarthritis of the temporomandibular joint organ and its relationship to disc displacement. *J Orofac Pain* 15(3):193–205.

Chapter 5
Occlusion

Foroud Hakim DDS, MBA, BS

Jessie Vallee DDS, BS

The study of occlusion has been a topic of interest in dentistry for many years. The complexity of the topic has led many learned individuals to devote a lifetime to its investigation with the aim of improving understanding of it. Occlusion and its relationship to gnathostomatic function and dysfunction has been and will continue to be a topic of controversy. Mastication, phonetics, and esthetics all relate to the position of the teeth within the dental arches. A clear understanding of some universally accepted concepts within the subject of occlusion, particularly those best supported scientifically, is paramount for a doctor to practice complete dentistry.

The intent of this chapter is not to provide a comprehensive review of all concepts relating to occlusion. Certainly, thousands of pages of text have been devoted to the subject. Several recommended texts are suggested for reference and further study at the conclusion of this chapter. Considering the context of this writing, this chapter is devoted to reviewing some basic principles of occlusion that are integral to the practice of restorative dentistry and thus esthetic dentistry.

Too often, the relevance of occlusion to routine dentistry is forgotten. The notion that a profound understanding of occlusal principles and mastery of occlusal schemes is reserved only for complex restorative rehabilitation is incorrect. Sore teeth, structural breakdown, periodontal issues, and restorative failures may all be related to occlusion. These problems are encountered daily in dental practice. The fundamentals of occlusion are the same whether considering traditional or esthetic dentistry. Violation of these principles may lead to the early demise of all genres of esthetic restoratives ranging from a simple class V resin to a full-mouth ceramic reconstruction. Understanding occlusal principles and employing these from the start of diagnosis and treatment planning through smile design and eventual restoration delivery undoubtedly leads to improved esthetic outcomes, harmonious and comfortable patient function, long-term occlusal stability and restoration endurance, practitioner gratification, and decreased stress.

To facilitate a meaningful discussion of one of the most relevant principles of occlusion, and then to relate these to esthetic restorative design, the following topics will be addressed:

1. Occlusal disease
2. Determinants of occlusion
3. Centric relation
4. Mutually protective occlusion and guidance
5. Envelope of motion and function

Occlusal Disease

For the sake of nomenclature, Dr. Gordon Christiansen's definitions of the "Six Pathologic Conditions of Occlusion" (2001) are a good foundation.

Bruxism

Also called excursive grinding, bruxism is a prevalent condition that some believe affects up to one-third of the population. Destructive to a degree at any level, bruxism in severe forms often leads to prematurely mutilated dentition at an early age. Identification with subsequent prevention or protection are paramount when a subject demonstrates signs and symptoms of active bruxism. There are many implications associated with active bruxism that may affect how and when to perform esthetic restorative procedures.

The etiology of bruxism has been a subject of debate for many years. Consensus identifies the two most likely causes as odontogenic (relating to occlusion) and psychological. We will not delve deeper into the subject for the purpose of this text other than to recommend to the reader to seek continued education on this subject. Certainly, if esthetic dentistry is to be performed on a patient with a history of active bruxism, adaptations for case design, removal, or minimization of possible etiologies (structural or psychological) and splint protection should be considered (fig. 5-1).

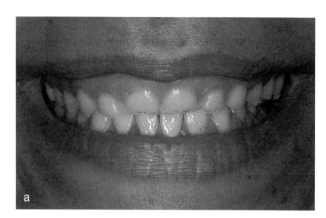
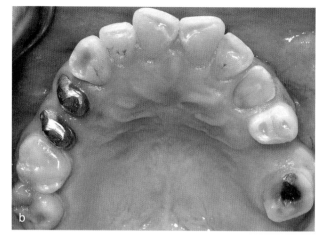

Figure 5-1. Severe bruxism.
a. Note the tremendous incisal wear of patient's anterior teeth due to a chronic, protrusive path parafunctional habit.
b. The debilitated arch of a patient with a history of severe nocturnal bruxing. Note significantly worn enamel, large areas of exposed dentin, ceramic delamination from metallic copings, and even tooth loss attributed to parafunction.

Clenching

Also referred to as static grinding, clenching may occur alone or in combination with bruxism. When clenching occurs independently of bruxism, it may result in steepening anterior guidance. Some studies have demonstrated nocturnal biting forces approaching 300 lb/in^2 created by clenchers on their molars. Esthetic restorations as well as natural dentition should be protected in clenchers. This is most typically done with full-coverage splints.

Abfractions

Historically, abfraction lesions have been attributed to facio-lingual flexure of teeth leading to cervical tooth structure loss at the point of fulcrum. Recently, compelling evidence has been delivered by Dr. Abrahansen identifying the cause of abrasion as dentrifices delivered via toothbrushing (Dawson 2007). Because of the impossibility of controlled in-vivo studies of this subject, and inconsistencies between the results of Dr. Abrahansen and clinical findings, it is difficult to cite a definitive etiology at this time. It is likely that both mechanical abrasion as well as bending stresses contribute to the formation of abrasion lesions. As these lesions develop, loss of resistant enamel exposes dentin. Dentin and cementum are softer and more vulnerable to dentrifice-related abrasion. The undermined fulcrum point of affected teeth left thinner and less resistant to flex further supports a mechanical stress explanation.

From a restorative perspective, it is perhaps more important to acknowledge when abfractive lesions are

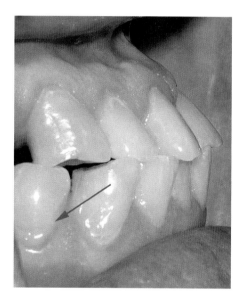

Figure 5-2. Abfraction lesion occurring on a tooth coincidental with significant incisal wear.

present and react accordingly rather than debate the etiology. Consider that these lesions occur in areas where esthetic restoration margins often terminate. No matter the etiology, if abfraction leads to marginal breakdown, crowns and veneers may fail prematurely. The prudent esthetic dentist looks for evidence of occlusion-related stress on the dentition as well as evaluates for possible overzealous brushing with abrasive dentrifices and takes measures to protect and instruct patients to minimize the occurrence of abfractions (fig. 5-2).

Primary Occlusal Trauma

Primary occlusal trauma occurs as a result of abnormal occlusal loads landing on otherwise healthy teeth. Most often, this is a result of newly placed restorations, esthetic restorations being no exception. Early detection and appropriate equilibration are important for reversing the harmful impact of functional or parafunctional occlusion on such premature contacts.

Secondary Occlusal Trauma

Secondary occlusal trauma occurs when the element of periodontal disease is added to the previous scenario. Thus, treatment not only involves equilibration but also periodontal therapy and possible splinting.

Temporomandibular Disorder (TMD)

More than any other topic, TMD has been a source of controversy within the literature. It has even been difficult for the profession to adopt a universal glossary and terminology relating to this subject. Only brief mention and differentiation is merited with the context of this text.

TMD can be broken down into two categories, those relating to masticatory muscle dysfunctions and those relating to joint or intracapsular disturbances. Identification, diagnosis, and if necessary, treatment of TMD can begin with general practitioners and escalate to specialist referral, pending complexity. Ultimately, irreversible or elective dentistry (esthetic dentistry) should not be initiated on a patient with undiagnosed TMD. Joint and occlusal stability must be a prerequisite or anticipated consequence of esthetic restorative rehabilitation.

Determinants of Occlusion

The determinants of occlusion are commonly broken down into two components: anterior and posterior. Comfortable and efficient physiological function of the gnathostomatic complex hinges on structural harmony between these two components. In other words, harmony between the occluding teeth and the temporomandibular joints (TMJs) is essential.

Posterior Determinants

The TMJs are considered the posterior determinants of occlusion. Evaluation of joint health, anatomy, stability, and function shall proceed occlusal anylysis. Joint pathology, dysfunction, or instability are red flags to haphazard initiation of esthetic dentistry.

The anatomy of the articular fossa, the descending articular eminence, and the medial walls in large part determine the path traveled by the condyles and thus the mandible during function. The impact of joint anatomy and function on occlusion cannot be ignored. The combination of joint guidance coupled with mandibular geometric precursors such as jaw size, the Curve of Spee, and the Curve of Wilson affect tooth anatomy and occlusion significantly. This impact is more significant on posterior teeth and most significant in the absence of dominant anterior guidance.

Anterior Determinants

The anterior determinants of occlusion are defined in short by the interocclusal relationship of the teeth. This can be further divided into posterior and anterior teeth impact. The role of posterior teeth is to provide vertical stops utilized in mastication as well as protection from deflective, off-axis loading of anterior teeth. Posterior occlusion should not interfere with joint harmony or anterior guidance. Conversely, anterior teeth play a key role in the protection of posterior teeth through eccentric movements. This concept of "mutually protected occlusion" will be addressed further throughout the chapter. Anterior teeth also serve in phonetics, socialization via esthetic reveal, and incising and tearing food. When in optimal position, the anterior teeth perform these functions with appropriate relation to the tongue, lips, and occlusal plane. Dr. Dawson (2007) refers to this phenomenon as the "anterior teeth being in harmony with the envelope of function."

The intertwined relationship between joint guidance, anterior teeth position, and contour as well as posterior teeth position and anatomy is essentially what determines the geometric proportions, inclinations, and relative positions of proposed esthetic restorations. Parameters such as occlusal plane radius, anterior tooth height, anterior tooth inclination, anterior lingual contours, posterior cusp height, and posterior groove width and direction are among the features predicated by the aforementioned relationship.

Centric Relation

Centric relation (CR) refers to a musculoskeletal position relating the mandible to the maxilla. CR originally gained popularity as a useful concept in removable prosthodontics due to repeatability. In the absence of teeth, a mechanism of determining the maxillo-mandibular relationship was needed. Its universality led to crossover into the fixed prosthodontic arena, and CR has remained conceptually throughout the years within dental literature and

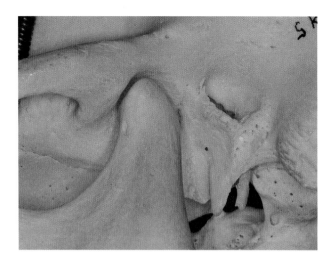

Figure 5-3. CR position of TMJ on teaching skull. Note the space between the condyle and superior fossa where the articular disk would be transposed in a live subject.

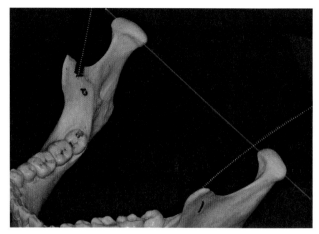

Figure 5-4. Line bisecting the condyles depicting the hinge axis of pure rotational movement in CR prior to translation.

text. The ever-evolving definition of CR has led to confusion on the subject and even led to doubt regarding its usefulness or validity in diagnostic and restorative dentistry. It is important to clarify that CR, as a skeletal position, has absolutely not changed. Better understanding of joint physiology and anatomy has simply led to a more descriptive and accurate definition.

A modern definition of CR consistent across most literature, including leading textbooks and *The Glossary of Prosthodontic Terms*, may read as, "CR is a musculoskeletally stable position where the condyles are braced in the most supero-anterior position of the eminentiae with a properly interposed disk assembly" (fig. 5-3). Dr. Dawson has added two additional modifiers, the release of inferior lateral pterygoid contraction and the absence of pain or discomfort to loading, both of which are very useful for added clarification. In other words, CR not only infers the position but also the relative health of the condylar-disk assemblies. CR exists irrespective of the position or even presence of teeth. Twenty to twenty-five millimeters of free rotation about a fixed horizontal axis can occur before the condyles move out of the CR position and begin translation (fig. 5-4).

Determination and verification of CR (or the conclusion of unverifiability) should play a significant role in all occlusal treatment, including restorative and esthetic rehabilitation. Does this mean that all restorative esthetic dentistry should be designed with occlusion coincidental to CR? Is this always prudent or even possible? What are the exceptions? When should esthetic dentistry be postponed or not performed at all? These are some of the questions related to occlusion asked by practitioners seeking to increase their participation in the esthetic

restorative field. This chapter will answer some of these questions as well as outline a strategy that practitioners can employ to make prudent decisions regarding the design of occlusion for their esthetic restorations.

Decision Points

Condition of Temporomandibular Joints

A critical red flag when considering esthetic restorative dentistry is unstable TMJs. Symptomatic and progressive TMD, progressive joint deformation and corresponding interocclusal fluctuations, and unverifiable CR are all contraindications to irreversible restorative treatment. As a matter of practicality, it is certainly acceptable to perform necessary restorative dentistry on isolated teeth. Such permanent or interim restorations can be placed with esthetically acceptable outcomes in mind, but the primary goal in these circumstances is tooth structure stabilization and elimination of pain, caries, or infection. Care should be taken to place such restorations in occlusion that does not lead to further progressive dysfunction or instability. Restorations creating unstable circumstances such as the absence of occlusal stops or proximal contacts, deflective inclines, premature contacts, or eccentric interferences should be avoided.

The goal with unstable TMJs is the diagnosis of joint pathology or derangement, halting the progression, and eventual stabilization. Only then can any significant restorative or esthetic dentistry be considered.

Extent of Case

More specifically, this refers to the number of teeth involved. As a general rule, when the majority or all teeth present are planned for restoration, maximum intercuspation (MI) should be coincident with stable and verifiable CR. If MI does not equal CR preoperatively, careful analysis allows mapping of the interferences or prematurities leading to the discrepancy. Through new restoration anatomy, occlusal equilibration, or a combination of both, patients undergoing esthetic restorative dentistry can predictably be restored to coincidental CR and MI. With all other factors being equal, this approach to occlusal design leads to long-term joint and dental arch stability and increases restorative success rate and longevity.

On the other hand, the restorative needs of a patient are often limited to one or a few teeth only. In such cases, similar to the more complex, larger scope cases, if MI and CR are equal preoperatively, care should be taken to not interfere with this harmony. Conversely, when MI does not coincide with CR, simple duplication of the preoperative occluso-incisal anatomy may in fact be opportunity sacrificed. For example, beyond simple esthetic improvements, careful modification of esthetic restoration form such as incisal edge length, lingual incline, or cusp anatomy may lead to more favorable eccentric interarch tooth relationships.

Ultimately, in limited or single-tooth cases where MI does not equal CR, some additional thought is required. If occlusal analysis reveals that the tooth or teeth to be restored are solely or in large part responsible for the discrepancy, it is logical to eliminate this discrepancy when developing restoration anatomy. If this strategy eliminates a significant source of the CR–MI interferences, occlusal equilibration can also be employed to eliminate additional interferences present on teeth not being restored. In essence, even in cases that are considered simple to intermediate in scope, practitioners must be aware of opportunities to increase occlusal balance, stability, and harmony and take advantage of these opportunities when restorative esthetic dentistry is planned.

In the event that a preoperative CR–MI discrepancy is largely unrelated to the tooth or teeth to be restored, there is a decision to be made. If the discrepancy is not progressively increasing, the patient's TMJs are stable, and asymptomatic and clinical judgment shows no significant benefit from additional treatment, it is quite acceptable and even commonplace to simply restore the involved tooth or teeth to conforming occlusion. In other words, the new restorations are in harmony with both the patient's CR and conforming MI and do not impart any interferences within that span.

Centric Relation Validity

Despite its proven reliability and absolute necessity in occlusal diagnostics, CR and its value in dental diagnostics and treatment has periodically come into question.

In most cases, misunderstood definition, difficulties in manipulation and location, or confusion about its relation to restorative and esthetic dentistry have led to doubt or criticism by opponents of CR.

Regarding location of CR, with a small amount of training and practice, even the novice practitioner can be trained in CR manipulation. This is proven yearly when second-year dental students at the University of the Pacific Arthur A. Dugoni School of Dentistry reliably verify and repeatedly locate and record CR on each other during an exercise in their class on occlusion. In most cases, with the help of some muscle deprogramming using an anterior discluder like a leaf gauge, and bimanual technique, even patients deemed "difficult" can be repeatedly manipulated in CR. It is also diagnostic to know when CR identification is not possible as mentioned earlier in this chapter.

It may be useful to interject a subclassification of CR. In the event that a TMJ has undergone deformation and remodeling as a result of disease or trauma but has settled to a stable, comfortable, and reproducible position, decisions regarding treatment are not any different than when traditional CR is identified. Such a reformation has been coined "adapted centric posture" by Dr. Dawson. This nomenclature satisfies a previous void in terminology and should help to eliminate some of the confusion faced by practitioners regarding esthetic treatment planning related to occlusion and TMJ status. Table 1 serves as a quick reference for triage of esthetic treatment planning as it relates to joint status and CR.

Mutually Protected Occlusion and Guidance

In an optimized occlusal scheme, when a patient closes in CR, simultaneous, equal-intensity contacts occur on all teeth. On posterior teeth, these contacts should occur on cusp tips to corresponding flat opposing surfaces. Variations of this scheme, such as tripodization, are also acceptable as long as vertical loading leads to force vectors along the long axis of teeth, eliminating lateral deflection.

Anterior teeth should ideally have an incisal edge to lingual fossa relationship that minimizes splaying or lateral deflection. Even so, the presence of definitive, multitooth posterior stops is in large part responsible for protection of anterior teeth during centric biting, mastication, and clenching. The moment the mandible moves forward or laterally and condyles translate, anterior teeth should engage in "ramping" that immediately separates the posterior teeth. When anterior teeth shoulder this burden of load in eccentric movements,

Table 5-1.   Treatment planning triage.

MI = CR or Adapted CR	MI ≠ CR or Adapted CR	CR Unverifiable
Characteristics: • CR verifiable and repeatable • No TMD tx needed • Harmonious jaw closure without interferences • No discomfort to loaded TMJs	**Characteristics:** • CR is verifiable and repeatable • Condyles displace from CR or adapted CR position for MI to occur • Any pain is related to muscular dysfunction and not joint derangement	**Characteristics:** • Impossible to manipulate TMJs to a repeatable position due to muscular dysfunction, joint pain, or pathology
Restorative Implications: • Occlusal equilibration does not need to occur prior to restorative treatment • Restorative esthetic treatment should not alter CR/MI harmony and maintain or improve ideal anterior guidance • Occlusal splint may be prescribed after esthetic restorations are delivered to protect ceramics in patients with history of active bruxism	**Restorative Implications:** • Prognosis improves as interferences are eliminated • Symptoms may be alleviated with preoperative splint therapy and/or equilibration • Optimal goal with restorative treatment is to have MI = CR (may occur with adjunctive ortho treatment) • Anterior esthetic rehabilitation should optimize guidance • Postoperative splint protection	**Restorative Implications:** • TMD triage and treatment needed prior to restorative treatment • Based on TMD etiology, treatment may range from simple splint therapy to address muscle spasm to synovial joint therapy to address a variety of internal derangements • Simple restorative treatment permissible to address decay, pain, or infection • Complex esthetic treatment delayed until joint stability and verifiable CR achieved

Note: MI = maximum intercuspation; CR = centric relation; TMD = temporomandibular joint disorder; TMJ = temporomandibular joint.

posterior teeth are shielded from lateral and deflective forces for which they are not ideally suited. A number of geometric and physiologic factors make anterior teeth better suited to tolerate eccentric loading, including greater distance from power vectors (muscles of mastication), increasing inefficiency of the gnathostomatic lever systems, bony anatomy, and proprioceptive capabilities.

This exquisite relationship between anterior and posterior teeth is commonly referred to as "mutually protected occlusion" (fig. 5-5).

Whenever esthetic dentistry is planned for anterior or posterior teeth, duplication (if preoperatively present) or creation of optimized protective occlusion is considered an overriding goal. Acceptable exceptions to this general scheme are directed by individual patient circumstances. Factors such as parafunction, complicating periodontal status, or partial edentulism (corrected with fixed, removable, or implant-retained prosthodontics) may lead to consideration of alternative schemes such as lateral group function.

While esthetic restorations are placed throughout the dental arches, esthetic smile design and corresponding restorative treatment prevails in the anterior segments and most often occurs in the maxillary arch extending distally to the bicuspids. Incisal edge length and inclination not only impart esthetics, but when combined with lingual fossa anatomy and interincisal relationships, maxillary anterior restorations affect function and protective disclusion.

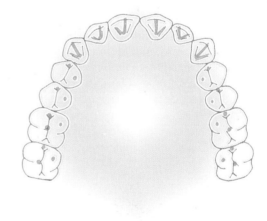

Figure 5-5.   Diagram of idealistic occlusal scheme consisting of equi-density centric contacts between cusp tips and flat fossae of all teeth coupled with eccentric guidance patterns exclusively on anterior teeth: "mutually protective occlusion."

It is worthwhile to discuss some nomenclature that defines the interincisal relationship of anterior teeth. The terms *functional horizontal overlap* (FHO) and *functional vertical overlap* (FVO) are quite useful. FVO is measured in millimeters as the distance between the maxillary and mandibular incisal edges. This follows the traditional orthodontic measurement and can be measured at incisors or canines. For example, if tooth #8 vertically over-laps #25 by 4 mm, it is said to have an FVO of 4 mm. Conversely, if these same teeth are in an anterior open bite relationship of 2 mm, FVO = −2 mm (fig. 5-6). FHO measurements as they pertain to occlusion differ from the traditional orthodontic evaluation. In orthodontics, FHO refers to the hortizonal overjet from the maxillary incisal edges to the facial profile of the corresponding mandibular anterior tooth. With regard to occlusal clas-sification, FHO refers to the horizontal distance between the facioincisal edges of the mandibular anterior tooth and the corresponding lingual profile of the maxillary anterior tooth. Figure 5-7 demonstrates this difference in measurement based on respective definitions. One quickly sees the impact of FVO and FHO on occlusion and disclusion. An FHO measurement of zero indicates proximity of incisors that make them available for immediate guidance and disclusion of posterior teeth upon any protrusive movement. Likewise, an FHO of zero for canines indicates their availability for immedi-ate lateral guidance and disclusion. It follows that FVO measurements indicate the amount of vertical rise that incisors and canines provide upon eccentric mounts. Using these parameters, anterior guidance can then be defined as ideal, absent, steep, shallow, immediate, or delayed simply based on the observed or prescribed FVO and FHO of anterior teeth.

By definition, anterior guidance is imparted by ante-rior teeth. Since esthetic dentistry most often involves the restoration and reformation of anterior teeth, the esthetic dentist must take advantage of opportunities afforded when placing elective or need-based anterior esthetic restorations to optimize anterior guidance. Well-designed anterior guidance promotes tooth and restoration longevity, TMJ health, and occlusal balance. Ideal anterior guidance often overrides complications that exist when joint guidance is the primary determi-nant of occlusion. Complex considerations of posterior restoration morphology such as cusp height, fossa, and groove width, or ridge and groove path, are often sim-plified when incisors and canines are well positioned with appropriate FVO, FHO, and inclination.

Regarding specific design and guidance parameters of anterior esthetic restoration, some acceptable variations exist based on the path traveled by the mandible.

Protrusive Guidance

The important concept to keep in mind when designing protrusive guidance is bilateral balance. It is desirable to spread the protrusive guidance across as many of the anterior teeth as possible. Arch geometry, orthodontic position, and relative incisal edge length differences between central and lateral incisors are unique to each patient and their specific smile design. When the protru-sive guidance must be limited to fewer than six teeth, the four incisors or even the two central incisors may and often do provide the majority of the protrusive guidance. This variation is of course case specific, but the concept of maintaining roughly equal load on either side of the midline and to even numbers of teeth is desirable.

Lateral Guidance

Two acceptable alternatives are recommended when designing the lateral guidance features of anterior restor-atives. Again, specific case parameters often dictate which is the best choice for a given patient. In a canine disclusion design scheme, the moment the mandible begins a lateral movement, the working-side opposing canines engage so that the facioincisal edge of the man-dibular canine guides against the lingual fossa of the maxillary canine through completion of the lateral movement at an edge-to-edge position. All other teeth in both arches are discluded by virtue of this working canine guidance. In a group anterior guidance scheme, the canines of the working side again provide lateral guidance, but the load is also shared with the lateral and central incisors on the working side. Thus, the working-side anterior teeth share the guidance for much, if not the entire length, of the lateral stroke (figs. 5-8 a through d).

Decisions regarding which anterior teeth shoulder the various eccentric movements often come down to the position of the inciso-occlusal plane and the relative orthodontic position of the lower anteriors to the pro-posed incisal stepping in length of the maxillary central incisors, lateral incisors, and canines (determined through wax-up and smile design.) Of course, limita-tions are eliminated when lower anteriors are also scheduled for esthetic rehabilitation. Factors that require additional thought when deciding if a tooth is a candi-date for bearing, sharing, or not participating in guid-ance may include periodontal status and crown-to-root ratio. When the tooth in question is part of a bridge, splinted units, or supported by an implant, additional consideration is also required.

Ultimately, the esthetic dentist must synthesize all the clinical circumstances and go forward with a best prac-tices approach through the diagnostic wax-up and smile design process. Through articulation, photographic ref-erences, and an understanding of patient desires, a pro-posed smile design is developed in wax. However, only after this template is transferred to the mouth via tem-poraries can proposals regarding guidance, disclusion, and occlusion be tested and then perfected through interim wear and adjustments.

Vertical overlap	Functional horizontal	Anterior guidance	Posterior disclusion
4mm	0mm	Ideal	Good
4mm	1mm	Delayed	Poor
1mm	0mm	Shallow	Minimal
0mm	0mm	none	none
-2mm	0mm	none	none

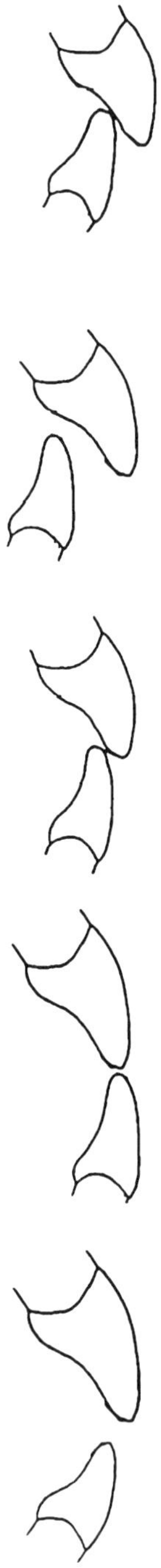

Figure 5-6. This table clearly illustrates the effects of varied FVO and FHO on anterior guidance and posterior protection.

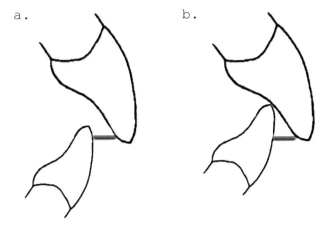

a.

b.

Figure 5-7. While both diagrams a and b would have an equal horizontal overjet measurement by traditional orthodontic evaluations, from an occlusion and guidance perspective, the difference in FHO is dramatic.

Upon confirmation of esthetic, phonetic, and functional success of provisional restorations, this tested and approved scheme must be transferred accurately to the laboratory. This step should not be underemphasized. Photographs, silicone templates, impressions of the perfected prototypes, and incisal guide tables are all valuable aids for ensuring the duplication accuracy of the final restorations with regard to the provisionals.

Envelope of Motion and Function

After lengthy discussions of the role of anterior teeth in esthetics, phonetics, guidance, and protection, it is logical to examine some physiological parameters that may set boundaries on effective positioning of anterior teeth whether through esthetic dentistry, orthodontics, or a combination of both.

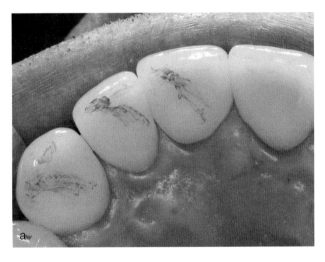

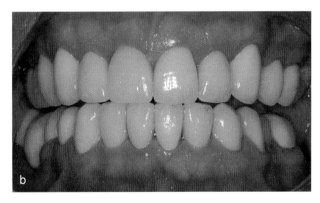

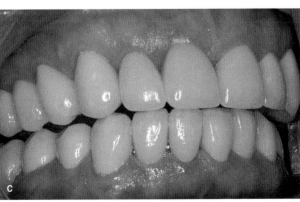

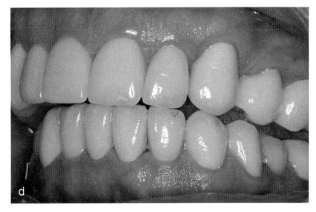

Figure 5-8. Well-designed guidance on an all-ceramic rehabilitation case.
a. and d. Anterior group guidance (involving teeth 9, 10, and 11) was the prescription of choice for left lateral movements.
b. Bilaterally balanced protrusive guidance was achieved on incisors.
c. Canine guidance was prescribed for right lateral movements.

The coordinated and simultaneous function of the orbicularis oris muscle and the tongue combine to develop the "neutral zone" for anterior teeth. For posterior neutral zone definition, the buccinator muscle replaces the orbicularis oris. Esthetically restored teeth positioned in conflict with the neutral zone are more likely to exhibit postoperative instability. This may manifest through orthodontic relapse, periodontal distress, or muscular dysfunction. While subtle or minor repositioning of anterior teeth may result in neutral zone adaptation and restorative and esthetic success, dramatic violations of neutral zone–dictated tooth positions are certainly contraindicated. The esthetic dentist must be aware of the patient's neutral zone and justify significant restorative repositioning through provisional testing and patient observation. In the event that the anterior neutral zone needs to be identified, traditional phonetic methods can be used. Circumstances where this determination may be needed include esthetic restoration of anterior teeth as pontics of a fixed partial denture, restoration of anterior implants, or simple replacements of previous restorations where neutral zone violation is suspected.

Simple neutral zone modification can often be accomplished through orthodontics, but more extreme surgical approaches such as tongue reduction, peri-oral muscle lengthening, or vestibuloplasty may be necessary in select cases.

Through phonetics and lip closure paths, labial and incisal position of maxillary anterior teeth are developed. Likewise, the lingual surfaces of the maxillary anterior teeth are developed through prescribed anterior guidance. All that remains is to determine the interincisal relationship of the maxillary and mandibular anterior teeth. To understand this process, a review of the "envelope of motion" is required.

Since the mandible is the only moving jaw, movements made by the mandibular teeth have historically been studied by gnathologists. The most extreme possible movements of the mandible, including maximum opening, translation, protrusion, and lateral excursions are defined as border movements. These are determined by musculoskeletal and ligamentous relations. Instrumentation can be employed to measure a patient's border movements, and this can be transferred precisely to an adjustable articulator. Two-dimensional tracings of mandibular movements in all their planes can be developed; these are referred to as Poussett's tracings.

While understanding the envelope of motion is important for understanding mandibular function, in reality, normal physiological mandibular movements associated with mastication, speech, and social expression fall within a narrower range. Dawson refers to this as the "envelope of function."

A common mistake made in fabricating anterior crowns or veneers is making them too long or too far labially. This mistake violates the neutral zone, may interfere with phonetics and often leads to poor esthetics. Conversely, placing incisal edges too far back interferes with the envelope of function. Consequences may include tooth collision during function, a feeling of restriction or being "locked in" for the patient, and resulting muscle dysfunction, occlusal imbalance, and periodontal and restorative damage.

In summary, a clear understanding of the neutral zone and the envelope of motion is required when considering smile redesign or any significant esthtetic dentistry for anterior teeth.

Recommendations

After highlighting some of the principles of occlusion most related to smile design and esthetic dentistry, it is important to reiterate that this writing has in fact only been a superficial review. The author emphasizes the importance of continued education for all practitioners seeking to increase their involvement in esthetic restorative dentistry, particularly as the scope and complexity of cases increase. Two texts that are excellent resources for questions about occlusion and TMJ function are *The Clinical Management of Temporomandibular Disorders and Occlusion*, 6th ed., by Jeffrey P. Okeson, and *Functional Occlusion: From TMJ to Smile Design* by Peter E. Dawson. For doctors seeking advanced training and education on these topics, a host of reputable institutes and organizations offer a variety of continuing education curriculums related to occlusion and restorative and esthetic dentistry, including the Pankey Institute (www.pankey.org), the Seattle Institute (www.seattleinstitute.com), and the Dawson Academy (www.dawsoncenter.com).

It should also go without saying that whenever performing esthetic dentistry through indirect restorations, appropriate instrumentation and articulation should be utilized. This includes face-bow registrations for maxillary position, recording of centric relation, and the use of semiadjustable articulation. While semiadjustable articulation is generally adequate for even the most complex restorative rehabilitation, fully adjustable articulation and pantographic records are recommended by some advisors.

Regarding postoperative protection and care of esthetic cases, some experts feel that splint wear is imperative, while others argue that perfected and stable occlusion and protective disclusion eliminate the need for splint protection. The author takes a somewhat moderate position on this matter. While perfected occlusion is always the goal in all restorative care, splint protection may be a prudent choice for patients with a history of nocturnal parafunction. Even when a new and improved occlusal scheme is delivered via restorations and is postulated to increase stability, there is never a guarantee that parafunction will cease or that ceramics will endure. In particular, nocturnal splint wear is recommended when due to esthetic requirements, the envelope of function has been restricted or steepened to any degree. An occlusal splint with flattened anterior guidance relative to the restorations may go a long way toward maintaining restorative and periodontal stability. Recommendations on types and wear of occlusal splints can be found in chapter 20.

Works Cited

Christensen G. 2001. Now is the time to observe and treat dental occlusion. *Journal of the American Dental Association* 132(1):100–102.

Dawson P. 2007. *Functional Occlusion from TMJ to Smile Design*. St. Louis: Mosby.

Chapter 6
Esthetic Case Design

Gabriela Pitigoi-Aron DDS

Marc Geissberger DDS, MA, BS, CPT

Esthetic treatment planning is the process of gathering information and developing a plan to address both dental disease and the patient's chief complaint. As described in chapter 4, the process can be broken down into two phases: information gathering and consultation. Case design is the process of developing the actual appearance and function of the proposed treatment plan. It can be accomplished between the initial appointment and the consultation, or following the consultation appointment once the patient has selected the treatment plan that most closely addresses his desires. Simply stated, treatment planning allows the practitioner to discuss the possible; case design allows the practitioner to construct the probable.

This chapter will outline the necessary steps to achieve predictable esthetic results by outlining the case design process. Although most dentists abandoned their waxing skills shortly after their formal training was completed, utilizing these skills can assist the practitioners in fine-tuning their esthetic eye. The design process will help practitioners develop an achievable, three-dimensional wax template that can be shared with the patient, laboratory technician, and other involved parties. This chapter will demystify the design process and describe a sequential, predictable process that can be incorporated into any esthetic practice.

Conceptualizing the Esthetic Case

Definition

Case design is a complex part of the esthetic treatment. To properly perform it, different skills are required, ones in which mathematics and art must find a common ground. Case design enables the clinician to develop treatment strategies and identify possible difficulties and solutions. Additionally, several preparation guides can be developed from the designed case that will greatly enhance the quality and efficiency of the preparation phase of treatment. The case design process must

marry both esthetics and function. These two guiding principles must be viewed as inseparable entities.

The term *smile designer* was introduced more than twenty years ago (Golub-Evans 2003) and has seen a resurgence of popularity following the identification of the importance of both micro and macro design concepts in esthetic dentistry (Morley and Eubank 2001).

Devoting the appropriate time to the design process of all esthetic cases will prevent the unexpected. The protocols used in esthetic treatment in years past rarely utilized prepreparation design. Rather, a treatment plan was developed, teeth were prepared for restorations, a final impression was obtained, and the lab was instructed to fabricate definitive restorations. This so-called "prep and pray" modality left much of the esthetic success to chance. Depending on the complexity of the proposed treatment and the number of teeth involved, the case design process can range from basic to very complex; in some cases a significant amount of time and effort must be dedicated to the process.

General Principles

Technological advances in the last thirty years have revolutionized how we look at the world, and the dental field is no exception. Many options are now available, some not even imagined before. Esthetic dentistry often occupies the front cover of many dental journals, and the number of publications dedicated solely to esthetic dentistry has increased dramatically. Developers and manufacturers of dental products have designed many new esthetic materials and related procedures, making them available to a wider array of patients (Hewlett 2007). The informed patients show an increased desire to benefit from these new esthetic solutions (Christensen 2000). This trend has been enhanced by vigorous marketing of esthetic dental products and procedures and by the public's desire to look younger and "beautiful." Currently we have entered an era of "unprecedented demand for appearance-related dental treatment" (Hewlett 2007). This phenomenon has led to practices that have been inundated with esthetic treatment requests. The migration from solely treating acute dental pain and needs to enhancing facial appearance as an integral part of comprehensive care affords the practitioner the opportunity to assist the patient in different ways.

Patients may be unable to differentiate between dental treatment that is mandatory or optional (Christensen 2000). Furthermore, many patients will present for treatment to address an isolated principal complaint. Esthetic treatment may only be a consideration after the initial problem has been addressed. Still other patients will be acutely aware of their esthetic targets, often fuelled by a very clear cosmetic problem. Many patients may have a clear sense of what they wish they looked like but are inadequate at assessing the treatment modalities necessary to achieve their desired outcomes. This phenomenon should come as no surprise. Patients lack the skills required to determine the etiology of their perceived esthetic deficiency. Smile design requires a "wealth of knowledge and experience in order to make appropriate treatment recommendations" (Snow 2007). Life experience teaches us that a good deal of study, work, and dedication is essential to design and deliver exceptional esthetic results. Without significant patient education, very few patients, if any at all, can grasp the complexity of the issues we address during the design and implementation phases of esthetic treatment. Consequently, the clinician must create opportunities to "introduce" patients to the exciting and complex world of smile design before initiating treatment (Snow 2007). In general, patients love to be educated, and that should be a privilege and a pleasure for the dental practitioners and their teams.

The patient must be well informed about the difference between "the need" and "the want" during the treatment planning process to arrive at an informed decision (Christensen 2000). In today's information age, patients are constantly bombarded from several sources of media, not all of which are accurate. Online sources of information have become so pervasive that it is not uncommon for a patient to present for a consultation armed with several treatment options and opinions regarding esthetic dental services. A simple search of "cosmetic dentistry" on the Internet will yield several millions of sources of information. In addition to this source of information, patients are ill-equipped to differentiate information found on TV, in magazines, through direct mail, in internal dental marketing information, or even books about esthetic dentistry, all of which are designed to appeal to the lay person (Golub-Evans 1994). Most of these sources of information are actually various forms of advertising and are intended to influence the patient's perceptions about esthetic den-

tistry and selective dental treatment. It is essential that patients be well informed. If unrealistic expectations go unchecked, the final cosmetic result may not satisfy the patient. A well-designed case, shared with the patient, is the most effective way to ensure that patient expectations and achievable results are closely matched.

Because of the subjective nature of most cosmetic procedures, it is not uncommon for patients to receive different treatment plans aimed at satisfying their chief concern. Although this may lead to confusion and frustration on the part of the patient, we must recognize that several approaches can and often do accomplish the desired result. "As an example, a patient might be told by one dentist that he or she 'needs' 16 veneers, and by another dentist that he or she does not need any treatment. These situations are extremely confusing for the patient, and in the long run, bad for the profession" (Christensen 2000). Each practitioner must strive to defend his or her approach and not discredit another's. This approach can help to diffuse a potentially uncomfortable situation.

"Dentists or technicians traditionally have made choices about esthetic treatment as they believed best, without consulting patients to any large degree. However, dentists need to investigate what patients want and determine if it is feasible" (Van Zyl and Geissberger 2001). In recent years, patients have become increasingly involved in the design and selection process. As patients have become more knowledgeable regarding esthetic dental options, their expectations have correspondingly risen.

The patient perception and approval must be considered an integral part of the smile design process (Johnston et al. 2005; Moore et al. 2005; Wakefield 2006). It is important to note that "aesthetic perception varies from person to person and is influenced by their personal experience and social environment. For this reason, professional opinions regarding evaluation of facial aesthetics may not coincide with the perceptions and expectations of patients or laypeople" (Flores-Mir et al. 2004). For example, tooth shape is very important in the esthetic smile. The perception of the tooth size can be altered to meet the patient's expectations of pleasing tooth shape (Javaheri 2004).

The preference for the tooth shape varies among restorative dentists, orthodontists, and laypeople (Anderson et al. 2005). The same study showed both of the following: that "laypeople tend to be less critical than dental professionals," and with some specific tests, "restorative dentists tended to be more critical than both laypeople and orthodontists" (Anderson et al. 2005). Earlier studies showed significant differences between dental professionals and patients (Brisman 1980).

The importance of smile design cannot be underestimated. The following list of observations supports the need to devote substantial time and effort to this process:

1. Western society places a large amount of importance on facial beauty.
2. An attractive smile is an integral part of facial beauty.
3. Esthetic materials and procedures have expanded exponentially, complicating the selection process.
4. "Yet, foundations of health, proper function and sound scientific principles also must prevail" (Morley 1999).

Key Components of a Successful Esthetics Case Work-up

Although beauty may have more to do with personal preferences and perceptions, certain ageless principles and mathematics can still be applied when attempting to create dental beauty. When designing a case, the practitioner is charged with providing potential esthetic patients with adequate information and education to make an informed decision. In today's busy society and in this age of immediate information, it may be unrealistic to engage in a lengthy instruction process, although some might enjoy it! Luckily, the busy practitioner has a very effective way to transfer the information to his busy patient: showing in real life the new, proposed smile design.

There are various techniques available that enable the practitioner to provide visual aids designed to allow patients to preview their new smiles. Each carries its own drawbacks and benefits. No one technique is flawless. The following are just a small sampling of available techniques:

1. Adding composite directly to the patient's teeth
2. Showing a wax-up to the patient
3. Displaying before-and-after pictures of completed cases
4. Simulating possible results by means of computer/video imaging software
5. Simulating the potential smile through a simulated smile design process

"Belser and colleagues, Magne and colleagues and Adar described a self-curing acrylic mask placed on the patient's teeth to help both the technician and the patient see the proposed incisal edge position. This 'mock-up' technique required the direct addition and sculpting of flowable resin-based composite to the anterior teeth to determine tooth shape and position" (Van Zyl and Geissberger 2001).

Collect All Necessary Data

The smile design process begins with the collection of data. The following is a list of the items one should collect to begin the design process. Generating a checklist is an effective tool to ensure that all necessary information is gathered prior to the design process. At a bare minimum the checklist should include the following:

1. A clear understanding of the patient desires
2. A complete medical and dental history
3. Diagnostic radiographs
4. Photographs
5. High-quality study casts mounted on the articulator (Rosenstiel, Land, and Fujimoto 2006)
6. Facial landmark registration (stick bite or the "T" reference)
7. Periodontal evaluation (Magne, Magne, and Belser 1996)
8. Orthodontic evaluation
9. Oral surgery evaluation (possible implants or other surgical procedures)

Study All the Data

Prior to beginning the actual design process, the practitioner must review all gathered material. The initial conversation about the patient's desires, coupled with your clinical findings, should be the primary driving force behind the design process. Several parameters must be explored during this step. Does the desired change necessitate a modification in the occlusal scheme? How many teeth must be involved to accomplish the esthetic goals? What other specialties of dentistry must be involved to accomplish the desired results?

Study the Smile

This stage is very important, and different perspectives should be considered. This can be accomplished by a specialist with advanced training, the general dentist, or with the use of computerized methods. In the last couple of years, the smile analysis with the aid of computer imaging has become a key element in esthetic dentistry (Brooks 1990; Gianadda 2001; Ackerman and Ackerman 2002; Strub, Rekov, and Witkovski 2006). A comparison was also done by Basting, Trindade, and Florio (2006) between the subjective and computerized methods. Their study highlighted the importance of the "use of digital photographs for facial analysis." The smile can be classified as "social smile" or "enjoyment smile" and should be studied in detail and from different angles (Moskowits and Nayyar 1995; Phillips 1999; Paul 2001). Deciding how the new teeth will fit within the frames of references (discussed in chapter 2) is a key component in the process. Pleasing tooth shapes must blend harmoniously with the lips and gingiva to be deemed esthetic.

Present the Tentative Treatment Plan

Prior to embarking on the design process, it is important that both the practitioner and patient have agreed on a tentative treatment plan. This is essential, as it will drive the case design process. Having a relatively well-defined game plan will help direct the practitioner during the design phase.

Designing the Case

Ultimately, esthetic success of any case is a melding of art and mathematics. A gifted designer can simultaneously blend these apparently juxtaposed concepts into a harmonious result. Knowledge of the mathematical principles alone will not lead to success. Rather, the ability to create subtle deviations from those principles can, in fact, create pleasing results. The mathematic principles of tooth size must be viewed as design tools, not design goals. This chapter will describe the design technique to create harmonious predictable results.

The association of dental esthetic with numeric values has a long-standing history. The golden proportion has been used in the past (Lombardi 1973; Levin 1978; Ricketts 1982) and is still used today, even with numerous controversies noted in the literature (Preston 1993; Mahshid et al. 2004; Hasanreisoglu et al. 2005). The golden proportion is a ratio (1:1.618) that has been described by Fibonacci, or Leonardo of Pisa (ca. 1200 AD). Variations from the golden proportion have been proposed, for example, the golden percentage (Snow 1999, 2006), the recurring esthetic dental (red) proportion (Ward 2001) or the grid analysis system (Naylor 2002). The preferences for each vary among dentists (Rosenstiel, Ward, and Rashid 2000; Ward 2007).

Case design must start with the position of the maxillary two central incisors (Spear, Kokich, and Mathews 2006). The position of the central incisors will be established utilizing the frame of references described in chapter 2. The midline of the face, interpupillary line, lips, and gingival contour must be assessed in the placement of the maxillary central incisors. Additionally, phonetics must be factored into the placement of the maxillary central incisors. Several key factors must be assessed when commencing the design process:

1. Soft tissue positions: The practitioner must assess the position of the lips and gingiva. If the desired tooth position and appearance can be improved by the repositioning of the lips and gingiva, it is imperative to involve specialists in the design process.

Generally speaking, if the gingival position and lip support are deemed appropriate, the complexity of the case is decreased. If, however, the patient desires can only be met with the modification of soft tissue components, the complexity of the case is increased and must involve other members of the treating team. Developing several approaches to complex cases during the treatment planning process that the patient can select from will help guide the design process.

2. Occlusal scheme: A critical step in the design process is determining if the existing occlusal scheme will be modified. This will have a significant impact in the overall design process. If occlusal modification is indicated or desired, a determination of how it will be accomplished will also impact the design process. If orthodontics will simultaneously address soft tissue and occlusion issue, it should be considered as a reasonable treatment option. If the occlusal issues can be corrected utilizing a restorative approach, the design process will take an entirely different path.

3. Missing teeth: Missing teeth can pose significant esthetic challenges and must be addressed during the treatment planning process. The practitioner must decide if implants, removable partial dentures, or fixed partial dentures will be used to replace missing teeth. This decision must be made prior to initiating the design process as it can directly affect the esthetic result.

4. Tooth color: If the chief goal of the patient is to obtain whiter teeth, then the number of teeth involved can change dramatically. It must be recognized that the correction of tooth size and shape issues in a dental arch is far easier when individuals like the existing color of their teeth. Patients who want to change not only the size and shape of the teeth but the color may require the involvement of several additional teeth.

Once the aforementioned topics have been explored, the practitioner, a trained assistant, or a laboratory technician must wax the case. This process will be outlined in detail in the following portion of this chapter.

Present the Designed Case

Once the wax-up is completed, it is essential that the patient views the design, clearly understands the level of involvement necessary to accomplish the result, and approves the initial design before treatment should commence. Allowing the patient to preview the case prior to commencing affords the practitioner the opportunity to uncover any concerns or hesitations on the part of the patient.

Perform a Simulated Smile Design for the Patient

In most cases, the wax-up can be transferred to the patient to allow them to preview the potential esthetic modifications. This is an extremely rewarding process for the practitioner. The results are often quite dramatic and can be life changing. The process of simulation allows the patient to reflect upon the design and provide feedback to the practitioner. This process can also help identify patients with unrealistic expectations.

Establish the Final Treatment Plan

After the simulation is complete, the process of finalizing the treatment plan can be accomplished. Having the patient review the designed case will allow the practitioner to clarify the tentative treatment plan. Any questions or concerns may be addressed at this phase. The waxed case should be viewed much like the architectural drawings for a new building. The waxed case becomes the three-dimensional rendering that will drive the case forward.

Case Studies

The remaining portion of this chapter will be devoted to exploring the case designs of three cases. These cases will help illustrate the principles discussed earlier in this chapter. The first case will demonstrate the use of computer software to simulate a simple diastema closure. The second and third cases are far more involved. Both had significant restorative and esthetic issues coupled with a loss of occlusal stability. The third case will be described in detail to clearly outline the design process. The purpose of showing the design process in detail is to demystify it.

Case #1: Diastema Closure

The presence of spaces between teeth can be managed with either an orthodontic or restorative approach. Next to yellow teeth, gaps or spaces in teeth are viewed as the least appealing esthetic issue for Americans. Therefore, it is not uncommon to have patients request the closure of spaces between their teeth. Software has been developed to assist practitioners in the design process and can be used for many relatively simple esthetic cases (Guess and Solzer 1988). The likelihood that the use of software can yield predictable results decreases as the complexity of the case increases. Generally speaking, with simple diastema closures, no major modifications of occlusion scheme are required (figs. 6-1 and 6-2). When designing

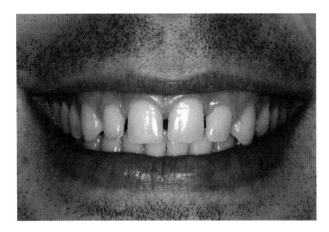

Figure 6-1. Preoperative view of patient with spaces between anterior teeth.

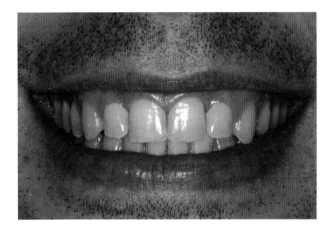

Figure 6-2. Computer-imaging simulation of the diastema closure for the same patient.

a diastema closure case, it is critical to consider the etiology of the space "rather than just the space" (Oesterle and Shellhart 1999). "The use of computer-imaging simulation enhances patient's understanding of a proposed treatment plan concerning maxillary anterior diastema closure" (Almog et al. 2004).

Case #2: Full-Mouth Rehabilitation

The next case to be discussed is far more complex and beyond the capability of simple software manipulation. The patient presented for treatment with an initial chief complaint that her teeth were too short. The clinical examination revealed a severely worn dentition for a female individual in her third decade of life. Additionally, her history of bulimia had contributed significantly to the rapid loss of tooth structure and the destruction of her dentition. Based on the patient's inability to chew, drink, and speak appropriately, the initial treatment plans included a full-mouth reconstruction utilizing fixed restorations with an increase of vertical dimension to create restorative space. Her current condition lacked sufficient space for an esthetic and reconstructive rehabilitation. Furthermore, all parties involved in treatment agreed that her teeth appeared far too short (figs. 6-3, 6-4, 6-5, and 6-6).

Because a significant change in the vertical dimension of occlusion was anticipated, the treatment plan also included a mandibular splint to be worn twenty-four hours a day to ascertain whether or not the patient could tolerate the new vertical dimension of occlusion. The case was opened to create restorative space for the anterior teeth utilizing golden proportions for both dental arches. A mandibular splint was fabricated and delivered to the patient to be worn for four months to confirm her ability to tolerate the new position. In a case like this,

the actual wax-up should not be undertaken until the new vertical dimension is established. Once confirmed, the practitioner must visualize the completed esthetic results before any wax is added to the study casts. Devices such as the Safident divider (fig. 6-7), waxing guides from Panadent (figs. 6-8 and 6-9), and Snow's

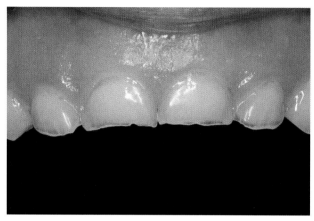

Figure 6-5. Case #2 maxillary incisors, facial view.

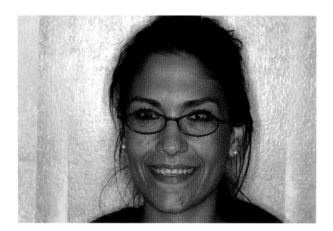

Figure 6-3. Case #2: patient's full face.

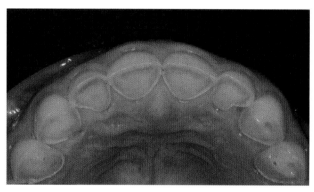

Figure 6-6. Case #2: maxillary incisors, occlusal view.

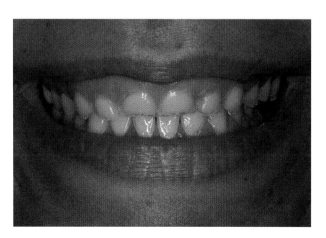

Figure 6-4. Case #2: patient's smile.

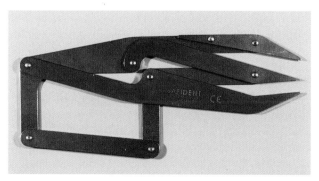

Figure 6-7. Safident divider.

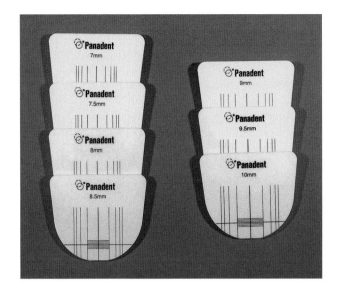

Figure 6-8. Panadent waxing guides.

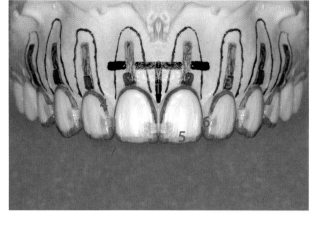

Figure 6-10. Key anatomic features for wax-up process: (1) T-reference (black), (2) axial inclination (blue-green), (3) zenith (dark red), (4) lines angles (blue), (5) incisal margins (light green), (6) contact areas (light blue), and (7) incisal embrasures (orange).

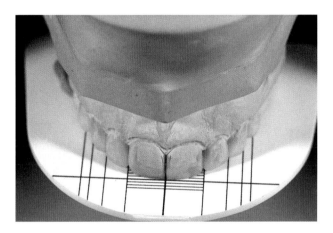

Figure 6-9. Panadent waxing guide in use.

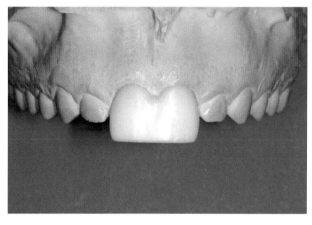

Figure 6-11. First step of the waxing process: create a "uni" tooth.

golden percentage concept are effective tools that should be utilized during the waxing phase of case design. The difficulty in applying the golden proportion is that the lateral incisor is used as the denominator to establish the ratio. This mathematical equation can prove exhausting. The golden percentage is a simpler concept to apply during the design phase (Snow 1999).

The Wax-up Process

There are several key anatomic features that must be incorporated during the design process. Without careful attention to these features, the designer runs the risk of esthetic failure (Schärer, Rinn, and Kopf 1982). These features, listed below and pictured in figure 6-10, are guidelines that must not be viewed as esthetic absolutes but rather as references that can enhance the result of all esthetic and restorative cases.

1. T-reference
2. Axial inclination
3. Zenith
4. Lines angles
5. Incisal margins
6. Contact areas
7. Incisal embrasures

Step One The design of any esthetic case should always begin with the maxillary central incisors. The process begins by creating a single flat surface along the proposed incisal edge at the new length of the central incisors. The incisal edge must be parallel to whichever horizontal reference point the practitioner has decided to parallel. Fill in wax between central incisors, creating a "uni" tooth (fig. 6-11). This step in the wax-up process is extremely important. Creating a continuous incisal edge allows the designer to place the midline perpendicular to this surface quite predictably. If the incisal edge of the two maxillary central incisors is not waxed along the correct horizontal plane, a cant will be introduced. The facial landmark registration should be placed on the mandibular arch to confirm that the incisal has been placed along the correct horizontal reference.

Step Two Once the incisal edge of the maxillary central incisors has been established, the vertical reference is established. The vertical reference is set at 90 degrees to the incisal edge. This "T-reference" should be parallel (see black line, fig. 6-12) to the midline of the face and perpendicular to the horizontal reference point (often the interpupillary line). The process of capturing the T-reference or facial landmark registration is described in chapter 2. This procedure should be done during the records appointment with the patient.

When establishing the dental midline, the reference point is always the facial midline. Whenever possible, the two should coincide. In cases where the position of the central incisors makes it impossible to achieve coincidental facial and dental midlines, the dental midline is set parallel to the facial midline. Figure 6-13 illustrates the transfer of the T-reference or facial landmark registration to the cast. These lines can be transferred to the cast.

Step Three The next step in the process is to create the facial embrasure between the two maxillary central incisors. This is the first step in creating central incisors that are mirror images of each other. As the carving takes place, careful attention to creating symmetry must be observed. During this process, the designer must maintain the T-reference (see fig. 6-14). Keeping the mesial buccal line angles relatively flat will create central inci-

sors that appear generally square. Rounding these line angles will create teeth that appear round. It is important that the designer has predetermined what tooth shapes will be used. Utilizing a measuring device will help ensure the proper dimensions are established and maintained. Wax-ups can be measured down to the 10th of a millimeter. When trying to establish symmetry of the central incisors, a measuring device is essential (fig. 6-15).

The incisal embrasure between the central incisors can vary in size dramatically. The incisal embrasures (orange in the figures) have specific relationships to each other. Regardless of the size of the embrasure placed between the central incisors, a critical relationship of all embrasures must be maintained. The incisal embrasures between maxillary teeth increase in size as one travels posteriorly in the dental arch. It is essential that the relationship of the embrasures is established and main-

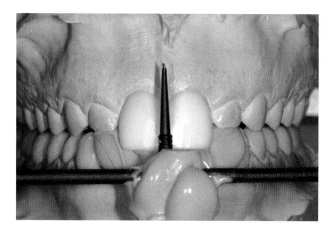

Figure 6-13.   The transfer of the T-reference or facial landmark registration to the cast.

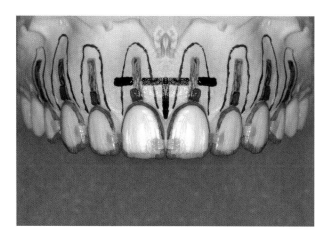

Figure 6-12.   T-reference: black line should be parallel with the midline of the face and perpendicular to the horizontal reference point.

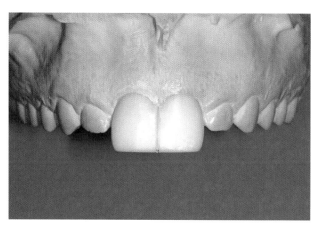

Figure 6-14.   Create the facial embrasures according to the T-reference.

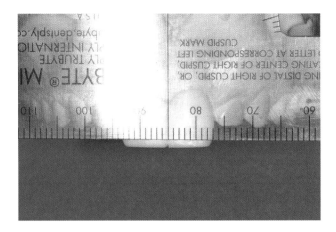

Figure 6-15. When trying to establish symmetry of the central incisors, a measuring device is essential.

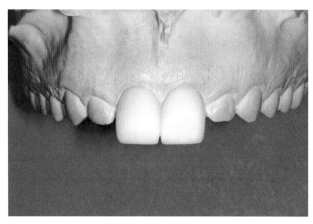

Figure 6-17. Wax-up of the two central incisors based on correct width-to-length ratios.

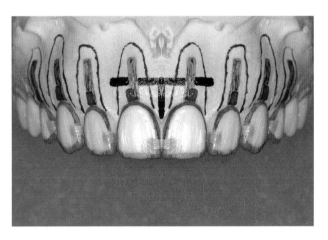

Figure 6-16. A simple reference is the small-medium-large relationship between the anterior incisal embrasures.

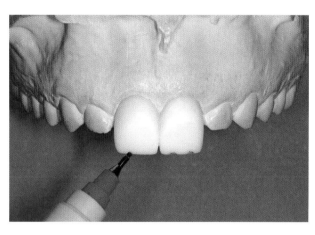

Figure 6-18. Wax-up continues with "Wax-Stop-Look-Assess-Modify" rule.

tained throughout the design process. A simple reference is the small-medium-large relationship between the anterior incisal embrasures (fig. 6-16).

Step Four As the design process proceeds, it is vital to reflect on the progress at regular intervals. This will ensure the design process delivers the best product possible. Successful designers always use the following rule: Wax-Stop-Look-Assess-Modify (figs. 6-17, 6-18, and 6-19).

Step Five The next step is to create the lateral incisors. The golden percentage is used to establish the width of the lateral incisors in relation to the central incisors. Wax is added to both lateral incisors creating the proper width-to-length ratio (fig. 6-20). Unlike the central incisors, the lateral incisors do not have to be perfectly

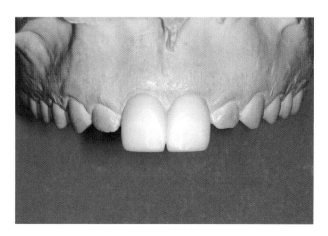

Figure 6-19. Wax-up completed for the incisors.

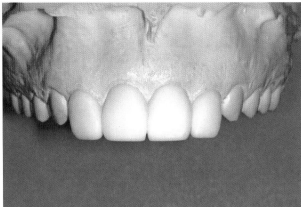

Figure 6-20.   Preliminary wax-up of lateral incisors.

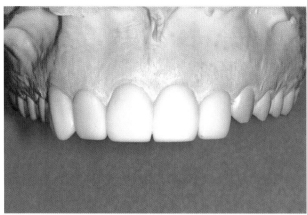

Figure 6-22.   Wax-up of the right canine.

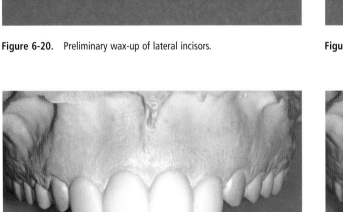

Figure 6-21.   Continued development of lateral incisor anatomy.

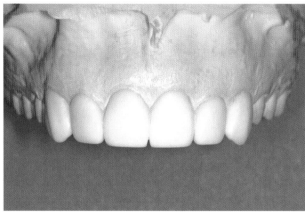

Figure 6-23.   When waxing the canines, symmetry should be considered as well.

identical. Variations in size and shape of the maxillary lateral incisors occur commonly in nature and are generally well tolerated by the viewing public. While total symmetry may be the goal of the case, subtle variations can decrease monotony. If fine variations are going to be incorporated in the design, the lateral incisors are the location to place them. Creating deviations between pairs of central incisors or canines is not advised. In nature, these teeth tend to be highly symmetrical and deviations will not be readily tolerated.

Step Six The designer must work back and forth between the lateral incisors to create shapes to establish bilateral symmetry (fig. 6-21). The embrasure between the central and lateral incisor must be larger than the embrasure between the two central incisors. Rounding the distal incisal corner of the central incisors will accomplish two things. First, it will open the incisal embrasure between the central and lateral incisors. Second, it will create the illusion of narrower and rounder central incisors. If

square teeth are desired, the incisal embrasures should be relatively small.

Step Seven Wax is added to the canines to establish anterior guidance, lateral guidance, and facial esthetics. Canines tend to be highly symmetrical teeth in nature. The designer must keep this fact in mind, striving to create canines that appear symmetrical (figs. 6.22 and 6.23). At this stage in the process, slight asymmetry can be observed in figure 6.23. This will be addressed in a later stage of the wax-up process. As the canines are finalized, it is critical that the incisal embrasure between the lateral incisor and canine is larger than that found between the lateral and central incisor.

Step Eight Wax is added to the first premolars. These teeth will serve as the transition teeth to the posterior region. As such, they must be designed with facial anatomy that is parallel to the surface of the canine. Too often the facial aspect of the canines is so bulky that they

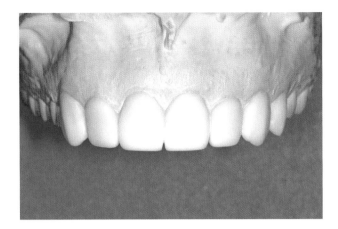

Figure 6-24. Wax is added to the first premolar.

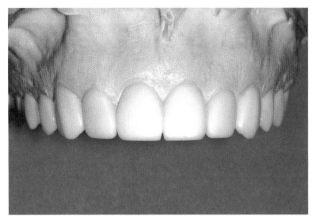

Figure 6-26. The wax-up process continues.

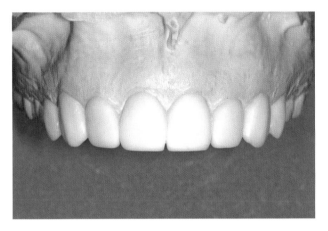

Figure 6-25. When adding wax to the premolars, attention has to be paid to creating a smooth transition from anterior to posterior teeth.

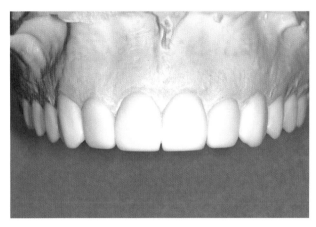

Figure 6-27. More details are added.

obscure the view of the first premolars. Particular attention must be paid to this area so that a smooth transition from anterior to posterior teeth is established (figs. 6.24 and 6.25).

Step Nine Placing the designed wax-up on a flat surface can aid the designer in assessing the incisal embrasures and symmetry of the anterior teeth. The Panadent waxing guides are excellent tools that can be used at this stage of the process. At this point, it is a good idea to set the case aside and take a break. Stepping away will help the designer see things he or she might have missed by continuing the process without stopping (figs. 6-26 and 6-27).

Step Ten While the facial surfaces of the central and lateral incisors are generally flat, the roundness of the facial aspect of the canines must be established. This will aid in the esthetic transition that occurs between anterior and posterior teeth. Carve canine to establish the proper

reveal and contours emphasizing the heights of contour (figs. 6-28 and 6-29).

The position of the proximal contacts is essential in maintaining gingival health and creating the appropriate incisal embrasures. It is important to note that the proximal contacts migrate gingivally as one moves distally in the dental arch. The location of the proximal contacts is displayed in light blue in figure 6-30.

At this phase of the design process the axial inclination of the teeth should be assessed. Lines drawn parallel to the long axis of the maxillary teeth involved in an esthetic design generally converge around the belly button. When the teeth are tilted too significantly, that convergence point migrates toward the head. If the teeth are designed too flat or vertically, the convergence point migrates toward the feet (vertical green lines on fig. 6-30). The appearance of the axial inclination can be easily modified by adjusting the facial line angles. Rounding the mesiobuccal line angle at the gingival portion and the distobuccal line angle at the incisal portion will

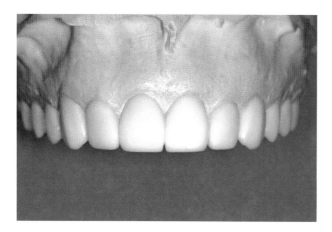

Figure 6-28. The roundness of the facial aspect of the canines is fine-tuned.

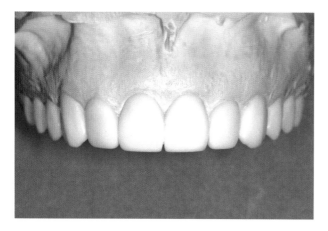

Figure 6-29. Carve canines to establish the proper reveal and facial heights of contour.

create the illusion that the incisal edge has migrated mesially.

Step Eleven As the design process continues, proper anterior guidance must be established. Designing the appropriate occlusal scheme must occur simultaneously with the esthetic design. The lingual surfaces of the anterior teeth are waxed to provide both protrusive and lateral guidance. The slope of the articular eminence can dramatically affect the design of the lingual surfaces of anterior teeth. Refer to chapter 5 for a complete discussion of occlusion as it relates to esthetic design.

Step Twelve Facial depressions on anterior teeth are placed to help with light reflection. These are generally placed along the long axis of the teeth. When an emphasis on length is desired, making these facial depressions relatively long and narrow is advised. If the designer would like to emphasize width rather than length, the depressions should be relatively broad and shallow. The use of facial depressions is an effective tool in creating desired illusions of length, width, or height. In general, the facial embrasures are deeper on lateral incisors and canines. They should be relatively shallow on central incisors and first premolars.

Step Thirteen Add age-appropriate incisal characteristics. These may or may not include mammelons. In figure 6-31, the left side of the arch has highly stylized incisal characteristics. The right side is relatively flat and nondescript. The use of flat incisal edges will have two effects. First, flat incisal edges will create teeth that appear generally square. Second, flat incisal edges will tend to age the appearance of the teeth. Rounder incisal edges will create rounder tooth shapes and help create a more youthful-appearing dentition (fig. 6-31).

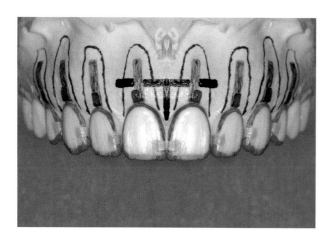

Figure 6-30. The location of proximal contacts is displayed in light blue and the green lines represent the long axis of the teeth.

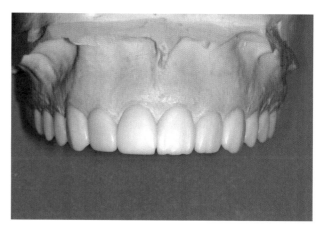

Figure 6-31. The left side of the arch has highly stylized incisal characteristics. The right side is relatively flat and nondescript.

The designer must also place the incisal edge in a proper faciolingual position so that the edge strikes the wet-dry line of the lower lip. This positioning is fundamental in helping the patient achieve appropriate phonetics. Phonetics is best assessed when the wax-up is transferred to the oral cavity during simulation. Figure 6-32 shows a simulation of the lips in relationship to the designed case. These were created using vinyl polysiloxane putty and acrylic paint (for esthetic purposes only). The light green line defines the parallelism of the lower lip line with the smile line.

Simulation Once the design process is complete, a putty/wash impression is made of the completed shapes. The impression will be used to simulate the design in the oral cavity. A bis-acrylic resin provisional material can be loaded into the impression and delivered to the unprepared arch for simulation. The impression is removed upon complete setting of the acrylic resin. Figures 6-33

and 6-34 demonstrate the before and after conditions for this patient. The after photo is of the simulation, not the definitive restorations.

Once the designed shapes have been transferred to the oral cavity, both the designer and recipient can assess the proposed design. Additionally, phonetics and lip support can be assessed. Modifications to the design may be made prior to the preparation appointment. The finalized design will become the source of provisional restorations.

Case #3: Rehabilitation of a Severely Worn Dentition

The final case is similar to the previous case. The patient, a young man in his third decade of life, complained of teeth "shortening" and presented for the fabrication of a nightguard. He has a medical history significant for acid reflux that is controlled by medication. He was moderately restored with several posterior resin restorations. Several areas of decay were noted on occlusal and proximal surfaces of his posterior dentition. The clinical examination also revealed several areas of erosion, attrition, and abrasion throughout the mouth. The general appearance of the hard tissue exam revealed unsupported enamel, pitting, and exposed dentin. His periodontal status was unremarkable (figs. 6-35, 6-36, 6-37, and 6-38). The lower incisors were spared from the effects of the acid. This is a common clinical finding in these cases. The tongue generally protects the lingual surface of the lower teeth.

Through the use of a diagnostic occlusal splint and measurement of the freeway space, the case was designed by opening the vertical dimension by 4mm. The maxillary central incisors measured 6mm in length.

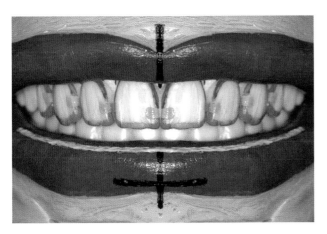

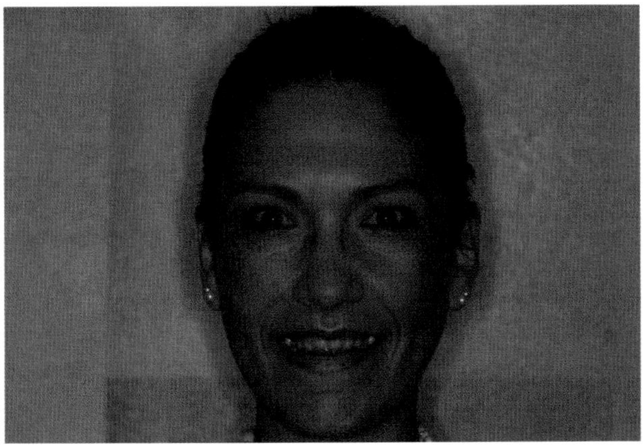

Figure 6-32. Simulation of the lips in relationship to the designed case. The light green line defines the parallelism of the lower lip with the smile line.

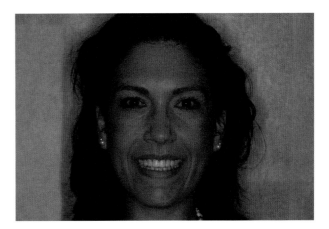

Figure 6-33. Case #2: patient before the simulated smile design.

Figure 6-34. Case #2: patient with the simulated smile design. This photo is of the simulation, not the definitive restorations.

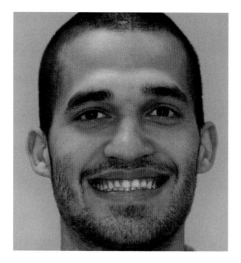

Figure 6-35.   Case #3: patient full face.

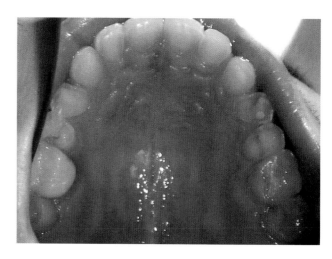

Figure 6-37.   Case #3: occlusal view of the maxillary arch.

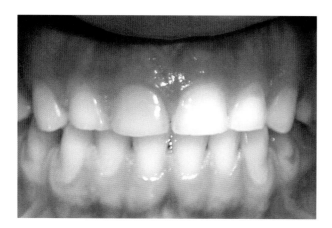

Figure 6-36.   Case #3: anterior teeth 1:2 view.

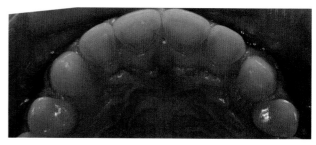

Figure 6-38.   Case #3: occlusal view of the maxillary anterior teeth.

An occlusal splint was worn for several months as the case was designed. The treatment plan included a full-mouth reconstruction to restore lost tooth structure, esthetics, phonetics, and masticatory function. The images that follow demonstrate various stages of the design process (figs. 6-39 through 6-43).

The initial wax-up only included six maxillary teeth. The patient was not yet fully committed to treatment. After a period of reflection, the patient consented to his restoration and the complete design was created. The initial wax-up was used to demonstrate the amount of tooth lost to his disease process. Figures 6-44 through 6-49 illustrate the complete design of the case. The groove placed on the cast just apical to the crest of the gingiva is an effective technique to aid in the trimming of excess material during simulation and provisional fabrication.

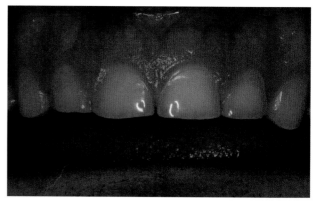

Figure 6-39.   Close-up view (1:1) of the maxillary anterior teeth, incisors at 6 mm length.

Figures 6-50, 6-51, and 6-52 illustrate the second smile design. During the simulation process, it was determined that additional esthetic modifications were needed. The patient felt that the central incisors appeared too long. An effective tool for simulating the removal of tooth

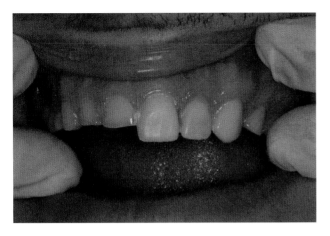

Figure 6-40. Showing to the patient the first steps of the wax-ups.

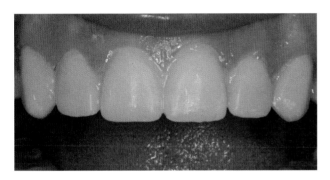

Figure 6-41. Incisors at 10 mm length.

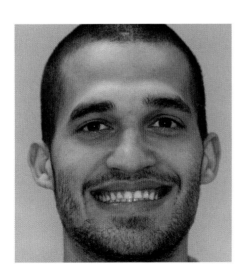

Figure 6-42 Case #3: preoperative full face before smile design mock-up.

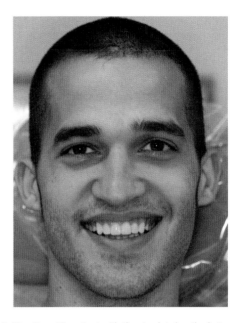

Figure 6-43. Case #3: patient with the simulated smile design canine to canine.

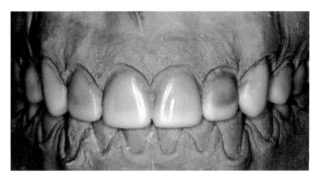

Figure 6-44. Case #3: wax-up on the cast, anterior view.

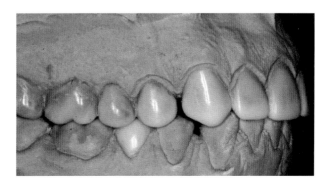

Figure 6-45. Case #3: wax-up, right lateral view.

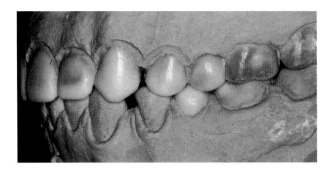

Figure 6-46.   Case #3: wax-up, left lateral view.

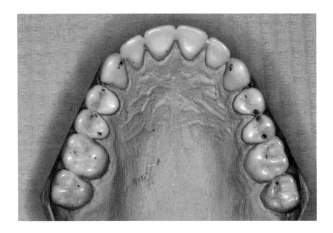

Figure 6-47.   Case #3: wax-up, occlusal view of the maxillary arch.

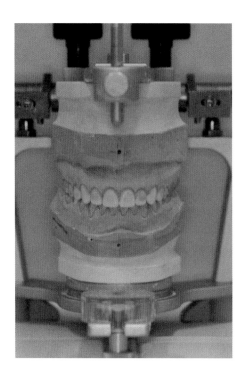

Figure 6-49.   Case #3: the completed wax-up on the articulator.

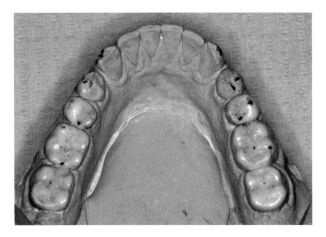

Figure 6-48.   Case #3: wax-up, occlusal view of the mandibular arch.

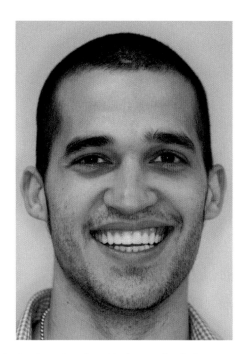

Figure 6-50.   Case #3: patient with the second smile design.

structure on a simulation or on natural tooth structure is the use of black ink. In this case, a Sharpie pen was used to mimic the shortening of the central incisors (fig. 6-52).

The following images (figs. 6.53 to 6.60) demonstrate the preoperative condition and the definitive results fol-

lowing the completion of treatment. It is important to note that the final results were developed using the design features developed earlier in the process. This case was restored using Lava crown restorations on all teeth.

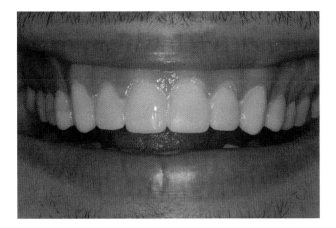

Figure 6-51. Case #3: close-up of the second simulated smile design.

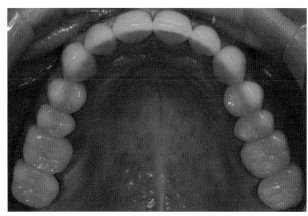

Figure 6-54. Case #3: view of the maxillary arch, fully restored.

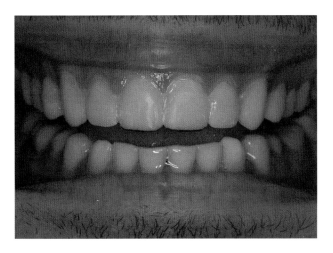

Figure 6-52. A Sharpie pen is use to mimic the shortening of the central incisors.

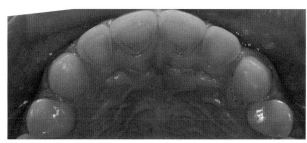

Figure 6-55. Preoperative occlusal view of the maxillary anterior teeth.

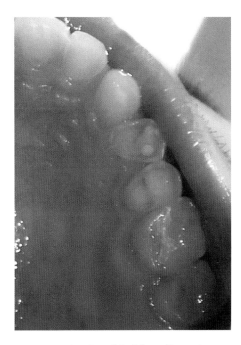

Figure 6-53. Preoperative view of the left maxillary arch.

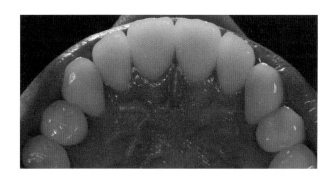

Figure 6-56. Occlusal view of the maxillary anterior dentition fully restored.

71

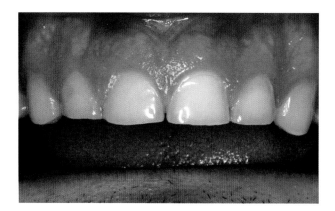

Figure 6-57. Close-up of maxillary anterior teeth, before treatment.

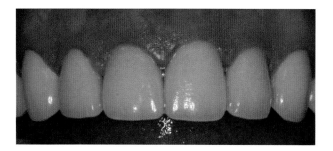

Figure 6-58. Close-up of maxillary anterior teeth, fully restored.

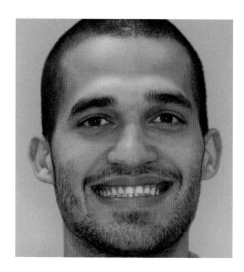

Figure 6-59. Case #3: patient before treatment.

Conclusion

The design phase of treatment is essential in establishing a blend of esthetics, function, and phonetics. The design phase should not take place after the preparation phase of treatment. Rather, it should occur as an integral part of the treatment planning process. Investing a significant amount of time during the design phase of any case will dramatically simplify the preparation, provisionalization, and delivery phase of treatment.

The design process will help prepare clinicians for the treatment phase of care, sharpen their esthetic eye, and provide personal satisfaction. The process will be highly rewarding to both the patient and practitioner.

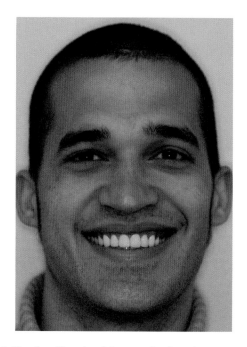

Figure 6-60. Case #3: patient fully restored and very happy.

Works Cited

Ackerman MB, Ackerman JL. 2002. Smile analysis and design in the digital era. *J Clin Orthod* 36(4):221–36.

Almog D, Marin CS, Proskin HM, Cohen MJ, Kyrkanides S, Malmstrom, H. 2004. The effect of esthetic consultation methods on acceptance of diastema-closure treatment plan: A pilot study. *J Am Dent Assoc* 135(7):875–81.

Anderson KM, Behrents RG, McKinney T, Buschang PH. 2005. Tooth shape preferences in esthetic smile. *Am J Orthod Dentofacial Orthop* 128(Oct):458–65.

Basting RT, Trindade RS, Flório FM. 2006. Comparative study of smile analysis by subjective and computerized methods. *Operative Dentistry* 31(6):652–59.

Brisman AS. 1980. Esthetics: A comparison of dentists' and patients' concepts. *J Am Dent Assoc* 100(Mar):345–52.

Brooks LE. 1990. Smile-imaging: The key to more predictable dental esthetics. *J Esthet Dent* 2(1):6–9.

Christensen GJ. 2000. Elective vs. mandatory dentistry. *J Am Dent Assoc* 131(10):1496–98.

Flores-Mir C, Silva E, Barriga MI, Lagravère MO, Major PW. 2004. Laypersons' perception of smile aesthetics in dental and facial views. *J Orthodontics* 31(3):204–9.

Gianadda R. 2001. Achieving an aesthetic smile design with integrated single- and multi-unit metal free restorations. *Dent Today* 20(6):42–46.

Golub-Evans J. 1994. Unity and variety: Essential ingredients of a smile design. *Curr Opin Cosmet Dent* 1–5.

Golub-Evans J. 2003. How to be a smile designer, part 1. *Dent Today* 22(11):66–68.

Guess MB, Solzer WV. 1988. Computer-generated diagnostic correction of anterior diastema. *J Pros Dent* 59(5):629–32.

Hasanreisoglu U, Berksun S, Aras K, Arslan I. 2005. An analysis of maxillary anterior teeth: Facial and dental proportions. *J Prosthet Dent* 94(Dec):530–38.

Hewlett ER. 2007. Selected topics in esthetic case management. *CDA Journal* 35(7):473.

Javaheri DS. 2004. Techniques for altering the perception of tooth size. *Dent Today* 23(Aug):50, 52–53.

Johnston DJ, Hunt O, Johnston CD, Burden DJ, Stevenson M, Hepper P. 2005. The influence of the lower face vertical proportion on facial attractiveness. *Eur J Orthod* 27(4):49–54.

Levin EI. 1978. Dental esthetics and the golden proportion. *J Prosthet Dent* 40(Sep):244–52.

Lombardi RE. 1973. The principles of visual perception and their clinical application to denture esthetics. *J Prosthet Dent* 29(Apr):358–82.

Magne P, Magne M, Belser U. 1996. The diagnostic template: Key element to the comprehensive treatment concept. *Int J Perio Rest Dent* 16(6):560–69.

Mahshid M, Khoshvaghti A, Varshohaz M, Vallaei N. 2004. Evaluation of "golden proportion" in individuals with an esthetic smile. *J Esthet Restor Dent* 16(3):185–92.

Moore T, Southard KA, Casko JS, Qian F, Southard TE. 2005. Buccal corridors and smile esthetics. *Am J Orthod Dentofacial Orthop* 127(5):528–29.

Morley J. 1999. The role of cosmetic dentistry in restoring a youthful appearance. *JADA* 130:1166–72.

Morley J, Eubank J. 2001. Macroesthetic elements of smile design. *JADA* 132(Jan):39–45.

Moskowits ME, Nayyar A. 1995. Determinants of dental esthetics: A rationale for smile analysis and treatment. *Compendium* 16(12):1164–81.

Naylor CK. 2002. Esthetic treatment planning: the grid analysis system. *J Esthet Restor Dent*. 2002 14(2):76–84.

Oesterle LJ, Shellhart WC. 1999. Maxillary midline diastema: A look at the causes. *JADA* 130(Jan):85–93.

Paul, S. J. 2001. Smile analysis and face-bow transfer: Enhancing aesthetic restorative treatment. *Pract Proced Aesthet Dent* 13(3):217–222.

Phillips E. 1999. The classification of smile patterns. *J Can Dent Assoc* 65(5):252–54.

Preston JD. 1993. The golden proportion revisited. *J Esthet Dent* 5(6):247–51.

Ricketts RM. 1982. The biologic significance of the divine proportion and Fibonacci series. *Am J Orthod* 81(5):351–70.

Rosenstiel SF, Land MF, Fujimoto. 2006. *Contemporary Fixed Prosthodontics*, 4th ed. Mosby Elsevier.

Rosenstiel SF, Ward DH, Rashid RG. 2000. Dentists' preferences of anterior tooth proportion: a Web-based study. *J Prosthod* 9(3):123–136.

Schärer P, Rinn LA, Kopf FR. 1982. *Esthetic Guidelines for Restorative Dentistry*. Chicago: Quintessence.

Snow SR. 1999. Esthetic smile analysis of maxillary anterior tooth width: The golden percentage. *J Esthet Dent* 11(4):177–84.

Snow SR. 2006. Application of the golden percentage in smile design and esthetic treatment success. *Contemporary Esthet*, Sept:30–37.

Snow SR. 2007. Strategies for successful dental treatment. *CDA Journal* 35(7):475–84.

Spear FM, Kokich VG, Mathews DP. 2006. Interdisciplinary management of anterior dental esthetics. *JADA* 137:160–69.

Strub JR, Rekov ED, Witkovski S. 2006. Computer-aided design and fabrication of dental restorations. *JADA* 137:1289–96.

Van Zyl I, Geissberger M. 2001. Simulated shape design: Helping patients decide their esthetic ideal. *J Am Dent Assoc* 132(8):1105–9.

Wakefield CW Jr. 2006. Porcelain veneers preliminary procedures before preparation. *Tex Dent J* 123(10):940–45.

Ward DH. 2001. Proportional smile design using the recurring esthetic dental proportion. *Dent Clin North Am* 45(1):143–54.

Ward DH. 2007. A study of dentists' preferred maxillary anterior tooth width proportions: Comparing the recurring esthetic dental proportion to other mathematical and natural occurring proportions. *J Esthet Restor Dent* 19(6):324–39.

Suggested Reading

Donovan TE, Cho GC. 1999. Diagnostic provisional restorations in restorative dentistry: The blueprint for success. *J Can Dent Assoc* 65(5):272–75.

Gürel G, Bistachacho N. 2006. Permanent diagnostic provisional restorations for predictable results when redesigning the smile. *Pract Proced Aesthet Dent* 18(5):281–86.

Marus R. 2006. Treatment planning and smile design using composite resin. *Pract Proced Aesthet Dent* 18(40):235–41.

Sarver DM, Ackerman MB. 2003. Dynamic smile visualization and quantification: Part 1. Evolution of the concept and dynamic records for smile capture. *Am J of Orthodontics* 124(1):4–12.

Sarver DM, Ackerman MB. 2003. Dynamic smile visualization and quantification: Part 2. Smile analysis and treatment strategies. *Am J of Orthodontics* 124(2):116–27.

Chapter 7
Considerations for Treating the Routine Esthetic Case

Noelle Santucci DDS, MA, BS

Marc Geissberger DDS, MA, BS, CPT

The most important skill that physicians of the orofacial complex must develop is sound oral diagnosis and treatment planning. Our clinical skills are irrelevant if our treatment plan is not appropriate, comprehensive, thorough, and properly executed. Oversights such as an improper occlusal scheme or function, neglected or poorly monitored periodontal treatment, improper treatment planning and sequencing, failure to refer to a specialist, or poor material selection could lead to subtle or major iatrogenic changes that could show up weeks, months, or years later.

"Single tooth" dentistry is appropriate in patients with good skeletal and occlusal schemes, proper vertical dimension of occlusion, and no posterior arch collapse. But as the patient's gnathostomatic system becomes more complex, the broader our diagnostic abilities need to be.

Dentistry has greatly evolved over the past ten to twenty years. Observe the new technology: rotary endodontics, CAD/CAM technology, digital radiography, digital impressions, evolution of the composition of porcelain and resins, and the explosion of the use of porcelain veneers. In addition, the patients coming to your office are more informed about the available technology, have higher dental expectations, and are even asking for procedures and materials by name. So how do we stay current and treatment plan properly in light of the new materials and technology?

The following three chapters will look at treatment planning from the basic or routine treatments, to the moderately difficult, and ending with comprehensive plans that include full-mouth rehabilitation. These chapters, although arbitrarily divided, should be viewed as a continuum in treatment planning methodologies.

Let's begin by defining the differences between an "ideal or minimally compromised case to one that is severely compromised both for the dentate and partially edentulous patient" (McGarry et al. 2002, 2004). The rationale for using these definitions is to aid the practitioner in feeling comfortable in selecting a dental case he or she wishes to treat. Once a practitioner is comfortable

in diagnosing and in treating the routine cases, he or she may move to the next level and feel more confident in the treatment planning decisions and outcomes. The American College of Prosthodontists (ACP) developed this classification system in 2004. Their "framework supports diagnostically driven treatment plan options" (McGarry et al. 2002) for both the dentate and partially edentulous patient (see table 7-1).

In this chapter, we will discuss the routine esthetic changes you can offer a patient and include the following topics:

1. Vital bleaching
2. Composite veneers
3. Peg laterals
4. Class IV composites
5. Ceramic veneers
6. Esthetic update of older crowns
7. All ceramic crowns
8. Three unit bridges
9. Orthodontic treatment to make a complex case routine
10. Unsuccessful outcomes

Any time an esthetic case is undertaken, whether simple or complex, your comprehensive examination should include photographic documentation, mounted diagnostic casts, esthetic wax-up, simulated smile design on the patient, thorough discussion of the risks, benefits, and alternatives, and informed consent. These topics are discussed thoroughly in other chapters in this text and should be referred to frequently as you go through the treatment planning chapters.

Bleaching/Tooth Whitening

In 2004 the American Academy of Cosmetic Dentistry asked Americans what they liked least about their smile. The most common answer was the color (darkness) of their teeth (AACD 2004). In 2000 Redbook asked Americans what feature in the opposite sex they found most

Table 7-1. American College of Prosthodontists classification system for diagnostically driven treatment.

	Class I	Class II	Class III	Class IV
Conditions creating a guarded prognosis:				
Severe oral manifestations of systemic disease				X
Maxillomandibular dyskinesia and/or ataxia				X
Refractory patient				X
Occlusal scheme:				
Ideal or minimally compromised	X			
Moderately compromised—anterior guidance intact		X		
Substantially compromised—extensive rest/same VDO			X	
Severely compromised—extensive rest/new VDO				X
Teeth condition:				
Ideal or minimally compromised—≤3 teeth in 1 sextant	X			
Moderately compromised—≥4 teeth in 1–2 sextants		X		
Substantially compromised—≥4 teeth in 3–5 sextants			X	
Severely compromised—≥4 teeth, all sextants				X
Partially edentulous patients only				
location and extent of edentulous areas:				
Ideal or minimally compromised—single arch	X			
Moderately compromised—both arches		X		
Substantially compromised—≤3 teeth			X	
Severely compromised—guarded prognosis				X
Congenital or acquired maxillofacial defect				X
Abutment condition:				
Ideal or minimally compromised	X			
Moderately compromised— 1–2 sextants		X		
Substantially compromised— 3 sextants			X	
Severely compromised—≥4 sextants				X
Residual ridge:				
Class I edentulous	X			
Class II edentulous		X		
Class III edentulous			X	
Class IV edentulous				X

Guidelines for worksheet:

1. Any single criterion of a more complex class places the patient into the more complex class.

2. Consideration of future treatment procedures must not influence the diagnostic level.

3. Initial preprosthetic treatment and/or adjunctive therapy can change the initial classification level.

4. If there is an esthetic concern/challenge, the classification is increased in complexity by one or more levels.

5. In the presence of TMD symptoms, the classification is increased in complexity by one or more levels.

6. It is assumed that the patient will receive therapy designed to achieve and maintain optimal periodontal health.

7. In the situation where the patient presents with an edentulous mandible opposing a partially edentulous or dentate maxilla, use class IV.

Note: VDO = vertical dimension of occlusion; TMD = temporomandibular joint disorder.

appealing. Of the top five most common responses, the smile was the only physical attribute mentioned. The smile is "an important part of the physical attractiveness stereotype (and) plays a significant role in the perception that others have of our appearance and our personality" and is one of the first things noticed about a person (Beall 2007). Unattractive teeth can have an "impact upon a person's self-image, self -confidence, physical attractiveness and employability" (Kelleher and Roe 1999; Pretty et al. 2006). It is not uncommon to see such a person with a guarded smile. A guarded smile is not a full smile and is observed when a patient refuses to show parts or all of their teeth when asked to smile fully. "The eye region is also important when identifying genuine, or sincere smiles. In 1862 the French neurologist, Duchenne de Boulogne, showed that the critical factor in distinguishing a posed from a genuine smile is contraction of the orbicularis oculi muscle, which surrounds the eye. Genuine (or 'Duchenne') smiles are accompanied by contraction of these muscles, causing wrinkles of the skin in the outer corners of the eyes, known as 'crow's feet' wrinkles" (Boraston et al. 2008). Since the orbicularis oculi is not under voluntary control, it generally does not contract in a posed or guarded smile.

The natural aging processes and extrinsic staining from drinking coffee, tea, cola, and red wine or from smoking are the most common causes of tooth discoloration. Intrinsic stains can have their etiology from pharmaceutical drug use, such as the antibiotic tetracycline, excessive fluoride ingestion during tooth formation, or from several systemic conditions or diseases (Pretty et al. 2006). Dental materials such as amalgam, composites, pins, and posts can also adversely affect the tooth's color.

Vital tooth bleaching is a safe and very conservative esthetic option for a patient (Heymann 2005). It is often a more viable "alternative therapeutic method … to crowning or veneering" or composites (Attin et al. 2003). It should be one of the first esthetic treatments offered to patients and the precursor to all esthetic restorative care whether it be a composite, crown, or veneer. Bleaching should be included in any esthetic treatment plan, discussed with the patient during the treatment plan consultation appointment, and completed prior to the commencement of any restorative care (See fig. 7-1). Of course, it is the patient's decision to accept or reject this recommendation.

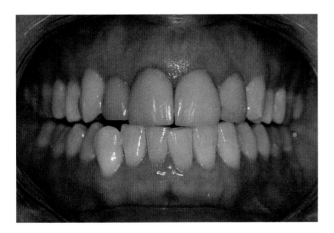

Figure 7-1. Preoperative photo after tooth whitening. The treatment plan to replace the existing anterior veneers is now ready to commence.

A thorough clinical dental examination is required prior to initiating bleaching therapy. Several clinical situations should be addressed prior to bleaching therapy. They include active caries, leaking, defective or failing restorations, and calculus removal (Heymann 1997). A provisional repair of defective restorations could be done until the whitening is completed and the definite restoration placed. This is recommended "in order to achieve an optimal seal of the pulp chamber … reducing the risk of adverse effects" from the bleaching agent penetrating through any open margins (Attin et al. 2004). Since whitening products have limited effects on dental restorative materials, the patient must be advised that any existing restorations will not whiten and may appear darker in contrast to the new tooth shade, necessitating replacement to match the new tooth color. Include the final replacement of those fillings in the treatment plan. The patient should also be scheduled for a complete prophylaxis to remove any plaque, calculus, and superficial staining prior to tooth whitening.

The etiology of the stain should be noted to assess if vital tooth whitening alone or in combination with a restorative procedure would be best employed (Pretty et al. 2006; Schwartz et al. 1996). The patient should also be encouraged to discontinue whatever habit contributed to the extrinsic staining process. Because vital tooth whitening reduces the enamel-composite bond strength (Barghi and Godwin 1994; Cvitko et al. 1991; Garcia-Godoy et al. 1993; McGuckin, Thurmond, and Osovitz 1992; Titley, Torneck, and Ruse 1992), it is "recommended to delay placement of restorations after termination of bleaching therapy for at least 1–3 weeks" (Attin et al. 2003; Heymann 1997a; Swift 1997). This allows time for any residual oxygen to escape and the color to stabilize. Patients should be informed of the slight color regression that occurs in the first week or two after whitening is discontinued.

Risks, benefits, and alternatives of bleaching should be discussed with patients and a consent form signed prior to commencing tooth whitening. According to Goldstein (1997), there has been no observed loss of tooth vitality in the past thirty years of vital tooth whitening. As with any dental procedure, there is some risk to bleaching, "but from the evidence it seems that bleaching teeth is comparatively safe" (Dadoun and Bartlett 2003). Tooth sensitivity is generally the most common side effect. Because whitening is time/dose-related, decreasing the concentration of the material being used or decreasing the time or frequency of use can aid in minimizing the sensitivity. The literature recommends that the patient be seen in the office one week after commencing treatment to check for progress or for any side effects or complications. Postoperative instructions should advise the patient to contact the treating dentist

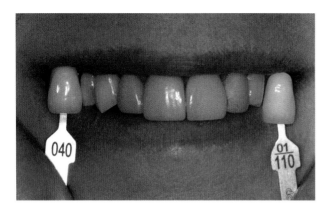

Figure 7-2. A photo of shade tab adjacent to the prewhitened teeth and postwhitened teeth is recommended as part of the permanent treatment record.

immediately if tooth sensitivity or gingival irritation or discoloration occurs. Again, remember to inform the patients that relapse in color occurs with every system and that touch-ups will be needed periodically.

Take a preoperative shade as a baseline to check for progress and color change. A clinical photograph with the shade tab adjacent to the prewhitened teeth and postwhitened teeth is recommended as part of the permanent preoperative treatment record (fig. 7-2).

There are three basic techniques for tooth whitening: over-the-counter (OTC) products, home bleaching, and power bleaching. The patients will get results with any of these techniques. The success of bleaching is based on two factors, the concentration of the bleaching solution and the length of time that the solution is in contact with the teeth. Additionally, the pH of the bleaching agent may have some effect on the speed of bleaching, but acidic bleaching agents present the potential for demineralization of tooth structure. Therefore, a neutral pH is generally used in all bleaching agents sold to dental practitioners.

OTC Home Bleaching

In 2001 hydrogen-peroxide whitening strips were first introduced. This OTC home bleaching technique involves using polyethylene strips impregnated with standardized doses of 6.5% hydrogen peroxide–based solution. The concentrations are low and the shelf life of the material is short. The professional-grade, office-dispensed strip was introduced in 2003 (Crest Whitestrips Supreme) with a 14% hydrogen peroxide concentration.

The effectiveness of this system has been documented (Gerlach, Gibb, and Sagel 2000; Gerlach et al. 2004;

Perdigao, Baratieri, and Arcari 2004; Sulieman et al. 2006; Swift et al. 2004). The advantage of this system is that it can give the patient an effective alternative to the dentist-assisted home bleaching method if cost is a concern. A disadvantage of whitening strips is that the strips cover only the anterior sextant. Other disadvantages include lack of dental supervision, use by patient of nonregulated materials, and the potential for overuse.

Instructions recommend placement of the strips over the facials of the anterior teeth and wrap lingually, twice daily for thirty minutes each time. Maxillary and mandibular arches can be done separately or simultaneously. Instructions from Crest advise that some people will have temporary and nonharmful tooth sensitivity or irritation of the gums and recommend using the strips every other day or discontinuing use if problems persist. Avoid contact with eyes, wash hands with soap and water after applying the strips, and do not eat, drink, smoke, or sleep while wearing a strip.

A second OTC home bleaching method available is tray-based teeth whitening products. These are not custom-fabricated bleaching trays, so they are not trimmed in a scalloped fashion ending at gum line with softened edges, so as to minimize contact of the peroxide with the gums. "OTC tray-based systems in particular must be used with caution because ill-fitting trays can lead to soft-tissue injury with the leaking of the bleaching solution, malocclusion problems if patient parafunctions on the appliance, and poor compliance" (Kugel 2003).

Dentist-Assisted Home Bleaching

Dentist-assisted home bleaching or take-home technique involves the use of a tray designed to hold whitening products against the dentition for a prescribed amount of time. The trays can either be a one-size-fits-all or custom made to the individual patient's dentition. The biggest advantage to trays is that all teeth or a selected number of teeth can be bleached. The biggest challenge for the patients is having the discipline necessary to be compliant at home each evening.

Most of the bleaching products are 10–28% carbamide peroxide or 2–5% hydrogen peroxide solutions in a glycerin base with carobopol as a thickening agent. Because whitening efficacy is based on a ratio of time and dose, higher concentrations decrease the time required to achieve results and lower concentrations require longer time frames to achieve similar results (Pretty et al. 2006; Sulieman et al. 2004). Patients are instructed to wear the trays from 1 to 4 hours each day. Some clinicians feel that overnight wearing of the trays can promote additional parafunctional habits and suggest that the patient remove the trays prior to going to sleep.

With the higher concentration of bleaching solutions, some patients may experience tooth sensitivity. This sensitivity can be manifested by twinges in the tooth, spontaneous pain, and/or increased sensitivity to cold (Heymann 1997). There are several ways to limit tooth sensitivity:

1. Utilize low-concentration bleaching agents (10%).
2. Utilize a bleach material that contains potassium nitrate, fluoride, or both.
3. Shorten the amount of time for bleaching.
4. Advise the patient to bleach every other day.
5. Consider the use of prophylactic anti-inflammatory agents.

To fabricate a custom tray, make good-quality maxillary and mandibular alginate impressions, pour in yellow stone, and trim properly. Studies show that a reservoir is not needed to keep the given amount of whitening material against the tooth (Javaheri and Janis 2000; Matis et al. 2002). Some manufacturers recommend the use of a reservoir. Generally this is accomplished by applying a light-cure block-out resin material on the mid-facial area of each tooth on the casts 1–2 mm in size and 1.5 mm short of the gingival margins. Using a vacuum former, fabricate the tray and trim following the scalloped contour of the gingival margin. If a reservoir has been used, then trim the tray so it will contact the gingiva lightly.

At the delivery appointment give verbal and written instructions that include the quantity of whitening gel to be placed in the trays, insertion and removal of the trays, time that the trays should be worn, and cleaning and storage of the trays. Most patients reach the desired color change in 7 to 14 days. For patients with tetracycline staining, treatment may need to continue for up to 6 months (Leonard et al. 2003; Pretty et al. 2006).

Appoint the patient in one week to check on progress. Advise the patient to call if he or she experiences any sensitivity or gingival irritation. If this occurs, make sure the trays fit well at the gingival crest, as "ill-fitting trays can lead to soft-tissue injury with the leaking of the bleaching solution" (Kugel 2003). The models can be given to the patient in the event that a tray needs to be refabricated due to loss or damage. Once the desired shade has been reached, wait two weeks to initiate any bonded restorative procedures. If no other treatment is planned, advise patient on how to initiate short-span touch-ups as needed, using the same trays.

Dentist-Assisted In-Office Bleaching

Dentist-assisted in-office bleaching utilizes a high concentration of hydrogen peroxide bleaching agent (15%–38%) left in contact with tooth structure for a relatively short period of time. The so-called power bleaches may or may not be used in conjunction with a light. The use of light-assisted power bleaching has grown substantially over the last decade with the introduction of products like BriteSmile® and Zoom®. There is conflicting literature on the effectiveness of light-assisted bleaching. According to research conducted by Gordon Christensen, the use of a light in addition to high-concentration bleaching agents had little to no effect on the overall bleaching results. This is in sharp contrast to the findings of Mary Tavares and colleagues' 2003 study of BriteSmile, which suggested significant improvement in the bleaching process with the use of light.

The major advantage of power bleaching is the immediacy of the results. This is very desirable with patients who feel that compliance with wearing trays will be an issue or who want or need immediate results.

There are several disadvantages to power bleaching.

1. Due to the use of high-concentration bleach agents, a rubber dam or soft tissue mask must be utilized to lessen the chance of a chemical burn to surrounding soft tissues.
2. The procedure requires an hour to an hour and a half of chair time.
3. Repeating the procedure may be required if optimal results are not achieved with the first treatment.
4. Many practitioners fabricate custom bleaching trays for their patient to take home with them so they can continue the process at home.

After a thorough comprehensive examination, prophylaxis, and consent obtained, a rubber dam or light-cured gingival mask (such as Opal-Dam by Ultradent) is placed to cover all exposed gingiva. This is imperative to prevent gingival irritation. The whitening gel is then painted onto the facials of the teeth and activated with the manufacturer's specifically designed light unit, such as a halogen, laser, plasma-activated curing, or LED. The light accelerates the degradation of the bleaching gel. After the designated time frame, remove the first gel application with high-powered suction and repeat the procedure once or twice more per manufacturer's instructions. Once the regimen is finished, using high-power suction, remove gel, rinse, and remove the rubber dam. Give written and verbal post-op instructions as mentioned above along with take-home trays for touch-ups. Advise the patient to call if sensitivity or gingival problems occur. The patient should be advised that tooth sensitivity could last up to 6 weeks after treatment.

Class IV Restorations

Class IV restorations by definition are those that involve the proximal and incisal edge of an anterior tooth (Roberson, Heymann, and Swift 2006) and result from an injury (Albers 2002) or extensive class III caries. The challenges to the placement of a class IV restoration include achieving proper color matching and anatomical contours, and maintaining a proper functional occlusal scheme. To maximize esthetic result and enhance longevity of the restoration, all of these features need to be in place.

Generally speaking, a relatively small class IV restoration can be done directly on the tooth with acceptable esthetic results. It should still follow the layering techniques to be described below. For large class IV fractures or extensive decay, four treatment modalities should be considered for these clinical situations:

1. Freehand direct resin restoration
2. Bonding the fractured piece of tooth back in place
3. Putty-assisted direct resin restoration
4. Indirect porcelain restoration

In a traumatic case where the fractured piece is retrieved, that segment can be bonded back to the remaining tooth. This can be done as the definitive restorative procedure, or as a temporary measure. The young patient in figures 7-3, 7-4, and 7-5 presented as an emergency following a playground fall. Clinical exam revealed class IV fractures of her maxillary right and left central incisors with no pulpal exposure. The fracture pieces were cleaned with a slurry of pumice and 0.12% chlorhexidine.

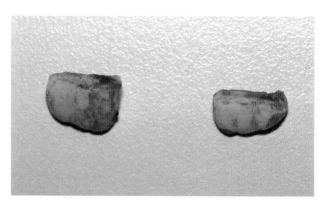

Figure 7-4. Recovered fractured segments.

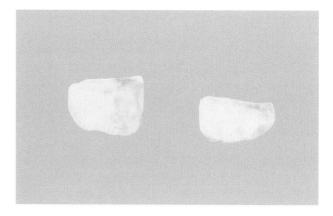

Figure 7-5. Recovered fragments cleaned prior to bonding in place.

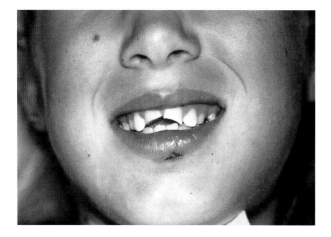

Figure 7-3. Preoperative photo following traumatic injury shows class IV fractures on maxillary right and left central incisors.

Confirm the fit of the fractured piece with the remaining clinical crown. A 1- to 2-mm bevel is placed circumferentially around both the tooth and the fracture segment. This will allow the composite resin used to bond the pieces back together to mask off the fracture line. The tooth and fragments are then etched for 15 seconds with 30–35% phosphoric acid, rinsed, and lightly dried without desiccating the tooth. Dentin bonding agent is applied to all etched surfaces but not cured. If cured, the segments may not fit together. Place a small amount of composite on the internal aspect of the fracture and immediately approximate the two segments and light cure. Composite is placed over the beveled areas of the tooth. Check the occlusion in all excursive movements to avoid any undue forces on the newly bonded fractured segment and finish and polish (fig. 7-6).

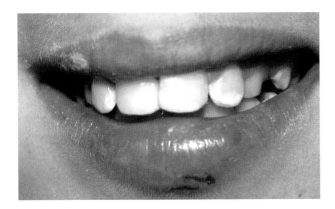

Figure 7-6. Repaired class IV fracture using actual fragmented pieces bonded into place.

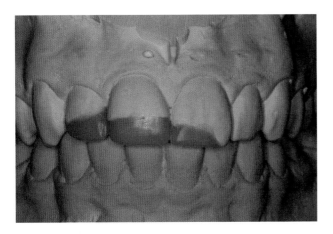

Figure 7-7. Mounted casts with full contour esthetic wax-up of the fractured area.

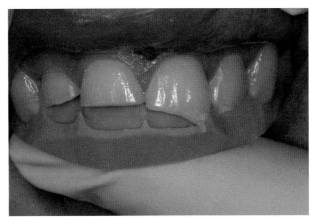

Figure 7-8. A putty matrix placed intraorally is used as an anatomical guide for the composite restoration as well as a template for the actual placement of the composite restoration.

A second technique for restoring a class IV fracture involves two phases. At the first appointment, after the assessments are completed, the emergency situation is stabilized, and the patient is out of pain, make alginate impressions of both arches. Mount the casts on an articulator and do a full contour esthetic wax-up of the fractured area (fig. 7-7). As discussed in chapter 6, the wax–up allows you to establish the proper contours, length, incisal width, and occlusal scheme. Take the articulator through all excursions during the wax-up process. The lingual anatomy of anterior teeth plays a significant role in tooth function and phonetics, and should be in harmony with the patient's occlusal schemes. Excessive occlusal forces can result in fracturing of the newly restored tooth. From the wax-up, a duplicate cast could be made and used to fabricate a putty matrix. It can also be fabricated directly on the wax-up, though you risk fracturing or dislodging the wax-up. The putty matrix can include all surfaces of the wax-up or can extend from the lingual to the facial

terminus of the incisal edge. A putty matrix placed intraorally is used as an anatomical guide for the composite restoration as well as a template for the actual placement of the composite restoration (fig. 7-8).

At the restorative appointment, shade selection is accomplished prior to anesthesia and rubber dam placement to avoid dehydration of the teeth during the shade selection process. Desiccation of a tooth surface can hinder shade selection. If a significant portion of a tooth is fractured, use the contralateral tooth as a guide for shade selection. Shade guides or digital spectrophotometer can be used as described in chapter 12. Because of the intricacy and polychromatic nature of teeth, several shades are selected to match the composite material to the enamel, dentin, and incisal translucency of the tooth for customization of the restoration. Always look for any unique tooth characteristics such as hypocalcification that you may wish to replicate in the restoration. A composite resin mock-up can be placed directly on the tooth and cured without the use of etchant or bonding agent to verify the shade(s) and obtain patient consent. This is a good proofing method of the shade because not all shade guides and resins match perfectly (Yap 1998). Once the shade is verified, this resin can be easily flicked off prior to tooth preparation. After shade selection is complete, try in the putty matrix to ensure proper seating and trim any excess material as needed. It is imperative that composite resin restorations be done under rubber dam isolation. "Rubber dam isolation significantly reduce(s) micro-leakage of resin" as "salivary contamination may affect the bond strength provided by some dentin bonding systems" (Christensen 1994; Hitmi 1999). In cases where a putty matrix is needed to complete the restoration, a slot-dam technique, described in chapter 19, should be utilized.

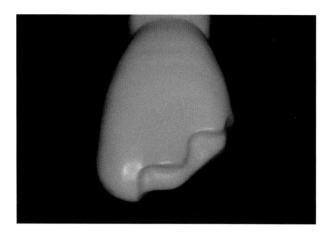

Figure 7-9. Stair-step preparation design to assist the masking of the restoration margin.

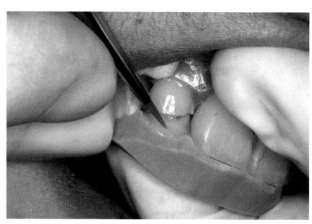

Figure 7-11. Placement of composite to shape the lingual anatomy as designed by the putty matrix.

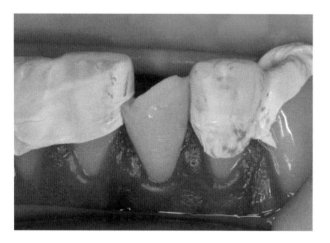

Figure 7-10. Teflon tape in place to protect adjacent teeth from etchant and bonding agent.

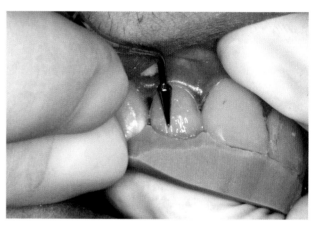

Figure 7-12. Placement of dentin layer with sculpting of mammalons into the resin.

To begin the preparation, any weakened or thin enamel is removed. Two types of margins can be used for the preparation. The chamfer margin that extends to half the length of the fracture and half the depth of the enamel is placed facially and lingually. Utilizing a stair-stepped design (fig. 7-9) "helps achieve a good esthetic result" (Bishara, Peterson, and Bishara 1984). A second option is the long, scalloped bevel placed with a tapered diamond. This design helps mask the margin of the fracture by allowing the color to blend gradually from fracture to natural tooth. On the lingual surface, where esthetics is not of a concern, place a 1- to 2-mm wide bevel or chamfer. Wide bevels do not increase strength but enhance esthetics. After pumicing the teeth, wrap Teflon tape, also known as plumber's tape, around the axial surface of adjacent teeth (fig. 7-10). Etch, rinse, and place a dentin bonding agent over the fractured area. After curing the adhesive, position the putty matrix against lingual sur-

faces. The matrix should extend at least two teeth on either side of prepared tooth, for stability of the putty matrix. Begin the layering of resin composites to address the variations in tooth color. Place a 0.5-mm-thin layer of body resin on the lingual aspect of the matrix from line angle to line angle forming the proximal contacts as well (fig. 7-11). Thin it to 0.3 mm as you approach the incisal edge to make room for the application of incisal resin. You will be packing against the matrix, which will shape your lingual anatomy. The next layer is the dentinal resin. Sculpt it just over the facial bevel toward the incisal edge. The incisal edge of this dentin resin should be scalloped into lobes to mimic the tooth's mammalons (fig. 7-12). The advantage of this shaping process is that it creates a more natural translucency in the incisal edge without it appearing as an obvious linear demarcation. The dentin resin should not be too thick facially, so as to leave room for a top layer of enamel resin.

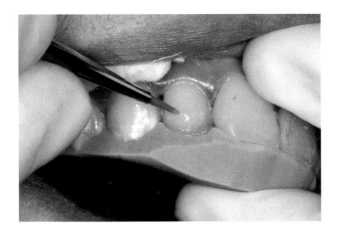

Figure 7-13. Incisal resin placement.

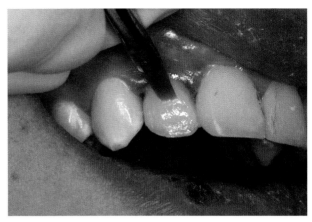

Figure 7-15. Application of enamel layer with instruments and sable brushes to bring out the final contour from incisal edge into the body enamel layer.

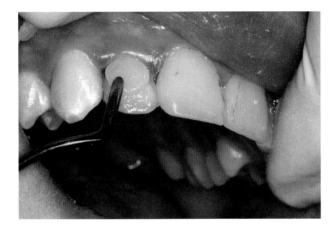

Figure 7-14. Final enamel layer.

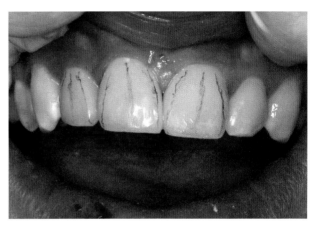

Figure 7-16. Pencil lines can be drawn on the tooth to confirm proper placement of line angles and embrasures.

Next, place the selected incisal resin in between the dentin lobes, under and to the incisal edge of the matrix. This allows for a deep and natural internal incisal translucency (fig. 7-13). Some clinicians recommend masking the fracture line at this point with a thin layer of diluted opaquer. Over the dentinal resin, layer the enamel shade starting at the cervical area and feathering it toward the incisal one-third of the tooth. A #4 artist's brush may be used to create a smooth surface.

The last step is to add the final enamel layer using instruments and sable brushes to bring out the final contour from incisal edge into the body enamel layer (figs. 7-14 and 7-15). Any anatomical facial characteristics should be sculpted in as the resin is being layered. At this point, the facial half of the putty matrix may be placed on the tooth to assess facial contouring based on the wax-up.

It is key to look at the tooth from every direction as the composite is being placed. Move between the 8

o'clock and the 12 o'clock position to give you the different perspectives needed to fully assess the anatomical contours from every direction. The shape of the tooth should mimic its contralateral counterpart.

When several teeth are to be restored, additional anatomical characteristics, confirmation of proper width, placement of line angles, facial-incisal embrasures, lobes, and developmental grooves can be enhanced with the use of fine grit diamonds. Then finish and polish the first tooth to completion. Teflon tape can now be placed on this fully restored tooth and the adjacent tooth is etched and bonded. Build its proximal contact directly against the first restored tooth using the putty matrix as your guide. Once all restorations are completed and the rubber dam is removed, check occlusion in all excursions and adjust as needed.

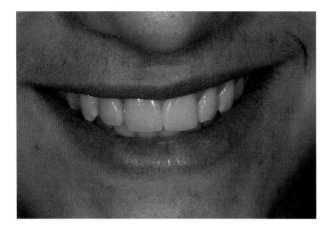

Figure 7-17.   The completed class IV restorations on the patient's maxillary right lateral and maxillary right and left central incisor.

Pencil lines can be drawn on the tooth to outline the position of the line angles, which were defined in the wax-up and transferred to the tooth with the putty matrix (see fig. 7-16). This can also serve as a guide for the restoration of the adjacent teeth. Figure 7-17 shows the completed class IV restorations on the patient's maxillary right lateral incisor and maxillary right and left central incisor.

Peg Laterals or Congenitally Missing Lateral

The Glossary of Prosthodontic Terms (1999) defines a peg lateral as an undersized, tapered maxillary lateral incisor. Hypodontia is one of the most common dental anomalies in the permanent dentition (Buenviaje and Rapp 1984; Endo et al. 2006; Ingervall, Seeman, and Thilander 1972). The maxillary lateral incisor is the most common anterior tooth to form with congenital anomalies, with prevalence for females over males. The peg lateral occurs in 1–2% of the population (Rowe and Johns 1981), and up to 3.7% in Americans (Buenviaje and Rapp 1984). The other variations include congenitally missing lateral incisors either unilaterally or bilaterally.

What would be the optimal way to handle this esthetic issue? There are several treatment options that may be considered:

1. Extraction of lateral incisors depending on the degree of malformation or periodontal problems

and implant placement with or without orthodontic treatment preceding implant placement.
2. Extractions and orthodontic treatment to mesialize the canines followed by recontouring of canines to make them appear to be lateral incisors
3. Extractions and two fixed partial dentures
4. Composite veneering of lateral incisors
5. Veneering or crowning of lateral incisors
6. Orthodontic treatment to eliminate the diastemas created by the malformed laterals and no restorative procedures
7. Orthodontic treatment to align the incisors in a favorable position for restoration with crowns or veneers

Exploration of these restorative paths must be examined. When the laterals are restorable and the adjacent teeth are unrestored or minimally restored, a porcelain veneer is a restorative option for the lateral incisors if the patient has reached developmental maturity.

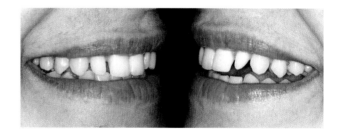

Figure 7-18.   The peg laterals have erupted on both the right and left sides into their natural position, leaving spaces mesially and distally.

Observe in figure 7-18 how the peg laterals have erupted into their natural position, leaving spaces mesially and distally. This advantageous position of both laterals allows for minimal preparation of the proximal surfaces for the porcelain veneers. One critical aspect in preparation is margin placement (see chapter 14 on preparation design). If the interproximal margin is supragingival or juxtagingival, your laboratory technician may have inadequate space to create a smooth emergence profile. This can result in a restoration that has an overhanging margin, an overcontoured margin, contributes to black triangles, gives the tooth an unnatural square appearance, or causes the restoration to impinge on the interdental papilla.

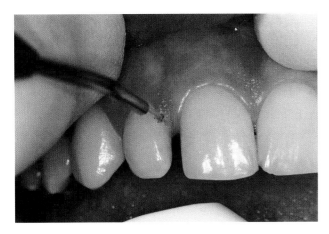

Figure 7-19. Soft tissue lasering to allow for apical margin placement. This allows the laboratory technician to create a more natural-looking emergence profile.

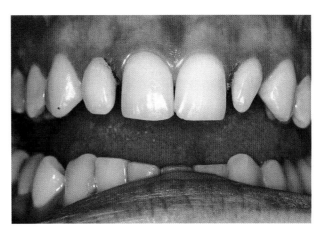

Figure 7-21. Immediate post-op following laser recontouring of the soft tissue.

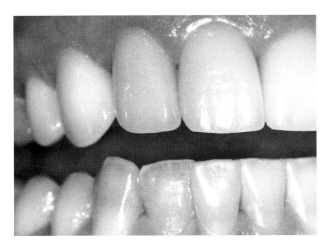

Figure 7-20. Veneer margin is visible on the mesial aspect of the maxillary right lateral incisor just below the gingival margin.

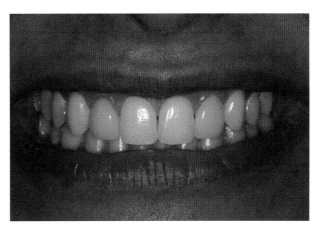

Figure 7-22. Ten-year post-op photo of original veneers placed over peg lateral incisors.

Soft tissue lasering is a valuable tool that allows for a slightly subgingival margin placement. This margin location allows your laboratory technician more space and freedom to adjust the emergence profile, giving the tooth a more natural contour while protecting the interdental papilla from impingement (fig. 7-19). Another common error is not moving the margin lingually sufficiently to help mask the margin placement. This is crucial if the restorations are placed to mask an unsightly tooth color. In figure 7-20, note how the veneer margin on the mesial aspect of the maxillary right lateral incisor is visible just below the gingival margin. In a clinical case where the goal was to mask the tooth's original color with a veneer, it would be crucial to move the margins lingually 1–2 mm so as to hide their location at cementation.

Figures 7-18, 7-19, 7-21, and 7-22 demonstrate a clinical case where peg laterals had naturally erupted in a favorable position and thus were restored with veneers. Slight laser recontouring of the soft tissue was performed to create space on the mesial aspects to allow for improved emergence profile in that area.

The ten-year postoperative photograph (fig. 7-22) shows original veneers that had been placed over the patient's peg lateral incisors. Note the healthy, stippled marginal and interdental papilla.

A second common treatment for peg lateral incisors has been to orthodontically move the anterior sextant to close the diastemas present. Let's look at some of the esthetic repercussions of this. In figure 7-23 where the teeth have been moved orthodontically, note the disproportional size of the maxillary left lateral and central incisor. The peg shape of the lateral is accentuated by its proximity to the larger central incisor. When teeth are not bodily moved but tipped orthodontically into position, the long axes are very steep distally. Gingival zeniths are now stepping up apically from central to canine rather than the central and canine zeniths being at the same height and the laterals positioned more incisally (fig. 7-23).

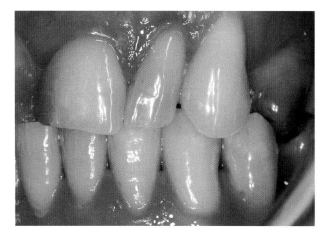

Figure 7-23. Postorthodontic treatment to close space around the peg lateral incisor. Its disproportionate size is accentuated by its proximity to the larger central incisor. Gingival zeniths step up apically from central to canine.

In the clinical case in figure 7-24, a female patient presented with large, stained composites on the central incisors, diastema on the mesial of the maxillary right lateral incisor, peg left lateral incisor, and a dark left maxillary first bicuspid. The canines were found to be in an appropriate occlusal position. View of the buccal corridor reveals palatally tipped bicuspids. This patient wished to have an esthetic makeover.

Several options could be considered to treat the esthetic issues and address the patient's chief concern:

1. Direct or indirect veneers on #7 through #10
2. Indirect restorations on #5 through #12
3. Indirect restorations on #4 through #13
4. Bleaching and any of the aforementioned options

Selecting direct or indirect restorations from #7 though #10 would require space redistribution to improve the size discrepancy present between the maxillary central and lateral incisors. By narrowing the centrals slightly and by moving the line angles of the laterals more to the proximals, achieving the golden proportion would have been possible. Six units should not be a consideration in this case. Placing veneers on the maxillary canines may have obscured the lingually displaced maxillary first bicuspids. Known as a dark corridor, negative space, or buccal corridor space, to the dental eye, this space is more esthetically pleasing the smaller it is (Roden-Johnson, Gallerano, and English 2005).

This case was extended to eight units to allow for the following:

1. Better distribution of space mesially-distally so as to more closely approximate the golden proportions.
2. Rotation of the right canine. As referenced in chapter 6, only the mesial half of the canines should be visible from a frontal view.
3. Buccal inclination of the first bicuspids with the restoration to eliminate the dark corridor.

As referenced in chapter 6, a diagnostic wax-up was completed applying all the aforementioned esthetic principles (fig. 7-25). Note the changes to width-length ratios, long axis inclinations, positioning of contacts, and the soft feminization of the teeth with the more rounded incisal embrasures, the rotation of the maxillary right canine, and the buccal inclination of the maxillary right first bicuspid. With the smile design in place, any modifications can be planned and treatment consent finalized (fig. 7-26). In this particular case, the patient did not reveal the cervical portion of her teeth or any supporting tissue; therefore, soft tissue contouring was not indicated.

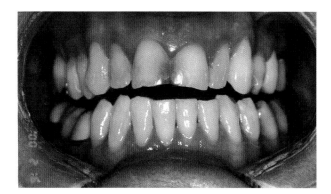

Figure 7-24. Note the diastema on the mesial of the maxillary right lateral incisor, peg left lateral incisor, a dark left maxillary first bicuspid, and the palatally tipped first bicuspids.

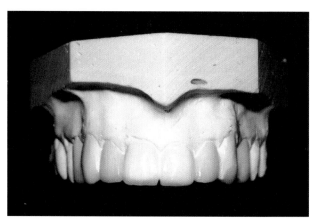

Figure 7-25. Diagnostic wax-up of eight units applying all the esthetic principles.

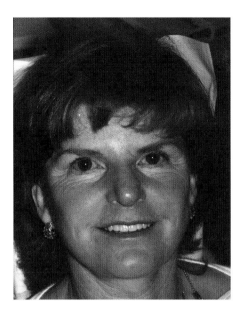

Figure 7-26.   Smile design.

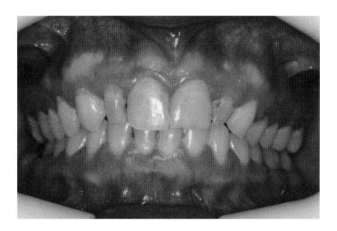

Figure 7-27.   Pre-op photograph showing post orthodontic closure of spaces from peg laterals, caries, and hypocalcification.

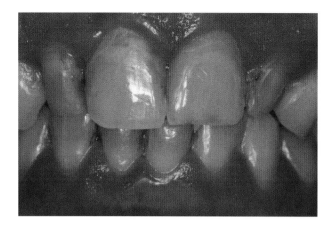

Figure 7-28.   Close-up view.

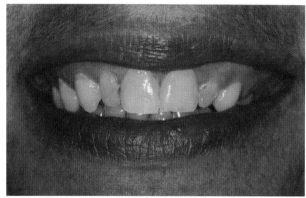

Figure 7-29.   Observe the lingual collapse of the posterior teeth, the inverse architecture of the gingival zeniths, and inverse curve of Spee.

Patients may present to you postorthodontic treatment wishing some esthetic enhancement. In this next case, the patient's chief concern was the decay around her anterior teeth and the disproportionate size of the maxillary central and lateral incisors (fig. 7-27). The decay and extensive hypocalcification is apparent. In the close-up photograph, observe the small lateral incisors, the overangulated left maxillary incisor and canine, and the reversed gingival architecture (fig. 7-28).

As we again move outward in our view (fig. 7-27), notice the severe lingual inclination of all the teeth beginning with the lateral incisors. As we observe the patient more fully (fig. 7-29), the collapse becomes more apparent in the patient's natural smile. Additionally, this patient has a significant amount of gingival display.

The bicuspids and molars are lost from view due to the position of the anterior teeth in relationship to them. The posterior teeth position has resulted in a reverse curve of Spee. Though this occlusal scheme may serve her functionally, the position of the teeth has compromised her esthetically.

The ideal esthetic treatment for this patient would have been to utilize orthodontics to retreat the case. The goals would have been the following:

1. Intrude the molars and bicuspids, reestablishing the proper curve of Spee.
2. Rotate the arch bucally to eliminate the dark corridor.
3. Redistribute the space of the anterior teeth to create space to restore the anterior teeth with indirect restorations at the correct golden proportion.

Esthetic and restorative results are optimized when the peg-shaped lateral incisors are moved orthodontically between the canines and centrals to facilitate the creation of the golden proportion. That position is "determined by the clinical requirements of the particular restorative or prosthetic procedure" (Kokich and Spear 1997; Oesterle and Shellhart 1999). Unfortunately with this case, the orthodontic results left inadequate restorative space to create a pleasing smile utilizing the concepts discussed in chapter 2.

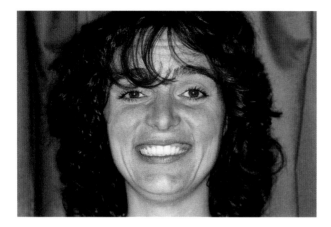

Figure 7-30. The newly placed four incisor veneers.

Having just completed orthodontic treatment, the patient declined orthodontic retreatment, not wishing to put additional time and cost into that option again. She opted to have the four maxillary incisors restored with porcelain veneers. Though far from ideal, the esthetic outcomes were an acceptable improvement. These four teeth had a better height-to-width ratio, long axis inclination, and zenith placement. Had treatment included the canines, the collapsed corridor would have been accentuated. It is important to note that the most distracting portion of this patient's smile is not the anterior teeth but the gummy smile and angulation around the maxillary posterior teeth (fig. 7-30).

A third option for treating hypodontic lateral incisors is to extract the lateral incisors if the following apply:

1. The periodontal conditions would result in guarded to poor prognosis if laterals were restored.
2. The degree of malformation results in a preparation for a fixed restoration with a poor crown-to-root ratio.
3. The remaining tooth structure is insufficient to properly support the chosen restoration.

A fixed partial denture to replace the extracted peg lateral incisors is a restorative option but could be deemed an aggressive procedure, especially if the central incisor and canines are in pristine condition. Implants should be considered as the primary means of replacing missing lateral incisors.

In patients younger than twenty-one years of age for whom skeletal development has not reached maturation, composite veneering of the existing lateral incisors should always be considered a viable option following orthodontics. Other treatment modalities, such as extractions and implants, should be delayed until full skeletal development has been reached. If the laterals are congenitally missing, the provisional treatment choices can include a flipper or stay plate, bonding a composite lateral to the centrals and canines, or a vacuum-formed orthodontic appliance with artificial teeth.

The orthodontic movement of maxillary canines into the space of a congenitally missing maxillary lateral incisor has a long-standing history. With the advent of implants and the dramatic improvement of esthetic procedures, that type of orthodontic movement must be reserved as an absolute last option. Though this treatment modality may solve one issue, it opens up other esthetic concerns. Figure 7-31 demonstrates a case in which the maxillary right lateral incisor was congenitally missing, the maxillary right canine had been orthodontically moved into the lateral position, and composite veneers had been placed on the maxillary right canine through to the maxillary left canine.

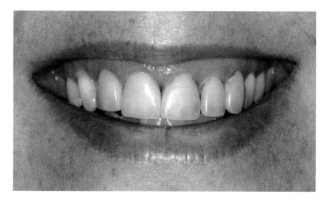

Figure 7-31. Preoperative photograph. Patient is congenitally missing the maxillary right lateral incisor. The maxillary right canine was orthodontically moved into the lateral position. Existing composite veneers are shown on maxillary right canine to the maxillary left canine.

Although the restorations served the patient for twenty years, the patient was not happy with the dark margins that had developed over time and desired a cosmetic refresher. There are several key points to be gleaned by analyzing this photograph. Since canines are longer, wider, and darker than laterals, the tooth size discrepancy poses an esthetic concern, especially in light of the golden proportions previously discussed. In this case, a composite veneer had been placed on the canine and shaped to look like a lateral incisor. In other situations, handpieces have been used to soften the cusp tip, flatten the facial profile, and reshape the lingual anatomy in an attempt to change the appearance without using a restoration. Reshaping them with a handpiece risks exposing so much dentin that a restoration is ultimately required (Miller 1995; Schmitz, Coffano, and Bruschi 2001).

Table 7-2. Natural angulations of the maxillary incisors and canines.

Tooth	M-D Angulation	F-L Angulation
Central incisor	<2 degrees	<28 degrees
Lateral incisor	<7 degrees	<26 degrees
Canines	<17 degrees	<16 degrees

Note: M-D = mesial-distal; F-L = facial-lingual.

All teeth have a natural labial and mesial cant (Okeson 1993; Dempster, Adams, and Duddles 1963; see table 7-2). In this next clinical case (fig. 7-32), the cant of the maxillary right second bicuspid, which was moved into the maxillary right canine position, is too distally inclined. It is also long and impinges, rather than lightly touching, the wet-dry border of the lower lip. Gingival crests are naturally higher on the central and canines in relationship to the laterals. In this situation (fig. 7-33),

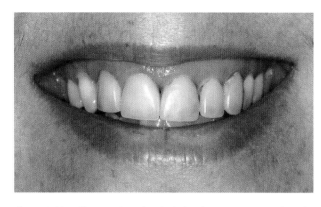

Figure 7-33. Close-up view. The gingival architecture is reversed on the right side in comparison with the normal architecture of this patient's left side.

the maxillary right canine, in the position of the maxillary right lateral incisor, does not have the normal gingival architecture of maxillary lateral incisors. The gingival architecture is reversed on the right side in comparison with the normal architecture of this patient's left side. In patients with gummy smile, this discrepancy can be very obvious. This alteration in the natural gingival contours, along with the gingival zeniths in the wrong anatomical position, detracts from the esthetic outcome.

Notice how the existing composite veneers are very square, contact points are long occluso-gingivally, and incisal embrasures are not well defined. The guidance normally provided by a canine is lost when it is mesialized. The treatment plan for this situation must include a plan to address the existing occlusal shortcomings. Additionally, several considerations need to be addressed to improve the esthetic outcome of this case. They include the following:

1. Tooth width-to-length ratio
2. Position of gingival height and zeniths
3. Midline position
4. Long axis of each tooth
5. Evaluation for periodontal surgery to address patient's gummy smile
6. A discussion of the general shapes of the new restorations

After discussion of all findings and treatment options, the patient decided not to have periodontal surgery and was comfortable with irregularities in gingival heights in spite of her gummy smile. With the final restorations of the right maxillary canine, central incisor through to the left maxillary canine, her desires of rounder, more proportionate teeth were achieved (figs. 7-34 and 7-35).

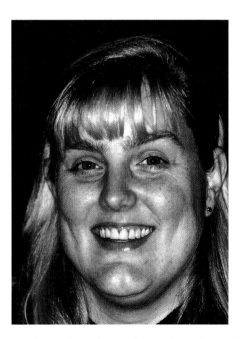

Figure 7-32. The maxillary right second bicuspid is in the maxillary right canine position.

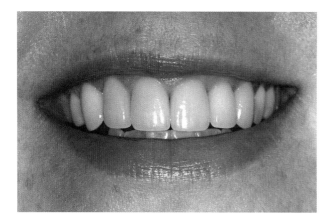

Figure 7-34. Postoperative photo of new porcelain veneers on the right maxillary canine, central incisor through to the left maxillary canine.

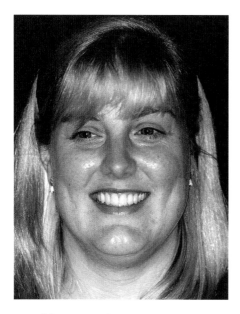

Figure 7-35. Full-face post-op photo. Patient was very happy with results and comfortable with irregularities in gingival heights in spite of her gummy smile.

The diagnostic wax-up is an effective tool in cases involving peg lateral incisors. The wax-up can serve as the guide for the orthodontist to place the anterior sextant in the most optimal position to ensure appropriate distribution of the teeth and corresponding spaces, proper tooth inclination, and occlusal scheme. This is true whether composites, veneers, crowns, or implants will be used for definitive restorative care.

Composite Veneer

Composite veneers are a viable alternative to indirect veneers for the esthetic restoration of anterior teeth. They are especially appealing for patients with limited resources, or as the primary esthetic treatment in young

patients. Composite resin veneers can be used to modify the appearance of peg laterals, close a diastema, or to mask an unaesthetic color.

In the appropriate situation, there are several advantages to the composite veneer. Composite veneers can provide a conservative, esthetic, and reversible treatment option, as little or no enamel is removed in the preparation process. There are no laboratory costs attached to the composite veneer, though they may require some preoperative planning and more chair time. There are several disadvantages that must be considered when contemplating the use of composite resin veneers. First of all, achieving esthetically superior results with composite resin veneers is technically challenging. Second, due to the tendency to stain over time, they cannot be deemed a color stable choice and may require upkeep.

Composite resin veneers are a better option in children or young adults than are porcelain veneers. "The interrelationships among clinical diagnosis, treatment planning, and facial growth expectations are important to understand for each patient ... as proper timing of treatment relative to growth expectations can provide a more desirable result" (Turchetta, Fishman, and Subtelny 2007). "The timing and magnitude of change in the various facial parameters differ during the same growth period as well between males and females" (Bishara, Peterson, and Bishara 1984). If permanent restorations are placed during a growth spurt, the margins of the restorations will end up being visible and retreatment will be required.

Placement of Composite Veneer

In any case where length or width will change with the composite veneer, a diagnostic wax-up should be completed prior to the restorative appointment. As discussed in chapter 6, the wax–up allows you to establish the proper contours, length-to-width ratio, and emergence profile. When accessing the height-to-width proportions in a case with peg laterals, you may find it necessary to add composite to the mesials of the canines or distals of the centrals as well. Be sure to look closely at the length of the teeth and assess whether some gingival recontouring with the laser will enhance the esthetic results from the perspective of length and width, as well as the location of the gingival zeniths.

Make a putty matrix of the wax-up or from the duplicate cast of the wax-up. It will serve two purposes: as the template for the smile design and the template for the placement of the composite resin to help establish the desired anatomic features.

The putty matrix as the template for the smile design or mock-up on the patient, gives the clinician, patient, and family member(s) the opportunity to consent to the design of the proposed treatment, and for the clinician to make changes as deemed necessary. These changes can be made either directly on the mock-up or on the wax-up itself. In a situation where a tooth is slightly rotated, placing any portion of the tooth outside the arch form, the smile design can help the clinician determine the amount of recontouring needed on that tooth prior to preparing it for the composite veneer. In a clinical situation where a dark tooth shade needs to be masked, additional removal of tooth structure is required to provide adequate space for layering of the composites.

Once the patient presents for treatment, color selection is paramount. Since teeth are not monochromatic, several shades are generally required to establish esthetic results. If dark colors need to be masked, an opaquing composite may be used as well. The various methods for shade selection are discussed in chapter 13. Color selection should be done prior to rubber dam placement as desiccation of tooth surface can alter tooth shade. A composite resin mock-up can be placed directly on the tooth and cured without the use of etchant or bonding agent, to verify the shade selected and to obtain patient approval. The advantage of proofing the shade is that not all shade guides and resins match perfectly (Kim and Um 1996, Yap 1998). In other words, a B-1 resin from a company may not match a standard B-1 shade tab. For direct resin veneers, a slot dam technique is indicated.

When multiple anterior teeth are being restored with composite veneers, it is essential to establish symmetry with the central incisors first. The canines can be restored next. Reserve the restoration of the maxillary lateral incisors for last. Any slight discrepancy should be placed on them. A bowley gauge or other measuring device may prove helpful in planning the restorations. A putty matrix generated from a diagnostic wax-up may prove the most efficient and predictable way to achieve outstanding esthetic results.

If the composite veneer is being placed to close a diastema or lengthen a tooth, little or no tooth preparation will be needed. A light chamfer may be placed. Surfaces to be veneered should be lightly roughened with a diamond bur. If the composite veneer is being placed to "effect a color change" (Aschheim and Dale 2001), then some enamel reduction is required. Generally, 0.3 mm of enamel reduction is recommended in the gingival third and 0.5 mm in the body area. These figures can be doubled in a situation where there is severe intrinsic discoloration.

Teflon tape is wrapped around the proximals of adjacent teeth to prevent etchant and bonding agents from altering those surfaces. The size of the diastema will dictate the location of the final finish line. The wider the diastema, the more subgingival the definitive margin should be placed. This is done to prevent the formation of any black triangles and to create a natural-looking emergence profile.

The layering technique is similar to that described for the class IV composite. Since creating the appropriate anatomical contours is a significant esthetic challenge, the use of a putty matrix will help establish the desired anatomic features. Several anatomic features must be established during the restoration phase of treatment:

1. Correct facial height of contour
2. Correct mesial and distal facial line angles
3. Appropriate facial depressions
4. Appropriate incisal characteristics
5. Appropriate shade transitions

Proper placement of the composite resin material will ensure the correct

1. Position of the long axis of the tooth
2. Position of the line angles and contact point
3. Emergence profile to minimize dark triangles
4. Replication of two facial anatomic planes
5. Point angles on the mesial and distal incisal edges
6. Incisal length, generally ½ mm shorter for the laterals than the centrals
7. Gingival zenith position maintained

Ceramic Veneers

This chapter will limit its discussion of ceramic veneers to cases involving between one and six restorations. Generally, the cases presented for discussion here will be relatively simple in complexity and design. More complex cases will be discussed in the following two chapters.

Porcelain veneers offer patients a conservative esthetic option for correcting issues of

1. Tooth color
2. Minor tooth misalignment
3. Diastemas
4. Congenital tooth malformations
5. Tooth fracture
6. Tooth wear

They may be contraindicated on patients with

1. Defective or insufficient enamel
2. Patients with oral habits such as nail biting, opening bobby pins with teeth, and biting on sewing pins, pencils, toothpicks, etc.
3. Short clinical crowns
4. Severe bruxing or parafunctional habits

If a veneer case is contemplated, a diagnostic wax-up is recommended to evaluate the need for orthodontic treatment, crown lengthening, gingival recontouring, and occlusal scheme evaluation and adjustments. Based on the clinical findings, both tooth whitening and orthodontics should be included in the treatment plan discussion. Teeth that are not repositioned through orthodontics prior to veneer restorations often require more tooth reduction. This process, incorrectly dubbed "instant orthodontics," can lead to the unnecessary loss of tooth structure in an effort to correct esthetic deficiencies. Completing veneer restorations following orthodontics is an excellent way to conserve tooth structure while enhancing esthetics.

A thorough understanding of the patient's occlusal scheme as well as the esthetic issues must be established prior to commencing treatment. If occlusal issues exist and canine guidance or appropriate group functions are not established, failure of the veneers due to fracture can be anticipated.

As discussed in chapter 6, a simulation from a diagnostic wax-up should be performed. If the design principles have been followed closely, then the patient should have a "Wow!" reaction. Evaluate the demeanor of the patient. If a patient's demands are too extensive, reconsider doing the case. The time-consuming nature of the patient's demands may not make the case cost effective. If minor changes to this mock-up are made intraorally, an alginate impression can be taken to fabricate another model and putty matrix for provisional fabrication. Additionally, the new model will serve as the diagnostic cast for the laboratory to follow when fabricating the veneers.

Take a digital photograph of the smile design. This photograph will serve as an excellent communication tool.

A copy can remain in the patient's record and a copy can be given to the patient to show the family what the proposed treatment would look like. Send your laboratory a copy as well.

The remaining portion of this chapter will be devoted to examining a few cases to point out several key concepts to consider when developing esthetic treatment plans on a limited number of teeth. The cases are designed to elicit thought on the reader's part and explore some foundational concepts in esthetic treatment planning.

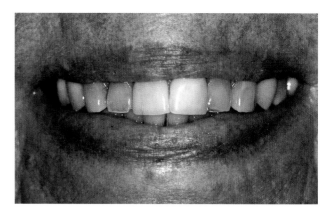

Figure 7-37. Veneers on central incisors no longer match patient's dentition.

Figures 7-36 and 7-37 show the preoperative condition of a female in her eighth decade of life. She had a history of esthetic treatment several years earlier but was not happy with the changes that had occurred with her teeth over the last decade. She was concerned that the veneers on her central incisors no longer matched her dentition. Additionally, she was concerned with the thin, worn appearance of her maxillary lateral incisors. At full smile, she does not display her molars, and she has existing porcelain-fused-to-metal (PFM) crowns on her maxillary right first and second bicuspids and her maxillary left first bicuspid. There are several approaches that could be used to enhance the esthetics of this case. They are as follows.

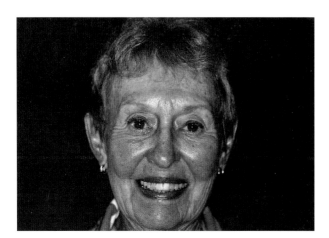

Figure 7-36. Preoperative full face and full smile.

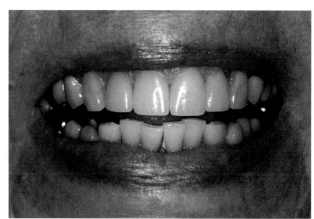

Figure 7-38. Post-op photos of age-appropriate conforming approach to esthetic case. New composite veneers on maxillary lateral and central incisors.

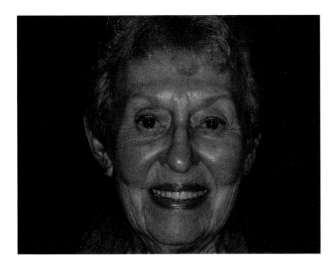

Figure 7-39. Full-face post-op photograph demonstrates the natural appearance of the age-appropriate veneers on the maxillary incisors.

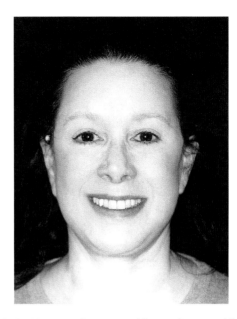

Figure 7-40. Younger patient presented for a replacement of four aging maxillary incisor veneers.

One choice is a full esthetic makeover. This treatment option is generally reserved for patients desiring a color and contour change on all teeth visible during a full smile. The second option could be to bleach all unrestored teeth. A decision must be made as to the final shade to match. Would it be to the shade of the existing veneers on the two central incisors? If so, then restoring from first molar to first molar with new crowns and veneers would be the treatment choice. But at her age, restorations of such a high value would stand out. In a conforming approach, we take into consideration the patient's natural tooth color in her existing oral environment. For this case only the four incisors were veneered. The final result is darker than the original veneers on the two maxillary central incisors, but they match her natural tooth color and blend esthetically overall (figs. 7-38 and 7-39).

In contrast to the treatment planning decision made on the above case, the younger patient in figure 7-40 presented for a replacement of four aging maxillary incisor veneers. She felt the shade of her natural teeth and existing veneers were too dark. She desired lighter teeth. Several treatment options should be considered with this type of case. They are placed in order from most conservative and practical to least conservative.

1. Bleaching would not significantly alter the appearance of any teeth restored with indirect restorations, necessitating the replacement of the existing restorations on the maxillary central and lateral incisors.
2. Porcelain veneers could be considered on the maxillary central and lateral incisors and on any additional teeth visible with a full smile at the new desired shade.

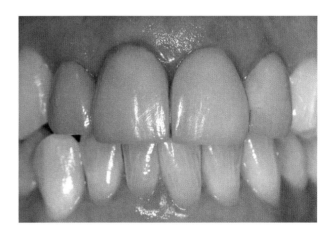

Figure 7-41. Preoperative photos after whitening. Note the marked contrast in color of the old veneers with the recently whitened teeth.

3. Bleaching of all teeth followed by the removal of existing veneers and replacement with composite resin veneers.
4. Bleaching of all teeth followed by the removal of existing veneers and replacement with full-coverage all-ceramic crowns.

The patient selected the first treatment option. In figure 7-41, the retracted preoperative photograph was taken after tooth whitening was completed. The color change was remarkable. Figure 7-42 shows a photograph of the selected shade tabs. This is an invaluable tool for the laboratory. The final outcome, pictured in figure 7-43, achieved the desires of the patient. When veneers are

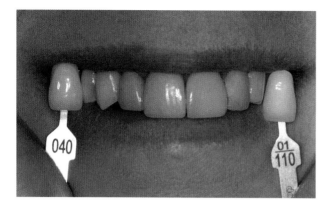

Figure 7-42. Send photograph of the appropriate shade tabs next to the recently whitened teeth to your laboratory to ensure color matching.

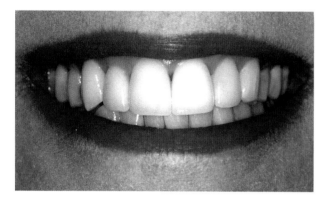

Figure 7-43. Postoperative photograph of four maxillary incisor veneers, matching whitened teeth.

selected in conjunction with tooth whitening, it is essential to advise your patient that periodic tooth whitening will be needed to maintain the color match between natural teeth and veneers.

Diastemas

A diastema is a space between two adjacent teeth in the same arch. Though midline diastemas are viewed by most as unattractive, the esthetic importance and frequency of occurrence can vary culturally and racially (Kerosuo et al. 1995; Oesterle and Shellhart 1999). The contributing factors should be diagnosed as part of the intake exam to create a better treatment outcome. Causes include the following (Chu et al. 2001; Oesterle and Shellhart 1999):

1. Normal occurrence in children during development until eruption of the canines

2. Tooth size discrepancies due to hypodontia
3. Excessive vertical overlap, which increases maxillary arch spacing and, if extensive,
   a. may create excessive maxillary or mandibular vertical alveolar overlap with or without inadequate vertical dimension of occlusion.
   b. then a key indicator of maxillary incisor vertical position is the amount of incisors exposed beneath the resting upper lip. This is generally 2–3 mm.
   c. treatment can include intrusion of maxillary teeth.
   d. then if there is excessive vertical alveolar development of the mandibular incisors, as in class II occlusion, orthodontic evaluation and treatment is indicated.
4. Lack of vertical dimension of occlusion due to short lower face
5. Wide spacing due to arch size vs. tooth size discrepancies
6. Angulations in either a labiolingual or mesiodistal direction of anterior teeth
7. Frenum pulls as a cause appear to be controversial in the literature and in some arenas are considered an outcome of the diastema rather than the cause
8. Pathology such as cysts or acromeglia
9. Tooth migration as a result of missing teeth, whether congenital or postextraction
10. Oral habits such as thumb sucking and tongue position at rest pushing against teeth
11. Periodontal disease that can lead to lack of support and splaying of teeth

The etiology of the diastemas will impact the treatment planning process and must be factored into any treatment decision. The following treatment options should be considered for small diastemas:

1. Placement of a proximal composite to close spaces
2. Invisalign or conventional orthodontics to close or redistribute spaces
3. Composite resin veneers to close spaces
4. Porcelain veneers to close spaces
5. A combination of resin bonding and orthodontics to close spaces

In cases involving larger spaces, all ceramic veneers or crowns in conjunction with tissue contouring can be added to the treatment planning considerations. The difficulty with larger diastemas is that there tends to be no interdental papilla, necessitating careful management of emergence design on the mesial and distal of all restorations.

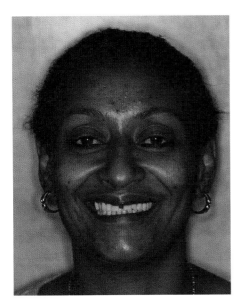

Figure 7-44. Preoperative photographs showing large diastema.

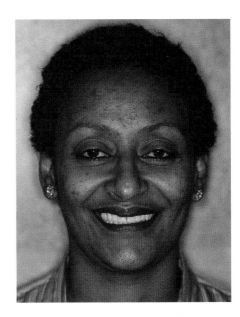

Figure 7-46. Postoperative photographs showing four new veneers.

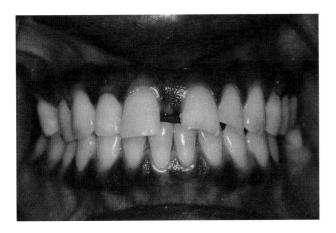

Figure 7-45. Retracted preoperative photographs showing large diastema.

The next case demonstrates one potential treatment option for a patient with a large diastema. The patient in figure 7-44 desires the reduction of the space between her central incisors and the repair of the fractures on her left central and lateral incisor. Clinical observation revealed a maxillary diastema of 7 mm (fig. 7-45). The mandibular midline was shifted to the patient's left. Her canine relationship was class III on the right and class I on the left. Additionally, the right lateral incisor was slightly lingually positioned and the two centrals bucally inclined. Initially, the only real consideration was a combination approach of orthodontics and resin bonding. The patient was not willing to undergo orthodontics and rejected the primary treatment plan. A complete diagnostic wax-up revealed that space redistribution between the four incisors would create an esthetic result and treat the patient's chief concern. The patient ultimately opted to retain a small diastema between the central incisors.

The case was treated with four Empress veneers on the maxillary incisors. To achieve this result, the preparations on the distal portion of the central incisors were more aggressive than normal to allow the laterals to be shifted mesially. Additionally, the laboratory moved the line angles medially to give the illusion of narrower teeth. Note that the centrals were tucked in lingually with the preparation. Gingival zeniths were repositioned as appropriate for each tooth and some gingivectomy done around tooth #8 to lengthen it slightly. Due to the limited number of teeth treated, the shade chosen for the veneers matched her existing tooth color, resulting in a natural appearance. To establish the illusion of an interdental papilla, the margins on the mesial of both centrals were placed subgingivally. This allowed the laboratory to create a natural and gradual emergence profile proximally (fig. 7-46).

In the second case, a fifty-five-year-old female wished to change the color of her four maxillary incisors to match the shade of her canines (fig. 7-47). The canines had been previously restored with crowns and she absolutely "loved" the color. The incisors were stained, and existing restorations had recurrent caries (fig. 7-48). The MI point angles of the centrals had been widened to close the diastema, but that only accentuated the black triangle above it. The patient had expressed her desire to maintain the diastema, as it had been a part of her all her life.

Tooth whitening was completed to lighten maxillary and mandibular teeth to match the color of her maxillary canines. Crowns were placed on the four incisors with appropriate midline placement and realignment of the long axis (figs. 7-49 and 7-50).

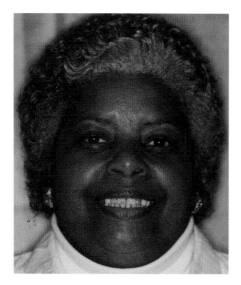

Figure 7-47. Preoperative photograph. Patient wishes to match her maxillary incisors to the shade of her canines and maintain the diastema in the final restorations.

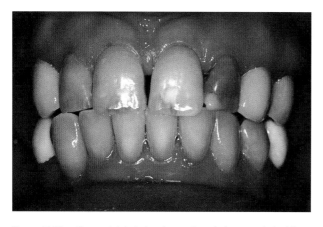

Figure 7-48. The mesial incisal point angles of the centrals had been widened to close the diastema, accentuating the black triangle above it.

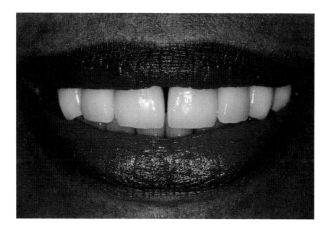

Figure 7-49. Postoperative photograph. Diastema is maintained in new restorations.

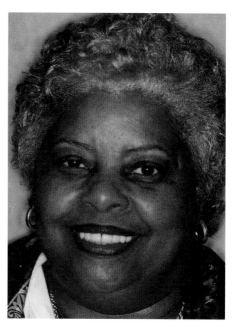

Figure 7-50. Retention of diastema maintains patient's natural characteristic.

Anterior Single-Unit Crowns and Esthetic "Update"

One of the most challenging dental situations is to place a single-unit crown on an anterior tooth, whether necessitated by a traumatic incident, caries, or replacement of an existing restoration prompted by a patient's desire for a more youthful appearance.

There is a plethora of new materials on the market to replace older PFMs. Procera, Inceram, Empress, Lava, Cerec, Cercon, OPC, and Captek are just a few examples of products commonly used in esthetic dentistry. These and other materials will be discussed in more detail in chapter 12. The esthetic challenge with any single-unit anterior restoration is to match the shade, contour, surface texture, light reflection/refraction, and incisal translucencies to the contralateral tooth. Figures 7-51 and 7-52 reveal a failing PFM crown on the maxillary left central incisor. The restoration had recurrent caries, a marginal discrepancy, an overhanging margin on the mesial surface, and root exposure secondary to gingival recession. The crown appears wide when compared with the width of the maxillary right central incisor.

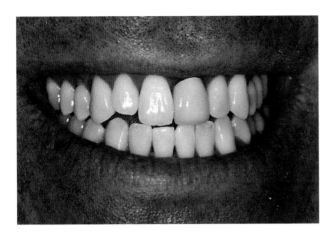

Figure 7-51. Postbleaching preoperative photograph. Note the mesial overhanging margin on the porcelain-fused-to-metal (PFM) crown on the maxillary left central incisor.

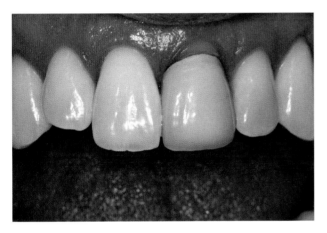

Figure 7-52. The PFM on the maxillary left central incisor is much wider than the maxillary right central incisor.

There are a couple of treatment options that can be considered for the restoration in a situation such as this. The first treatment option is to restore both central incisors and work out the width discrepancies between the two new restorations. This has the benefit of allowing the ceramist the opportunity to create symmetry and balance between two teeth. The second option is to fabricate a new single-unit crown and attempt to create the illusion of a narrower-appearing crown. The patient was unwilling to have an unrestored central incisor sacrificed for esthetic reasons and ultimately selected a single-unit restoration. The patient also desired lighter teeth and underwent an at-home tooth whitening procedure.

After tooth whitening, the tooth was reprepared, with the mesial margin placed slightly subgingival to ensure a smooth emergence profile. To address the black triangle on the distal side would have required restoring

more units in this case. Patient understood and accepted that outcome. Empress I was selected as the material for the new crown due to its excellent translucency, vitality, and fit. The single-unit anterior crown must be viewed as one of the most esthetically challenging restorative procedures and must be undertaken with that understanding.

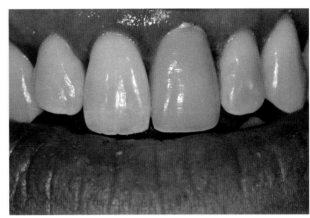

Figure 7-53. Try-in appointment. Crown color is too gray and lacks incisal translucency.

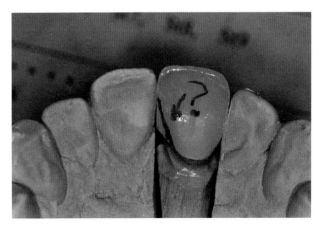

Figure 7-54. The crown on the die is marked with a Sharpie pen to show the laboratory the ledging and long proximal contact that needs correcting.

At the try-in appointment, two problems were apparent. First, the color was grayer, and it lacked incisal translucency (fig. 7-53). Second, the laboratory technician, in an effort to hide the black triangle, had created a ledge (fig. 7-54) with the abrupt emergence profile resulting in an inappropriately long contact occlusogingivally. The crown still appeared wide, as the line angles had not been sufficiently brought in medially to create a narrower illusion. The gingival zenith on the restoration was apical to the natural right central incisor (fig. 7-55). This was not an esthetic concern, as the patient did not show the margins in his full smile. The crown was returned to the laboratory for correction. Figure 7-56 shows the final Empress I crown in place. Compared with the preexisting PFM, the Empress crown has improved color, incisal translucency, contour, and width.

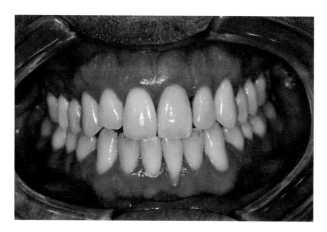

Figure 7-55. Gingival zeniths are higher than contralateral tooth but are not evident in patient's full smile.

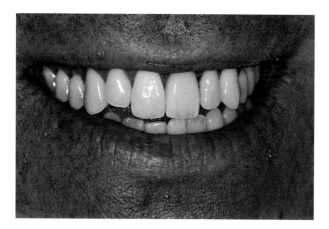

Figure 7-56. The crown color, incisal translucency, and width are more natural in appearance.

With a good quality laboratory and talented ceramist, a single-unit crown can match so well that it is difficult to distinguish from the natural tooth. In figure 7-57, the maxillary right central incisor needed to be restored with a crown due to extensive caries. It was restored with a PFM crown and matches very well with its contralateral tooth. Most important, it is conforming to the clinical situation of the patient.

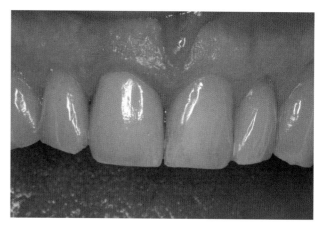

Figure 7-57. Highly esthetic and age-appropriate PFM crown on maxillary right central incisor matches well with contralateral tooth.

Posterior All-Ceramic Crown

Failing posterior porcelain-fused-to-metal or full-metal crowns can be replaced esthetically as well. The fifty-year-old patient in figures 7-58 and 7-59 presented with extensive recurrent caries around existing PFM crowns on her mandibular left second bicuspid and first molar. Upon removal of the crowns, the extensive decay on the mesial root of the lower left first molar left the restorability in question.

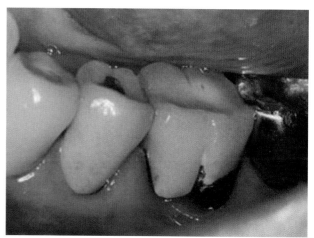

Figure 7-58. Pre-op photograph showing recurrent caries.

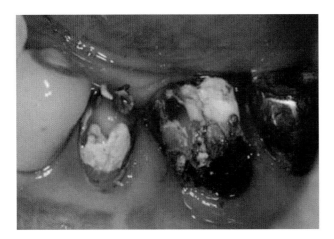

Figure 7-59. Crowns and caries removed and extent of caries accessed.

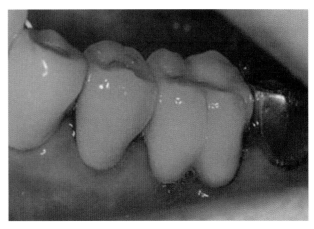

Figure 7-61. Final fixed partial denture in place.

Treatment options included the following:

1. Extraction of the lower left first molar and fabrication of a fixed partial denture from lower left second molar to lower left second premolar
2. Extraction of the lower left first molar and implant placement, followed by crown restorations on both adjacent teeth
3. Mesial root amputation of the lower left first molar and splinted crowns on both teeth

After discussion of the treatment options the patient elected to save the tooth at all costs. Endodontic treatment was initiated on the first molar followed by mesial root amputation. A post and core were placed to restore the distal root. For the first bicuspid, caries removal and build-up were completed as seen in figure 7-60. Splinted PFM crowns were fabricated and cemented on the two prepared teeth. The mesial root portion of the restoration was restored as a pontic. Figure 7-61 demonstrates

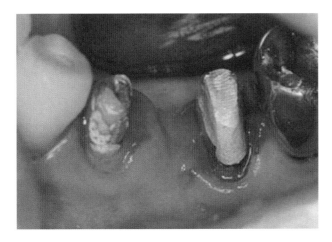

Figure 7-60. Cast post and core on the mandibular left first molar.

how the pontic was shaped to look like the mesial half of a molar tooth, with the natural fluting that would be visible on a tooth with some gingival recession. The outcome blended naturally with her other existing restorations.

Replacing the Single Missing Tooth

Providing restorative options for an extraction site must be looked at very carefully. Traditional options have included fixed or removable prosthetics. In recent years, implants have moved into the arena of viable options for the replacement of missing teeth. It is unacceptable not to offer them as an option to your patients, as implants are moving toward being considered standard of care. In many missing tooth situations, the single implant is often the most conservative and esthetic treatment option available.

If an unrestorable tooth is to be extracted, and an implant will be replacing the tooth, various consultations and radiographs need to be taken. The site has to be evaluated for acceptable parameters for implant placement. This includes evaluating the bone level, quality, and quantity. Bone grafting procedures may be necessary to augment the socket. Grafting procedures would avoid the creation of an extraction site defect. In consultation with your periodontist or oral surgeon, determine how long the site must mature prior to implant placement. Determine if a temporary splint or retainer should be used to maintain restorative space or prevent tipping. Restorative space must be large enough to accept the implant prosthesis. A good rule of thumb is 7mm of mesial-distal dimension from adjacent teeth, 7mm buccal-lingual bone dimension, and 7mm vertical bone ridge apically to the alveolar crest. Details on implant restorations are discussed at length in the next chapter.

Oftentimes a tooth deemed unrestorable may have had gross caries for many years, resulting in changes in the arch form. How would you address the following scenarios?

1. Opposing tooth has supraerupted into the carious space of the tooth to be extracted.
2. The adjacent teeth have tipped mesially or distally, encroaching on the tooth space.
3. Teeth have drifted out of alignment, affecting restorability.

These issues have to be addressed prior to the final restoration placement by analyzing a set of mounted diagnostic casts. If the opposing tooth has supraerupted, the change in the occlusal plane should be corrected prior to the restoration of the edentulous space. Long-standing edentulous spaces often necessitate more aggressive treatment modalities to correct the occlusal plane. Prophylactic endodontic procedures and crown lengthening procedures are often required in severely altered arches to reestablish the correct occlusal plane. If this option is being considered, you must ensure that the tooth with the new crown will have a crown-to-root ratio of 1:2 or minimally 1:1 and still maintain good periodontal health at the time of final restoration. If not, the longevity of the restoration will be compromised.

The use of new technologies in orthodontic treatment such as Invisalign, coupled with multidisciplinary approaches to esthetic needs, has led to more conservative and predictable treatment options for long-standing edentulous spaces. The use of orthodontics now provides an alternative to the aforementioned treatment options. Supraerupted and tilted teeth can now be corrected quite easily with orthodontic intervention.

Orthodontic treatment can create a more ideal restorative situation by recapturing space for an implant or fixed partial denture. Orthodontics facilitates the preparation on abutment teeth by aligning the abutments along a common path of insertion.

Orthodontic Treatment: Complex Cases Made Simple

Often, complex occlusal schemes are difficult to treat using solely a restorative approach. They can also lead to compromised esthetic results. Many complex cases can be greatly simplified with the use of Invisalign or minimal orthodontic intervention. Cases with any of the following clinical conditions may be dramatically simplified with orthodontic involvement:

1. Crowding or misalignment
2. Poorly aligned peg lateral incisors
3. Tipped molars
4. Rotated anterior teeth
5. Uneven gingival architecture
6. Irregular arch forms
7. Buccal corridor space issues

With anterior crowding, accessibility for direct or indirect restorations can be a challenging problem. To maximize an esthetic result, it is better to align the teeth in the most favorable position possible prior to restoring. Some aspect of the width-to-length ratio, midline location, or parallelism of dental to facial midline will be affected in the restorative outcome when crowding is present. Conservation of tooth structure has long been a tenet practiced by dentists since G. V. Black set restorative parameters for dentists. In anterior esthetic cases, once teeth are in a favorable position, the preparation design may be simplified from a full-coverage or three-quarter veneer preparation to a conservative facial veneer. The challenge facing the practitioner is to advise the patient of the need and advantages of orthodontic treatment to enhance the esthetic outcomes. If the patient is not aware of "invisible" braces, educate them. Invisalign technology has enhanced adult patients' willingness to accept orthodontic treatment as an adjunct to esthetic treatment. The age of the patient should not preclude you from offering orthodontic treatment as an option.

If a patient has retained primary molars and is older than twenty-five, with good periodontal health, those primary molars do not need to be extracted. Research has shown that these molars have a high percentage of retention for many years. On the other hand, if orthodontic treatment is needed to correct crowding or esthetic issues, then the primary molars can be extracted to aid in the creation of the required space.

If the laterals are congenitally missing, it is better esthetically not to mesialize the canines and then convert them to laterals via enamoplasty or with a fixed restoration. Keeping the canines in their intended position helps maintain the occlusal goal of canine disclusion, for which the tooth was designed. The laterals could be replaced with implants. Parents often ask what can be done in the meantime while their child is still in his or her developmental stage. During orthodontic treatment, especially with Invisalign, the aligners can have laterals inserted into them.

Once orthodontic treatment is completed, a removable stay plate is a viable option. Parents and patient must be advised that this will need to be redone periodically to keep pace with the child's cranio-facial development.

When patients are undergoing orthodontic treatment prior to other esthetic treatment, the general dentist must work closely with the orthodontist to ensure proper position of the teeth. Having regular personal conversations with the orthodontist about your treatment goals is an excellent way to ensure superior results. Mounted diagnostic models will aid in explaining why teeth need to be placed in a certain position, why a diastema must remain upon completion of orthodontics, and why the case must be finished with well-delineated canine guidance, as well as demonstrate the amount of restorative space required.

Unsuccessful Outcomes

Unsuccessful outcomes can be minimized with proper planning prior to the initiation of treatment. This requires a comprehensive intake exam, proper records including x-rays, photographs, stick bite, study models, diagnostic wax-ups, face bow transfers, and any necessary consultations with a specialist. Several treatment options and risks, benefits, and alternatives of treatment must be explained to the patient. A few situations that resulted in poor esthetic outcome and what was done to correct the situations will be discussed.

Ideally, the dental midline is coincidental with the facial midline. Studies have demonstrated that the dental midline can be as much as 2 mm off center for orthodontists and as much as 3.5 mm off for lay people to still be deemed esthetically pleasing (Cardash, Ormanier, and Laufer 2003; Johnston, Burden, and Stevenson 1999; Rosenstiel, Land, and Fujimoto 2006). More critical is the vertical alignment of the central incisors with the facial midline. Central incisors that do not parallel the facial midline can become very obvious even to the untrained eye. Orthodontics may be needed to resolve the discrepancy. If a restorative approach is selected to correct this situation, the problem should be resolved in the diagnostic wax-up prior to preparing the teeth for crowns or veneers.

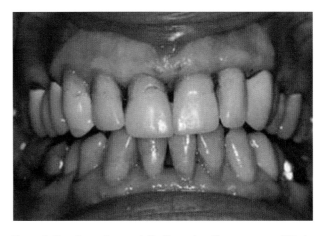

Figure 7-63. Composite material had been placed in an attempt to hide the visible margins.

If the clinician fails to maintain the long axis of anterior tooth preparations along the facial midline, a cant may inadvertently be introduced to the case. The patient pictured in figure 7-62 wished to have her anterior crowns replaced for esthetic reasons. The restorations had been placed many years ago, and several attempts to hide the visible margins had been made (fig. 7-63). The patient had a habit of tilting her head. This may have helped distract viewers from the obvious cant that existed between her dental and facial midlines.

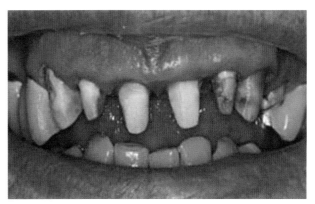

Figure 7-64. In assessing the original preparations, it is apparent that they are not parallel with the facial midline.

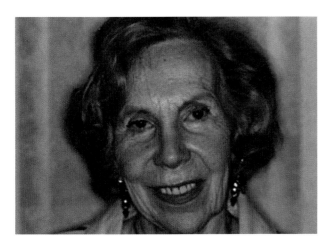

Figure 7-62. To help distract viewers from the obvious cant in her anterior restorations, the patient has a habit of tilting her head.

The reason for this cant was not fully understood until the restorations were removed. When the original preparations are assessed as seen in figure 7-64, it is apparent that they are not parallel with the facial midline. The preparations all lean to the patient's left. In all probability, no facial landmarks were recorded or sent to the laboratory technician. The laboratory technician likely fabricated restorations along the long axis of the preparations and created the cant. This situation can be prevented by aligning teeth (through orthodontics) or preparations (through restorative procedures) along the facial midline.

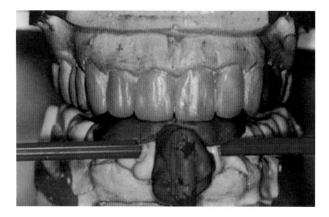

Figure 7-65. Diagnostic wax-up with the aid of the stick bite.

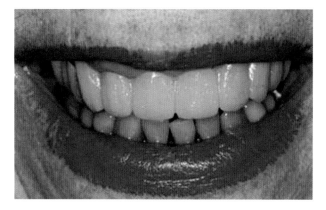

Figure 7-66. Smile design.

To correct this patient's situation, a facial landmark registration (stick bite) is used during the diagnostic wax-up phase to align the teeth along the facial midline (fig. 7-65). Once the teeth have been aligned vertically, the incisal edge can be placed perpendicular to that alignment. A simulated smile design can be done to assess the alignment of the proposed restorations. The smile design can be used as a surgical template as well,

if periodontal procedures are selected to correct the gingival tissue asymmetry (fig. 7-66).

The next case demonstrates a relatively conservative but unsuccessful attempt at an esthetic improvement of the maxillary dentition of a twenty-five-year-old male. Prior to veneer placement on the maxillary central incisors, a diastema of approximately 2 mm was present. Veneers were placed to address this patient's chief complaint, namely, closure of the space between his front teeth. Although the space was closed, a less than ideal result was obtained. Color aside, the two veneers appeared relatively wide, were diamond shaped, and appeared to have a poor width-to-length ratio. Additionally, the gingiva was inflamed due to the overcontured restorations (fig. 7-67). This case helps illustrate an unsuccessful esthetic outcome even though the chief complaint has been addressed. The chief complaint drives the decision-making process, but all esthetic cases should attempt to follow the guiding principles discussed in chapter 2. Attention to these principles will allow the clinician to simultaneously deliver outstanding results and address the patient's chief concern.

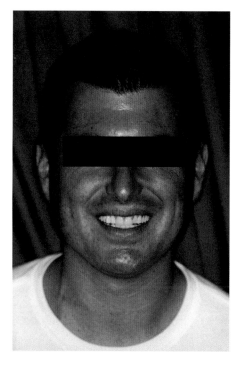

Figure 7-67. Existing veneers are wide, diamond shaped, and appear to have a poor width-to-length ratio.

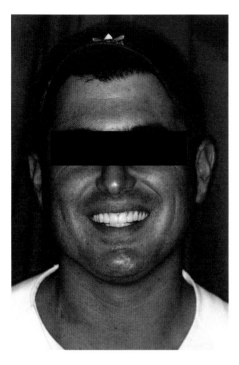

Figure 7-68. Postoperative photo of redone case. Four veneers were selected to allow for better space distribution.

Using the guiding principles and case design techniques, four veneers were selected to enhance esthetics and address the chief concern of the patient (fig. 7-68). Tissue recontouring was treatment planned to improve the gingival contours above the central incisors. The tissue response to the new restorations demonstrates a marked improvement over the former restorations.

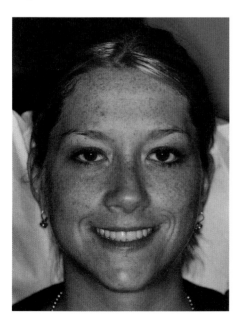

Figure 7-69. Preoperative photograph showing existing PFM crowns from the maxillary right first bicuspid to the maxillary left canine.

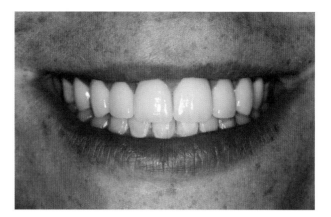

Figure 7-70. Close-up view of PFM crowns from #5 to #11. Note the dull color and overcontouring of crowns.

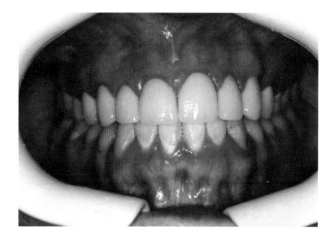

Figure 7-71. Note how the metal substructure has imposed a blue tinge to the marginal gingiva. The gingival zeniths cant toward the patient's right side and are not ideally positioned.

The next case demonstrates the necessity for patient involvement during the treatment planning process. Additionally, informed consent must allow the patient to reach his or her own decision from the information presented during treatment planning. Both clinician and patient must be comfortable with the prescribed course of treatment. The patient presented in this section (figs. 7-69, 7-70, and 7-71) had recently had treatment to restore badly damaged maxillary anterior teeth. The patient presented reporting that she was unhappy with the outcome for several reasons:

1. She was unhappy with the color and opacity of the restorations.
2. She was concerned with the gray appearance of the tissue around her new restorations.
3. She reported that the color was darker than the one originally agreed upon.

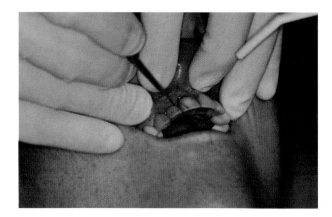

Figure 7-72. Gingivectomy performed to improve the tissue health and tooth width ratios.

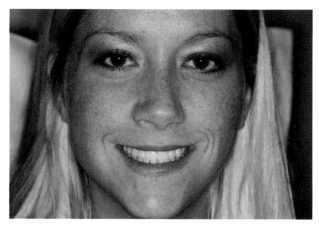

Figure 7-74. Natural smile with final restorations.

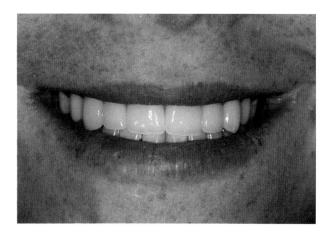

Figure 7-73. Close-up view of final restorations in place.

The information she provided allowed a new treatment approach to be developed. The revised approach included periodontal crown lengthening and replacing all PFM crowns with Empress restorations to improve esthetics and achieve the patient's desired shade. Crown lengthening was utilized to improve the tissue health and width-to-length ratios of the anterior teeth (fig. 7-72).

The final restorations are shown in figures 7-73 and 7-74. The new restorations achieved the desired results of improved translucency and a much brighter shade. Additionally, the width-to-length ratios, incisal characteristics, and tooth shapes achieved the esthetic result the patient desired.

Conclusion

This chapter has addressed basic esthetic parameters. Diagnosis, treatment, planning, and sequencing of a case are the foundation for esthetic results and must never be

overlooked. Generally speaking, esthetic failures often result from the lack of impeccable diagnosis, treatment planning, and sequencing. Esthetic treatments are not successful if they do not meet the expectations of the patient. If your treatment plan and the expectations of the patient do not coincide, or if an acceptable compromise cannot be met, then consider not continuing with treatment and referring the patient.

The principles and foundation information discussed in this chapter should be carried with you into the next two chapters as more complicated cases are discussed. Now that you are comfortable with these simple cases, let's challenge you to move toward the moderately difficult ones.

Acknowledgements

The authors wish to thank the following individuals for help in providing clinical cases highlighted throughout this chapter:

J. Fred Arnold III DMD, FAACD, Lexington, KY, figures 7-7, 7-8, and 7-11 to 7-16.
Harry Albers DDS, FAGD, Santa Rosa, CA, figure 7-9.

Works Cited

Albers HF. 2002. *Tooth-colored Restorative Principles and Techniques*, 9th ed. BC Decker.

American Academy of Cosmetic Dentistry. 2004. Can a new smile make you appear more successful and intelligent? Retrieved from www.aacd.com/press/consumerstudies.asp.

Aschheim KW, Dale BG. 2001. *Esthetic Dentistry: A Clinical Approach to Techniques and Materials*, 2nd ed. Mosby.

Attin A, Hannig C, Wiegnd A, Attin R. 2004. Effect of bleaching on restorative materials and restorations: A systematic review. *Dental Materials* 20:853–61.

Attin T, Paque F, Ajam F, Lennon AM. 2003. Review of the current status of tooth whitening with the walking bleach technique. *International Endodontic Journal* 36:313–29.

Barghi N, Godwin JM. 1994. Reducing the adverse effect of bleaching on composite-enamel bond. *Journal of Esthetic Dentistry* 6:157–61.

Beall AE. 2007. Can a new smile make you look more intelligent and successful? *Dental Clinics of North America* 51(2):289–97.

Bishara SE, Peterson LC, Bishara EC. 1984. Changes in facial dimensions and relationships between the ages of 5 and 25 years. *American Journal of Orthodontics* 85(3):238–52.

Boraston Z, Corden B, Miles LK, Skuse DH, Blakemore SJ. 2008. Brief report: Perception of genuine and posed smiles by individuals with autism. *Journal of Autism Developmental Disorders* 38(3):574–80.

Buenviaje TM, Rapp R. 1984. Dental anomalies in children: A clinical and radiographic survey. *ASDC Journal of Dentistry for Child* 51:42–46.

Cardash HS, Ormanier Z, Laufer, BZ. 2003. Observable deviation of the facial and anterior tooth midlines. *Journal of Prosthetic Dentistry* 89(3):282–85.

Christensen GJ. 1994. Using rubber dams to boost quality, quantity of restorative services. *Journal of the American Dental Association* 125:81–82.

Chu FC, Siu AS, Newsome PR, Wei SH. 2001. Management of median diastema. *General Dentistry* 49(3):282–87.

Cvitko E, Denehy GE, Swift Jr. EJ, Pires JA. 1991. Bond strength of composite resin to enamel bleached with carbamide peroxide. *Journal of Esthetic Dentistry* 3(3):100–102.

Dadoun MP, Bartlett DW. 2003. Safety issues when using carbamide peroxide to bleach vital teeth: A review of the literature. *European Journal of Prosthodontics and Restorative Dentistry* 11:9–13.

Dempster WT, Adams WJ, Duddles RA. 1963. Arrangement in the jaws of the roots of the teeth. *Journal of the American Dental Association* 67:779–97.

Endo T, Ozoe R, Yoshino S, Shimooka S. 2006. Hypodontia patterns and variations in craniofacial morphology in Japanese orthodontic patients. *Angle Orthodontist* 76(6):996–1003.

Garcia-Godoy F, Dodge WW, Donohue M, O'Quinn JA. 1993. Composite resin bond strength after enamel bleaching. *Operative Dentistry* 18(4):144–47.

Gerlach RW, Gibb RD, Sagel PA. 2000. A randomized clinical trial comparing a novel 5.3% hydrogen peroxide whitening strip to 10%, 15%, and 20% carbamide peroxide tray-based bleaching systems. *Compendium of Continuing Education in Dentistry* 121(29):S42-S43.

Gerlach RW, Sagel PA, Barker ML, Karpinia KA, Magnusson I. 2004. Placebo-controlled clinical trial evaluating a 10% hydrogen peroxide whitening strip. *Journal of Clinical Dentistry* 15(4):118–22.

The glossary of prosthodontic terms seventh edition. 1999. *Journal of Prosthetic Dentistry* 81(1):39–110.

Goldstein RE. 1997. In-office bleaching: Where we came from, where we are today. *Journal of the American Dental Association (supplement)* 128:11S.

Heymann HO. 1997. Conservative concepts for achieving anterior esthetics. *Journal of California Dental Association* 25 (6):437–43.

Heymann H. 1997. Nonrestorative treatment of discolored teeth: Reports from an international symposium. *Journal of the American Dental Association (supplement)* 128:Intro.

Heymann HO. 2005. Tooth whitening: Facts and fallacies. *British Dental Journal* 198(8):514.

Hitmi L. 1999. The rubber dam and shear bond strength. *Journal of Adhesive Dentistry* 1(3):219–232.

Ingervall B, Seeman L, Thilander B. 1972. Frequency of malocclusion and need of orthodontic treatment in 10-year old children in Gothenburg. *Swedish Dental Journal* 65:7–21.

Javaheri DS, Janis JN. 2000. The efficacy of reservoirs in bleaching trays. *Operative Dentistry* 25(3):149–51.

Johnston CD, Burden DJ, Stevenson MR. 1999. The influence of dental to facial midline discrepancies on dental attractiveness ratings. *European Journal of Orthodontics* 21(5):517–22.

Kelleher MG, Roe FJ. 1999. The safety-in-use of 10% carbamide peroxide (Opalescence) for bleaching teeth under the supervision of a dentist. *British Dental Journal* 187(4):190–94.

Kerosuo H, Hausen H, Laine T, Shaw WC. 1995. The influence of incisal malocclusion on the social attractiveness of young adults in Finland. *European Journal of Orthodontics* 17(6): 505–12.

Kim HS, Um CM. 1996. Color differences between resin composites and shade guides. *Quintessence International* 27(8):559–67.

Kokich VG, Spear FM. 1997. Guidelines for managing the orthodontic-restorative patient. *Seminars Orthodontics* 3(1): 3–20.

Kugel G. 2003. Over-the-counter tooth-whitening systems. *Compendium of Continuing Education in Dentistry* 24(4A): 376–82.

Leonard RH Jr, Van Haywood B, Caplan DJ, Tart ND. 2003. Nightguard vital bleaching of tetracycline-stained teeth: 90 months post treatment. *Journal of Esthetic Restorative Dentistry* 15(3):142–52.

Matis BA, Hamdan YS, Cochran MA, Eckert GJ. 2002. A clinical evaluation of a bleaching agent used with and without reservoirs. *Operative Dentistry* 27(1):5–11.

McGarry TJ, Nimmo A, Skiba JF, Ahlstrom RH, Smith CR, Koumjian JH, Arbree NS. 2002. Classification system for partial edentulism. *Journal of Prosthodontics* 11(3):181–93.

McGarry TJ, Nimmo A, Skiba JF, Ahlstrom RH, Smith CR, Koumjian JH, Guichet GN. 2004. Classification system for completely dentate patient. *Journal of Prosthodontics* 13(2): 73–82.

McGuckin RS, Thurmond BA, Osovitz S. 1992. Enamel shear bond strengths after vital bleaching. *American Journal of Dentistry* 5(4):216–22.

Miller TE. 1995. Implications of congenitally missing teeth: Orthodontic and restorative procedures in the adult patient. *Journal of Prosthetic Dentistry* 73(2):73–82.

Oesterle LJ, Shellhart WC. 1999. *Maxillary midline diastemas*: A look at the causes. *Journal of the American Dental Association* 130(1):85–94.

Okeson, Jeffrey P. 1993. *Management of Temporomandibular Disorders and Occlusion*, 5th ed. St. Louis, MO: Mosby.

Perdigao J, Baratieri LN, Arcari GM. 2004. Contemporary trends and techniques in tooth whitening: A review. *Practical Procedures & Aesthetic Dentistry* 16(3):185–92.

Pretty IA, Ellwood RP, Brunton PA, Aminian A. 2006. Vital tooth bleaching in dental practice: Part 1. Professional bleaching. *Dental Update* 33(5)288–304.

Roberson T, Heymann HO, Swift EJ Jr. 2006 *Sturdevant's Art and Science of Operative Dentistry*, 5th ed. St. Louis, MO: Elsevier.

Roden-Johnson D, Gallerano R, English J. 2005. The effects of buccal corridor spaces and arch form on smile esthetics. *American Journal of Orthodontics and Dentofacial Orthopedics* 127(3):343–50.

Rosenstiel, Stephen F, Land Martin F, and Fujimoto Junhei. 2006. *Contemporary Fixed Prosthodontics*. 4th ed. St Louis, MO: Mosby Elsevier.

Rowe AH, Johns RB, eds. 1981. *A Companion to Dental Studies: Dental Anatomy and Embryology*. Boston: Blackwell Scientific.

Schmitz JH, Coffano T, Bruschi A. 2001. Restorative and orthodontic treatment of maxillary peg incisors: A clinical report. *Journal of Prosthetic Dentistry* 85(4):330–334.

Schwartz R, Robbins JW, Summit JB, Sox Santos J. 1996. *Fundamentals of Operative Dentistry: A Contemporary Approach*. 3rd ed. London: Quintessence.

Sulieman M, Addy M, MacDonald E, Rees JS. 2004. The effect of hydrogen peroxide concentration on the outcome of tooth whitening: An in vitro study. *Journal of Dentistry* 32(4):295–299.

Sulieman M, MacDonald E, Rees JS, Newcombe RG, Addy M. 2006. Tooth bleaching by different concentrations of carbamide peroxide and hydrogen peroxide whitening strips: An in vitro study. *Journal of Esthetic and Restorative Dentistry* 18(2):93–100, 101.

Swift EJ. 1997. Restorative considerations with vital tooth bleaching. *Journal of the American Dental Association* 128: 60S-64S.

Swift EJ Jr, Miguez PA, Barker ML, Gerlach RW. 2004. Three-week clinical trial of a 14% hydrogen-peroxide, strip-based bleaching system. *Compendium of Continuing Education in Dentistry* 25(8, Supplement 2):27–32.

Tavares M, Stultz J, Newman M, Semith V, Kent R, Carpino E, Goodson JM. 2003. Light augments tooth whitening with peroxide. *Journal of the American Dental Association* 134(2): 167–75.

Titley KC, Torneck CD, Ruse ND. 1992. The effect of carbamide peroxide gel on the shear bond strength of a microfil resin to bovine enamel. *Journal of Dental Research* 71:20–24.

Turchetta BJ, Fishman LS, Subtelny JD. 2007. Facial growth prediction: A comparison of methodologies. *American Journal of Orthodontics and Dentofacial Orthopedics* 132(4): 439–49.

Yap AU. 1998. Color attributes and accuracy of Vita-based manufacturers' shade guides. *Operative Dentistry* 23(5):266–71.

Suggested Reading

Bloom DR, Padayachy JN. 2006. Aesthetic changes with four anterior units. *British Dental Journal* 10:542.

Dietschi D, Rossier S, Krejci I. 2005. In vitro colorimetric evaluation of the efficacy of various bleaching methods and products. *Quintessence International* 37:515–526.

Paravina R, Powers, John M. 2004. *Esthetic Color Training in Dentistry*, 1st ed. St. Louis, MO: Elsevier Mosby.

Summitt JB, Robbins JW, Hilton TJ, Schwartz RS. 2006. *Fundamental of Operative Dentistry: A Contemporary Approach*, 3rd ed. Chicago: Quintessence.

Touati B, Miara P, Nathanson D. 1999. *Esthetic Dentistry and Ceramic Restorations*. Singapore: Martin Duntz.

Chapter 8

Considerations for Treating the Moderately Difficult Esthetic Case

Ai B. Streacker DDS, BS

Marc Geissberger DDS, MA, BS, CPT

The increasing success of esthetic restoration of the anterior and posterior dentitions is largely due to advances in all-ceramic restorations and implant therapy. Beauty may be in the eye of the beholder, but if patients do not understand the physical limitations of their particular cases, failure may be imminent. Patient dissatisfaction with the outcome of esthetic care is largely due to poor communication and a poor understanding of the physical limitations of treatment (Samorodnitzky-Naveh, Geiger, and Levin 2007). Better communication regarding treatment outcomes requires a more thorough, sophisticated, and comprehensive examination incorporating photography, mounted diagnostic casts, diagnostic and esthetic wax-ups, and delivery of a smile design to the patient prior to embarking on esthetic restorative procedures. This will inform the patient by clearly demonstrating the possibilities of treatment outcome and make him or her a valued team member in care. This process will also help the practitioner decide if a multidisciplinary approach is needed to achieve the desired treatment results.

Anterior and Posterior Ceramic Restorations

Patients will present with a variety of esthetic concerns in the anterior and posterior areas of the mouth. The cases that will be classified as moderately difficult are those that do not require alteration of the vertical dimension of occlusion or correction of posterior arch collapse but that may involve removable prostheses with precision or semiprecision attachments. They may involve single tooth implants—especially in the esthetic zone—diastema closures, multiple single units, fixed partial dentures, and conventional removable partial dentures. Treatment must maintain or restore anterior guidance and proper occlusion. Preparation for a moderately difficult case requires the following:

1. A thorough assessment and discussion of the patient's esthetic goals (see chapter 4)
2. Preoperative photographs (see chapter 3)
3. Diagnostic study models mounted in a semiadjustable articulator using a face bow transfer with interocclusal records and a stick bite reference (see chapter 5)
4. A complete diagnostic wax-up (see chapter 6)
5. Tooth whitening (completed at least two weeks before treatment; Heymann 1997; Swift 1997)

Completion of these cases requires the following:

1. Postoperative photographs
2. An occlusal splint (night guard; see chapter 20)

Once the wax-up is complete, a silicone putty matrix can be formed over the waxed model of the proposed restorations. This matrix can then be used to demonstrate potential treatment outcomes to the patient. The silicone putty matrix is filled with bis-acrylic resin and placed in the patient's mouth. When the bis-acrylic resin has set, it is removed, leaving the proposed smile design in place over the patient's teeth. Chair-side modifications can be made by adding composite resin or removing bis-acrylic resin with a rotary instrument. The patient can wear it home to show their significant other, friends, or other family members, prior to committing to definitive treatment. The bis-acrylic material is not bonded to the teeth and peels off easily (Miller 2000).

In the posterior, hard tissue discrepancies, such as broken or missing teeth, can be addressed and occlusal modifications can be accomplished in wax. Silicone putty matrices can then be produced from this diagnostic wax-up and used to verify tooth reduction and to fabricate provisional restorations following the preparations (see chapters 5 and 16).

If a case involves a dental implant, the mounted casts can be a valuable adjunct in diagnosing the amount of available bone and placement angulations of the proposed implant fixture. The proposed prosthesis can be waxed up to reestablish the proper contours and function, followed by fabrication of a surgical template that will be used to guide the surgeon during implant placement.

Single-Unit Implants

For patients presenting with a single missing tooth, our first thought should be implant replacement, especially when the adjacent teeth are unrestored. A common situation with significant esthetic challenges is the patient with congenitally missing lateral incisors. In the past, orthodontic treatment was prescribed to close the space by moving the canines into the lateral incisor positions, often resulting in compromised esthetics and function. Today, due to the success of dental implant restorations, one should retain or create the needed space with orthodontic treatment prior to restoring with dental implants (Mayer et al. 2002; Romero et al. 2002; Naert et al. 2000; Schwartz-Arad, Hertsberg, and Levin 2005).

When treatment planning for a dental implant, careful planning of the extraction will make the esthetic and functional outcome more predictable. With the proper osseous volume, the surgeon can place the implant fixture in the optimal bucco-lingual, mesio-distal, and apico-coronal position, allowing for proper function and gingival esthetics.

The most appropriate position for the implant fixture is determined from a diagnostic wax-up, followed by fabrication of a surgical template. To ensure enough room for the transmucosal portion of the implant prosthesis, and to complete the transition from a round fixture to the morphology of the crown of the tooth it replaces, the fixture must be placed 3mm apical to the cemento-enamel junctions of the adjacent teeth. To ensure proper gingival stability and morphology, a buccal osseous crest thickness of 2mm should be maintained over the implant (Saadoun et al. 1994; Adell et al. 1990; Saadoun and LeGall 1992). If an osseous deficiency exists in a bucco-lingual or apico-coronal direction, an osseous augmentation or grafting procedure will be needed in order to achieve the necessary osseous volume prior to implant fixture placement.

Custom Provisional Prostheses (Phase I)

Producing and/or maintaining proper gingival morphology and emergence profile of the prosthesis are critical to the esthetic success of any anterior case. The transition from a round implant fixture to the prosthesis with the correct cervical shape and size must be accomplished. If a muccoperiosteal flap is made to place the fixture, an impression is made at this appointment for fabrication of a custom provisional prosthesis. The custom provisional prosthesis is fabricated to duplicate the form of the tooth/teeth it will replace, and to guide the healing and maturation of the gingival tissues (Touati 1997; Tauoti, Guez, and Saadoun 1999). This will help ensure that the proper morphology and emergence profile of the definitive prosthesis will be correct.

Delivery of Custom Provisional Prostheses (Phase II)

Exposure of the implant and abutment connection generally occurs three to six months following surgical placement. At this time the custom provisional prosthesis is placed. If routine surgical flap exposure is used, approximately two to six months of healing is necessary after implant exposure for the gingival tissues to reach full maturation. The definitive restoration can then be produced with predictable gingival results.

Restorative Phase (Phase III)

The final impression is made using a customized impression coping. The custom coping is fabricated from a silicone impression reproducing the transmucosal path occupied by the cervical contour of the custom provisional crown. This is done by removing the custom provisional crown and attaching it to an implant analog. The implant analog and custom provisional crown are inserted into silicone impression material as far as possible and should include the cervical portion of the provisional. When the silicone material has set, the provisional crown is removed from the analog and replaced with an impression coping. The cervical space around the impression coping is filled with an auto-polymerizing resin. After the resin has set, it is removed and contoured as needed. This procedure captures the transmucosal space produced by the custom provisional prosthesis. The assembly is now ready to be used to make the master impression for the definitive prosthesis.

The custom impression coping is attached to the fixture and exposed radiographically to confirm the accuracy of its placement. The definitive impression is made using an open tray technique (see chapter 15). The master cast produced from this impression accurately reproduces the cervical transmucosal space (Kois and Kan 2001).

With the aid of computer aided design/computer aided manufacture (CAD/CAM) technology, this custom transmucosal feature can be incorporated into a custom milled ceramic coping made of either alumina or zirconia. These achieve a more esthetic result due to their color and translucency. A traditional metal-ceramic technique can also be used to fabricate the custom coping, as discussed in the next section. The definitive restoration is constructed using all of the principals of esthetic dentistry discussed in previous chapters.

Immediate Custom Implant Provisionalization: A Prosthetic Technique

A healthy twenty-four-year-old female patient presented with multiple failing restorations throughout the maxillary and mandibular arches (figs. 8-1 and 8-2). The maxillary right and left lateral incisors had existing crowns with recurrent decay. Both teeth were structurally compromised with large oversized endodontic posts. A comprehensive examination was performed and treatment options were presented. Due to financial and time constraints, minimal treatment was requested. The treatment plan consisted of implant placement utilizing custom abutments for both maxillary lateral

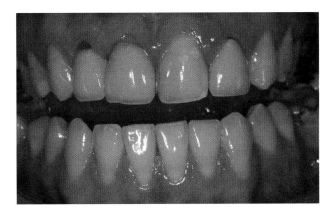

Figure 8-1. One-to-two view of twenty-four-year-old patient.

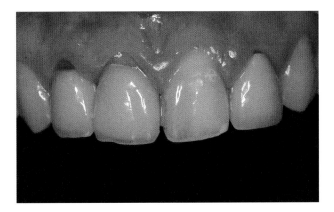

Figure 8-2. One-to-one view of twenty-four-year-old patient.

incisors, all-ceramic crowns for both maxillary central incisors, and whitening of all of the remaining anterior teeth. The patient also understood that additional treatment in the future would be necessary to restore her dentition to proper health.

To preserve bone during integration, platform switching (Kois and Kan 2001) was used with internal connection implants to shift the microgap medially from the periphery, in order to move the inflammatory cell layer from the fixture osseous interface to the fixture abutment interface. A diagnostic wax-up of both maxillary lateral incisors was created, and a putty matrix was used to facilitate chair-side fabrication of the customized abutments and restorations (see chapter 6). An esthetic provisional removable prosthesis was fabricated from the diagnostic wax-up in case immediate placement of the provisional was not possible due to implant instability.

Since necessary implant stability was not achieved at the time of surgery, the removable provisional restoration was adjusted and inserted so as to not traumatize the surgical site. A traditional six-month healing period allowed for osseointegration of the implants (Baumgarten et al. 2005; Anderson et al. 1995) Based on the expected definitive restorations' proportions and color, the removable provisional prosthesis was created from the diagnostic wax-up. Following six weeks of initial primary tissue healing of the surgical site, both maxillary central incisors were treated with minor laser gingival recontouring to establish a more esthetic soft tissue contour and zenith position, and restored with ceramic crowns. With the definitive restorations in place, a significant esthetic improvement was achieved during the remaining five-month healing period and allowed the patient to preview the projected esthetic outcome. After osseointegration and second-stage surgery was completed, the patient presented for the final implant restoration of the maxillary lateral incisors.

Clinical Technique

The patient presented with the second-stage healing screws in place (fig. 8-3). At this stage, the goal was to fabricate the customized provisional abutment and restoration. Once these were placed, the clinician could initiate fabrication of the definitive restorations. The purpose of the customized provisional abutment and restoration was to create the final tissue contours and emergence profile for the definitive restorations. Once they were created, an impression of the properly formed tissue contours was captured in the final impression, communicated to the dental laboratory, and reproduced in the all-ceramic restorations. Without the customized abutment, the final impression would simply capture

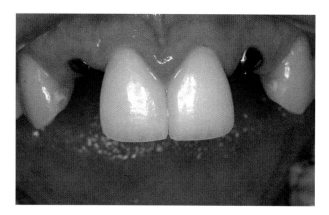

Figure 8-3. Healing screws in place in areas of maxillary right and left lateral incisors.

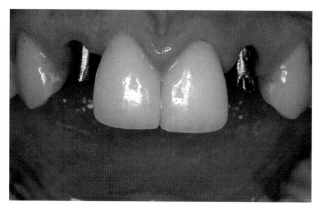

Figure 8-5. Provisional abutments prepared.

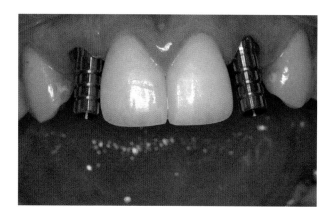

Figure 8-4. Provisional abutments in place.

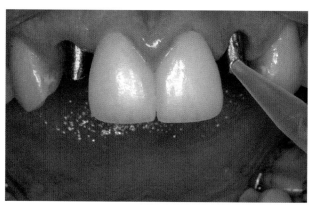

Figure 8-6. Block out material placement into provisional abutment screw channel.

the incorrect circular emergence profile of the surgical healing screws.

The healing screws were removed, and provisional abutments were placed to assess the alterations required to achieve appropriate tissue contour, support, and emergence profile (fig. 8-4). The provisional abutment was then prepared with a high-speed hand piece and significant water coolant to prevent any thermal transfer to the implants (fig. 8-5). Block-out material was placed in each of the screw access openings so the provisional material would not flow into them. Bisacrylic resin material was then injected around the prepared abutments (figs. 8-6 and 8-7). The putty matrix, fabricated from the diagnostic wax-up, was then filled with the bisacrylic resin material and seated intraorally (fig. 8-8). After initial curing of the resin material, the matrix was removed; the provisional abutment and restoration were removed to prepare for custom alteration and finishing (fig. 8-9).

The provisional restoration was contoured with flowable light-cured composite, which was placed around

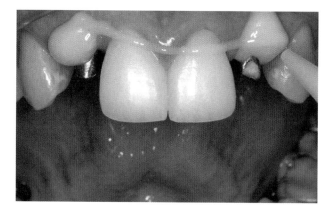

Figure 8-7. Placement of bisacrylic resin around prepared provisional abutments.

the abutment side of the provisional restorations (fig. 8-10). This process was repeated as each was contoured to create the proper emergence profile. Composite material was similarly added to the neck of each provisional abutment and contoured until the desired contours had

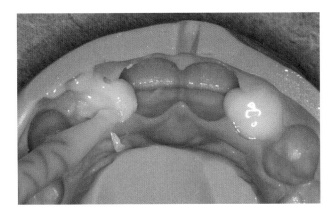

Figure 8-8. Bisacrylic resin placement into putty matrix, made from diagnostic wax-up.

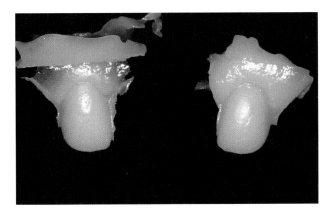

Figure 8-9. Provisional restoration removed prior to trimming and finishing.

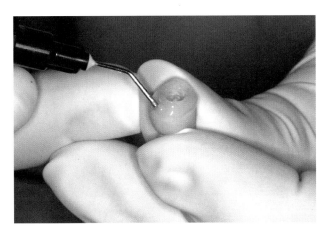

Figure 8-10. Placement of flowable light-cured composite resin around the abutment side of the provisional restorations.

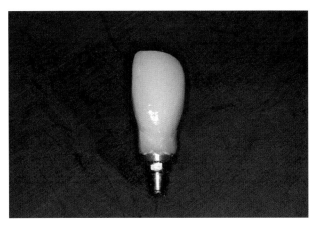

Figure 8-11. Completed custom provisional abutment with provisional crown.

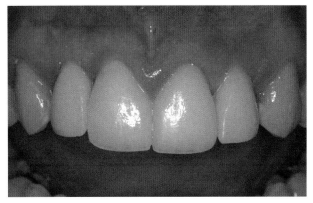

Figure 8-12. Custom provisional abutments and provisional crowns in place.

been achieved for the provisional abutment and restorations (fig. 8-11). The provisional abutment and restoration were subsequently tried in, and any final adjustments were made for tissue support and emergence profile.

The provisional abutment screw was placed and tightened to the proper torque, the provisional restorations were cemented, and the occlusion was adjusted (fig. 8-12).

The provisional restorations were allowed to remain in place for two weeks to provide time for the new tissue contours to stabilize. At the impression appointment, the provisional abutments and restorations were removed, and a conventional final impression was taken. The provisional abutments and provisional restorations were replaced as before, and the patient was reappointed for placement of the definitive restorations. A laboratory prescription was completed, and the definitive impression, occlusal registrations, facebow transfer, models with the provisional restorations in place, and photographs were forwarded to the laboratory. The laboratory technician was instructed to fabricate custom metal abutments and opaque them, as well as all-ceramic crowns (fig. 8-13).

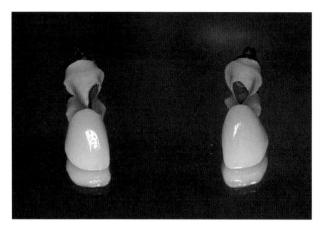

Figure 8-13. Laboratory-fabricated, custom porcelain-fused-to-metal abutments and all ceramic crown restorations, for the maxillary right and left lateral incisors.

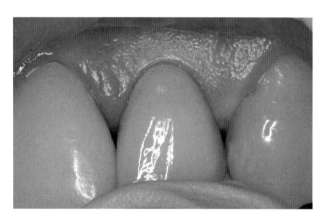

Figure 8-14. Try-in of ceramic crown on maxillary left lateral incisor.

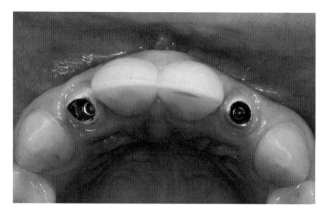

Figure 8-15. Incisal view of custom porcelain fused to metal abutments in place.

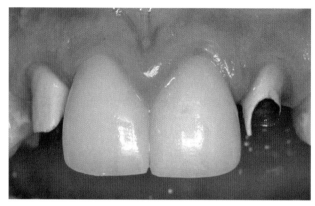

Figure 8-16. Facial view of custom porcelain-fused-to-metal abutments in place.

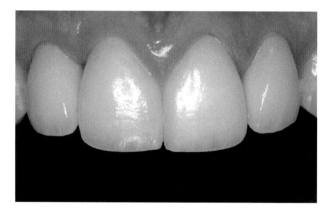

Figure 8-17. One-to-one view of maxillary right and left lateral incisor restorations in place.

At the delivery appointment, the provisional abutments and restorations were removed, and the customized implant abutments and crowns were tried in. Once the accuracy was verified, the definitive abutment screws were torqued to place. Polyvinyl block-out material was placed in the screw access openings, and the crowns were cemented with dual-cure composite cement (figs. 8-14, 8-15, 8-16, 8-17, 8-18, and 8-19).

While ceramic abutments can be used as the components for the definitive implant restorations, many of the abutments currently available do not allow for the custom subgingival contour of the ceramic. Similar to the surgical healing abutments, most prefabricated ceramic abuments produce a circular emergence profile rather than an anatomical one. In the authors' opinion, ceramic abutments may become compromised when extensive thinning of the ceramic is necessary, reducing the strength of the abutment. Further investigation may be necessary to establish ceramic abutment strength when extensive thinning of ceramic abutments is required, a relatively common occurrence with maxillary lateral and mandibular incisors. Alternately, custom-cast metal abutments maintain their strength following preparation and can be opaqued; a ceramic shoulder can be created to mimic the subgingival contour created by the provisional abutment. Ideally, the ceramic

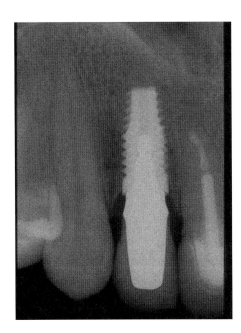

Figure 8-18. Radiograph of maxillary right lateral incisor, demonstrating platform switching.

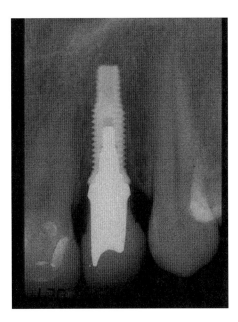

Figure 8-19. Radiograph of maxillary left lateral incisor, demonstrating platform switching.

shoulder should extend 0.5 mm subgingival to the free gingival margin.

Final Thoughts regarding Custom-Fabricated Implant Restorations

The utilization of a custom-fabricated provisional abutment and restoration following a six-month period of implant healing can aid in the preservation of hard and soft tissues. In many cases, the fabrication of an immediate, customized provisional abutment and restoration can be utilized to guide tissue contour and improve implant esthetics. This provisionalization technique can also be used in conjunction with immediate implant placement.

Porcelain Veneers

Patients will often present with the comment, "I want to improve my smile." Their condition may include one or more missing, fractured, misaligned, or discolored teeth in the esthetic zone. If a normal complement of minimally restored teeth is present with appropriate sizes and shapes, orthodontic treatment and whitening may be all that are required to satisfy the patient's esthetic concerns. If the teeth are heavily restored or the patient exhibits signs or symptoms of parafunctional habits, such as clenching or bruxing, full-coverage restorations should be considered to accomplish their esthetic desires. Missing teeth can be replaced with implants or fixed partial dentures.

The diagnostic wax-up is the key in determining if preprosthetic treatment, such as orthodontics, gingival recontouring, or crown lengthening will be necessary prior to restorative treatment. If it is determined that the golden proportions can be closely achieved and the patient's expectations met, a putty matrix can then be constructed. This matrix will be used to fabricate a chairside smile design for the patient, allowing the patient to visualize the proposed treatment outcome with greater clarity, before embarking upon the restorative phase of care. Figure 8-20 shows a simulated smile design for the restoration of four maxillary incisors.

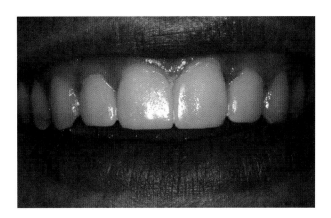

Figure 8-20. Simulated smile design in place, produced from diagnostic wax-up.

Diastema Closure

The patient in figure 8-21 presented having just completed orthodontic care. Diastemata were strategically positioned between the four maxillary incisors to allow correction of tooth width and arch size discrepancies using porcelain veneers. Since the lingual surfaces were not to be treated, existing anterior guidance was maintained, and the diagnostic wax-up was completed on a semiadjustable articulator (figs. 8-22 and 8-23).

If guidance were to be altered, the new guidance would be established in the diagnostic wax-up. Restoring canine guidance, when possible, is ideal because it elicits 30–40% lower muscle activity than group function (Manns, Chan, and Miralles 1987).

A duplicate cast can be made of the diagnostic wax-up and mounted on a semiadjustable articulator. The duplicate cast will allow for the fabrication of a custom incisal table and prevent damage to the fragile diagnostic wax-up. This custom incisal table can be sent to the prosthetic laboratory to be used to create the desired functional path and lingual surfaces of the definitive restorations.

Preparations

At the preparation appointment, a smile design, based on a fully contoured diagnostic wax-up, is placed and utilized as an aid during tooth reduction (fig. 8-24). Guide cuts are made through the bisacrylic resin into the enamel of the teeth to establish the proper amount of tooth reduction (fig. 8-25). This technique takes much of the guesswork out of preparation design and allows the practitioner to be as conservative as possible. Enough tooth structure is removed to allow sufficient room for proper shape and contour of the definitive restoration. Depending on the type of porcelain to be used, a porcelain thickness of 0.3 to 0.8 mm may be necessary (Malament and Socransky 1999; Touati and Nathanson 1999; Bloom and Padayachy 2006). Excessive removal of

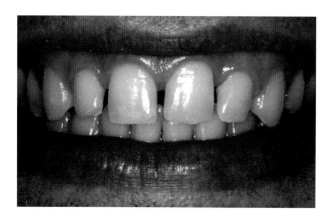

Figure 8-21. One-to-two view of patient, preoperative, postorthodontic treatment, demonstrating diastemata.

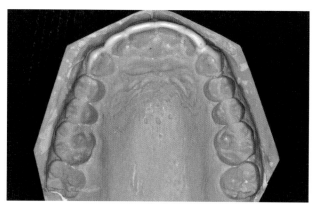

Figure 8-23. Incisal view of diagnostic wax-up on diagnostic casts demonstrating preservation of existing anterior guidance.

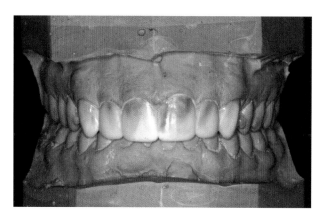

Figure 8-22. Facial view of diagnostic wax-up on diagnostic casts.

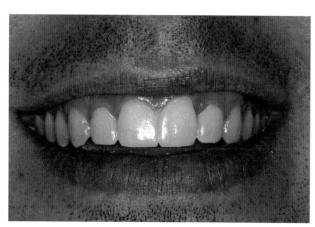

Figure 8-24. Smile design in place at preparation appointment.

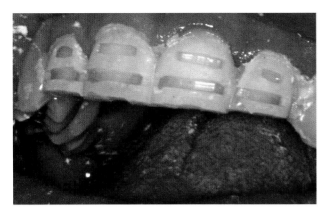

Figure 8-25. Reduction guide cuts placed through the bisacrylic smile design to maximize conservation of tooth structure.

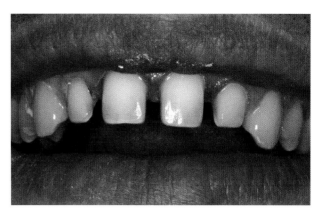

Figure 8-27. Facial view of completed veneer preparations demonstrating interproximal margin placement for closure of diastemata.

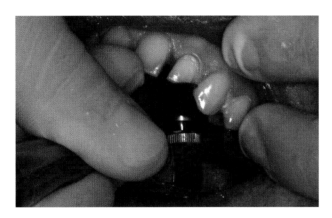

Figure 8-26. Refinement of veneer preparations for the four maxillary incisor teeth.

tooth structure can lead to pulpal trauma and a weaker bond of the veneer to the tooth (fig. 8-26; Nikaido et al. 2002; Sorensen and Munksgaard 1996; Magne 2000).

The preparations should maintain two facial planes and establish a definitive chamfer margin. Because diastema closure is one of the restorative goals, the chamfer margin is established at or slightly below the free gingival margin in the areas where space will be closed. This will allow the laboratory technician to create appropriate emergence profiles in the proximal areas. The mesial and distal proximal margins must extend through the proposed contact area and terminate at the mesiolingual and distolingual line angles. Failure to do this may lead to improper interproximal morphology and improper gingival embrasure form, and may create interdental dark triangles. The incisal edge is reduced 1.5 mm to allow for the incorporation of translucent porcelain. A butt joint margin is placed on the lingual of the incisal edge at approximately 45 degrees to the facial incisal plane of reduction. When diastema closure is not a

concern, gingival margin placement is kept juxtagingival or slightly supragingival to allow for ease of hygiene and increased gingival esthetics (fig. 8-27).

Impressions

Impressions can be taken with either a reversible hydrocolloid, polyvinyl siloxane or a polyether material. As always, care must be taken to minimize trauma to the gingiva; conservative margin placement should allow accurate impressions to be made without tearing the epithelial attachment; this helps ensure that there will be no changes in the gingival contour between the preparation and cementation appointments.

Shade Selection

Translucent restorations require that an extra piece of information be relayed to the dental technician. In addition to the choice of a shade or shades closest to the desired outcome and comments describing variations of surface characterization, the technician needs to know the color of the prepared tooth (dentin shade). This can be compared with shade tabs on a designated "stump shade" guide or simply compared with other tabs on a standard shade guide.

Provisional Restorations

Provisional restorations for veneer preparations are made in much the same way that the smile design is made. Unlike provisionals for full-coverage restorations, veneer provisionals are made in a single unit whenever possible to enhance overall retention. Precise fit at the gingival margins is crucial to minimizing gingival inflammation and the potential for recession.

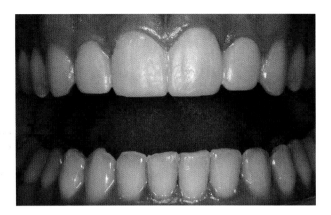

Figure 8-28. Provisional veneers for the four maxillary incisor teeth in place.

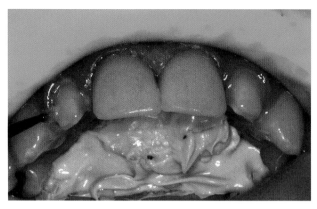

Figure 8-29. Slot dam in place demonstrating the use of interocclusal registration material to form the lingual seal.

When retention is good, provisionals may be cemented with clear or translucent eugenol-free provisional cement. For conservative preparations, it may be necessary to bond the provisionals to the teeth with a dental adhesive (fig. 8-28). An area of approximately 1.5 mm by 1.5 mm in the center of the preparation is etched with 37% phosphoric acid for approximately 10 seconds, then rinsed and dried. Adhesive is painted on the inner surface of the provisional veneers. The restoration is then put into place and light cured for 40 seconds. When removed, the provisional will most likely be destroyed, and any remaining bonding resin must be removed with a rotary instrument prior to trying in the definitive restorations. In patients with limited sensitivity, the provisional restoration may be constructed to be removable, allowing the patient the ability to remove the provisional for optimal hygiene and gingival health. The patient needs to maintain proper oral hygiene to ensure a stable gingival architecture and blood-free environment for the delivery appointment.

Restoration Placement

Try In

The first step in veneer placement is verifying fit and esthetics. These two steps are carried out without the use of a rubber dam. Fit checker or a silicone wash impression material is placed on the intaglio surface of each veneer, one at a time. The intaglio surface is moistened with water while the preparation is dried. The veneer is seated completely and the silicone material is allowed to set. When the veneer is removed, the set silicone material should remain on the dried preparation, identifying any high spots as an area of show through. These high spots are removed from the preparation only; adjusting the intaglio surface of the porcelain veneer may result in microcrack formation and the ultimate failure of the veneer (Griffith 1924; Munz and Fett 1999) After the

internal fit is verified, the marginal adaptation is checked and verified with an explorer. Then the interproximal contacts are checked and adjusted as needed using fine diamond instruments or abrasive polishing instruments. When all of the veneers fit accurately, all are placed with an appropriate shade of try-in paste, for color verification and patient approval. At this time, minor alterations in the porcelain can be made to effect subtle contour changes. After the patient approves, the resin bonding process can begin.

Bonding Procedure

The bonding process requires proper rubber dam isolation, as moisture contamination, even from the patient's breath, can reduce the bond strength. A slot-dam technique is used, which allows all of the teeth in the operative site to be isolated without rubber dam material being present between each tooth. When possible, rubber dam clamps are placed two teeth distal to the last prepared tooth. A hole is punched for each of these two teeth, and a slit in the form of the arch is made connecting the two holes. The dam is then placed and the lingual flap of rubber dam material is sealed with a silicone interocclusal record material (fig. 8-29). The intaglio surface of the veneers are washed with 37% phosphoric acid for 10 seconds, rinsed and dried. A silane-coupling agent is applied to the etched surface and allowed to sit for 60 seconds, after which it is air dried. The prepared tooth surface is etched with 37% phosphoric acid for the amount of time recommended by the manufacturer, rinsed, and air dried. For most contemporary bonding agents, the surface of the teeth should remain moist and not be desiccated. Adhesive is applied to the etched tooth surface and the intaglio surface of the veneers. The veneers are coated with cement of the chosen shade and seated fully on to the preparation. Light curing the cement for about 3 to 5 seconds will tack the veneer in

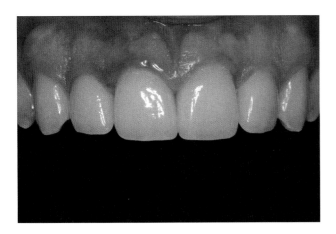

Figure 8-30. Maxillary porcelain veneers bonded in place on the four maxillary incisor teeth.

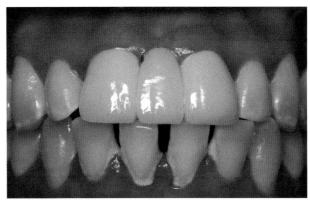

Figure 8-32. One-to-two view of maxillary and mandibular incisor regions.

place while allowing for the removal of excess with an explorer and dental floss. The cement is then light cured for the amount of time recommended by the manufacturer. The above sequence is repeated for each veneer. After all have been placed, the occlusion is verified, ensuring that the distal incisal edges of the lateral incisors are free of contact in lateral and laterotrussive movements. This is a common area of ceramic failure. Any remaining excess cement can be removed with fine diamond rotary instruments and polished with porcelain polishing instruments and compounds (fig. 8-30).

The next appointment will be for the fabrication of a maxillary night guard appliance, to protect the new restorations from any parafunctional activity.

Smile Correction Using Orthodontics, All-Porcelain Crowns, and Veneers

The next patient presented with a chief complaint of an unnatural looking bridge (fig. 8-31). The patient's history

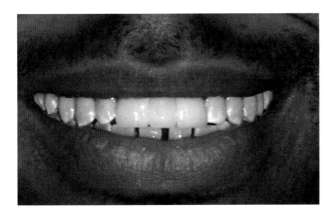

Figure 8-31. Preoperative view of unnatural-looking maxillary anterior bridge.

revealed that he had gone to a dentist to have a large diastema closed. At that time, the two central incisors were prepared as abutments for a 3-unit fixed partial denture to close a large midline diastema, with the obvious unaesthetic outcome (fig. 8-32). The patient presented with a photograph of himself that revealed his smile before any dental treatment had been performed. Records and diagnostic aids were obtained. They included facebow transfer, interocclusal records, stick bite, and preoperative photographs. Additionally, casts were mounted on a semiadjustable articulator. A diagnostic wax-up was done to recreate the patient's original diastemata to facilitate the treatment planning and diagnosis process.

The course of treatment was explained to the patient in great detail. The treatment would consist of removing the unaesthetic fixed partial denture, fabricating provisional crowns to recreate the original diastemata, and orthodontic tooth movement to close the space using either conventional wires and brackets or the Invisalign system. Invisalign (Align Technology, Inc., Santa Clara, CA) is a system of clear invisible aligners that can help position the teeth to prepare for restorative or cosmetic procedures. With Invisalign, patients wear clear removable aligners at all times, for a total of about 20–22 hours per day, removing them only for eating, drinking, and performing oral hygiene. Patients wear each aligner for a period of approximately two weeks, and then move on to the next aligner until treatment is complete (Bollen et al. 2004).

Many adult patients will choose the Invisalign system for obvious esthetic reasons, as did this patient (Meier, Wiemer, and Meithke 2003; Nedwed and Miethke 2005). Upon completion of orthodontic treatment, teeth whitening was proposed in conjunction with the restoration of the maxillary central incisors with all-ceramic crowns and the maxillary lateral incisors with porcelain veneers.

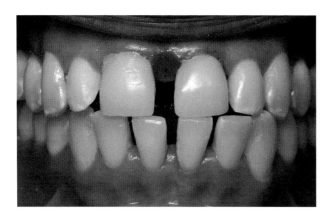

Figure 8-33. Anterior bridge removed and bisacrylic provisional crowns bonded on the maxillary central incisor teeth, restoring the pre-existing diastema.

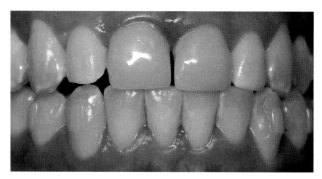

Figure 8-34. Maxillary and mandibular teeth post-Invisalign treatment.

First Restorative Appointment

At the first restorative appointment, the fixed bridge was removed and two bisacrylic resin provisional restorations, produced from the diagnostic cast, were bonded to place (fig. 8-33). Then elastomeric impressions and centric jaw relation record were made and sent to Align Technology, Inc. The Panorex and digital photos of the patient were submitted online through Invisalign's case management Web site.

In approximately three weeks, a three-dimensional computerized graphic analysis called ClinCheck was available on the Web site that depicts the expected movements of each aligner. Both dentist and patient can use this tool to visualize the sequencing of movement and preview the total number of aligners that are required for treatment, adjusting the predictions according to their specific clinical goals. Each aligner is designed to move the teeth between 0.125 and 0.25 mm per tray (Vlaskic and Boyd 2002). In this case, it was determined that the entire course of orthodontic treatment would require 15 aligners.

This patient was seen every six weeks to monitor the orthodontic treatment. At each visit, the patient was dispensed the next sequence of three aligners; the total orthodontic treatment time was approximately seven months.

Postorthodontic Treatment

Following Invisalign treatment, new records were taken, including new photographs and mounted study models. The teeth were then whitened using an in-office procedure supplemented with a take-home product for a period of two weeks (fig. 8-34).

A new diagnostic wax-up was created, factoring in the height-to-width ratios and the golden proportion. A

matrix was created for fabrication of the new provisional restorations for all four maxillary incisors.

Second Restorative Appointment

The provisional crowns were removed from both maxillary central incisors, and these were prepared to receive bonded all-ceramic crowns. The lateral incisors were prepared to receive feldspathic porcelain-bonded veneers, requiring only 0.3 mm of total reduction. Provisional restorations were then fabricated using a bisacrylic resin and delivered to the patient. The patient was allowed to wear and use the provisional restorations to verify function and proposed esthetic outcome. Once the restorations were approved, an alginate impression was made and study model produced for the laboratory to use as a guide during fabrication of the definitive restorations. The definitive impression and interocclusal records custom incisal guide table are made, and the case was sent to the dental laboratory for fabrication.

Case Delivery

Upon their return from the laboratory, the restorations were tried in, and after approval by the dentist and patient, were placed with a resin luting medium. In this case, the patient was made a clear Essix retainer, post-orthodontics; it also serves as an occlusal guard. The patient was instructed in the proper care of esthetic restorations (figs. 8-35, 8-31, and 8-36).

The Buccal Corridor

An inexperienced practitioner will often overlook subtleties about esthetic cases that may be clearly revealed by the diagnostic wax-up and smile design. One very important subtlety is the buccal corridor, the space occupied by the buccal soft tissues and teeth distal to the

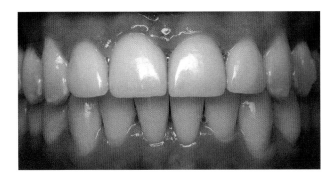

Figure 8-35. Completed case.

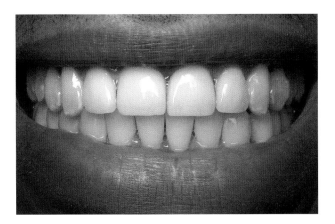

Figure 8-36. Postoperative view of patient.

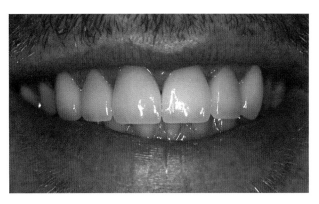

Figure 8-37. One-to-two view of the treated maxillary anterior teeth.

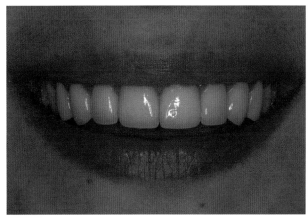

Figure 8-38. One-to-one view of patient in which the maxillary first and second premolars as well as the six anterior teeth were restored to maintain the buccal corridor.

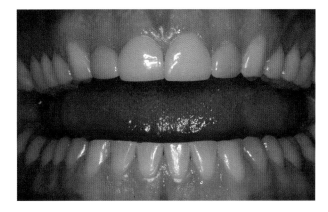

Figure 8-39. Preoperative view of patient requiring restoration of anterior guidance as well as cosmetic restoration.

canines. Patients will often refer to their smile in terms of the six anterior teeth, without any thought to the areas distal to the canines.

The next case is an example where only the six anterior teeth were treated (fig. 8-37). Notice how the buccal corridor seems constricted, and the six anterior teeth seem to jump out. The reason for this unaesthetic effect is that too few teeth were considered in the overall smile design. When one considers altering a patient's smile, one must consider restoring teeth in groups, as indicated by the diagnostic wax-up and smile design. The practitioner wishing to maintain, restore, or enhance the buccal corridor will usually need to restore at least eight or more teeth. There are very few smiles in which six anterior restorations are adequate to solve buccal corridor issues. Figure 8-38 shows a case in which premolars were restored to prevent such buccal corridor issues.

Restoring the Smile and Anterior Guidance

The patient in figure 8-39 presented with a chief complaint of dissatisfaction with his smile. Four com-

posite resin veneers were present from the maxillary right to the maxillary left lateral incisors, placed to close diastemata after orthodontic treatment. They were poorly proportioned and unaesthetic; the buccal

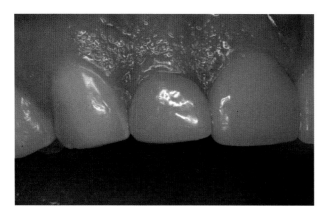

Figure 8-40. Preoperative view showing gingival zenith discrepancies of the maxillary right lateral and central incisors.

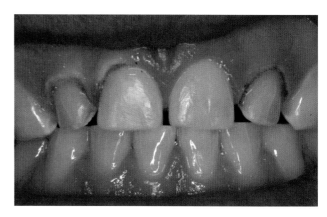

Figure 8-42. Immediate postoperative view of the maxillary right lateral, central, and left lateral incisors after gingival zenith correction with a diode laser.

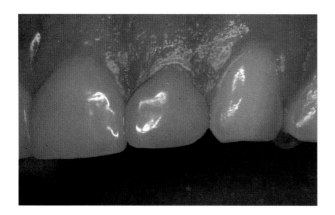

Figure 8-41. Preoperative view showing gingival zenith discrepancy of the maxillary left lateral incisor.

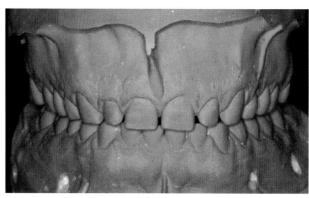

Figure 8-43. New diagnostic casts, post–gingival zenith correction mounted on semiadjustable articulator, prior to diagnostic wax-up.

corridor appeared collapsed. Anterior attrition and posterior wear facets were present due to lack of proper anterior guidance. A protrusive and lateral slide was present from centric relation to maximum intercuspation. Additionally, gingival zenith discrepancies were noted above both maxillary lateral and right central incisors (figs. 8-40 and 8-41). To design this case properly, complete preoperative records were taken and diagnostic casts were mounted on a semiadjustable articulator.

First Restorative Appointment

Interferences from centric relation to maximum intercuspation were identified and removed clinically. An occlusal equilibration was performed to eliminate the slide and stabilize the occlusal forces, creating simultaneous bilateral contacts on all posterior teeth in maximum intercuspation. The existing four veneers

were removed, and gingival recontouring was accomplished with a diode laser (fig. 8-42).

Diagnostic Wax-up and Smile Design

New impressions were made for new diagnostic casts upon which the case was designed and waxed up. A custom incisal guide table was fabricated to guide the prosthetic laboratory in developing the proper lingual contours for anterior guidance (figs. 8-43 and 8-44).

The diagnostic study casts revealed that additional gingival contouring would be necessary for all four mandibular incisor teeth in order to create more ideal proportions. It was determined that a total of sixteen porcelain-bonded veneers would be necessary to correct the patient's esthetic concerns and correct the anterior guidance (figs. 8-45 and 8-46).

Silicone putty matrices were made from the diagnostic wax-up and used to create the simulated smile design

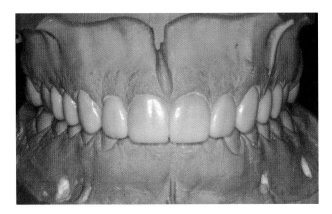

Figure 8-44. Diagnostic wax-up of maxillary anterior teeth. Notice that the maxillary first and second premolars have been included to restore the buccal corridor.

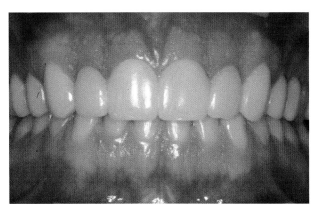

Figure 8-47. Simulated smile design delivered to the patient. Smile design is delivered via a putty matrix that is made from the diagnostic wax-up.

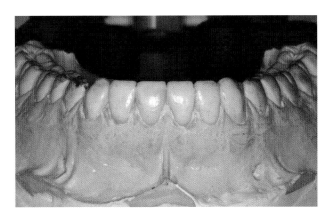

Figure 8-45. Diagnostic wax-up of the six mandibular anterior teeth.

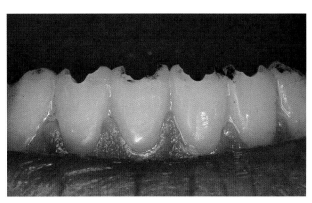

Figure 8-48. Simulated smile design in place and used as a guide for proper incisal reduction for the six mandibular anterior teeth.

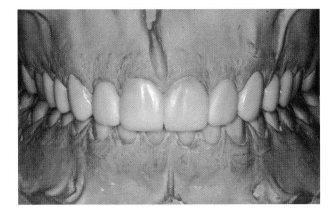

Figure 8-46. Completed diagnostic wax-up of the case restoring the patient's esthetic concerns as well as the anterior guidance.

(fig. 8-47). The amount of information this one procedure conveys to the patient is tremendous. The patient now clearly understands what he can expect from the treatment and precisely what is necessary to achieve it.

At this point, modifications can be made to the smile design, satisfying any esthetic concerns that the patient may have. The patient can wear it home to gain the approval of family and friends before committing to definitive treatment. Impressions are taken as additional study models are made to aid the prosthetic laboratory during fabrication of the definitive restorations.

Second Restorative Appointment

The smile design was left in place and used as a template for the veneer preparations. This allows for very predictable and precise preparations, minimizing loss of tooth structure (figs. 8-48, 8-49, 8-50, and 8-51). The preparations margins were kept slightly supragingival (fig. 8-52). Impressions were taken and provisional restorations constructed and delivered in the manner discussed earlier in this chapter. The stump shade and restoration shades were selected, in this case using the

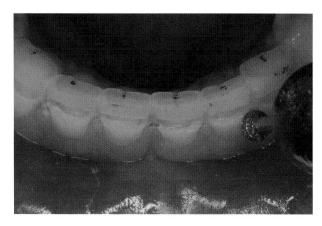

Figure 8-49. Simulated smile design in place demonstrating its use to determine proper facial reduction for the six mandibular anterior teeth.

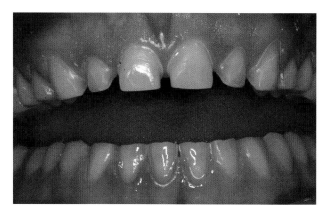

Figure 8-52. Supragingival margin placement of the maxillary and mandibular preparations.

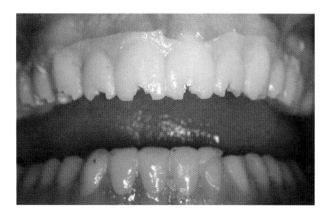

Figure 8-50. Simulated smile design in place demonstrating its use as a reduction guide for the incisal reduction for the maxillary teeth.

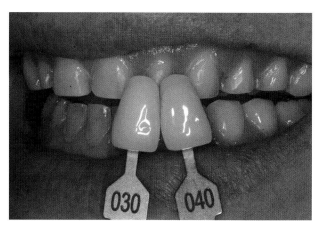

Figure 8-53. Shade selection for the maxillary lateral incisors.

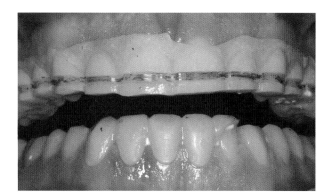

Figure 8-51. Simulated smile design in place demonstrating its use as a reduction guide for the facial reduction for the maxillary teeth.

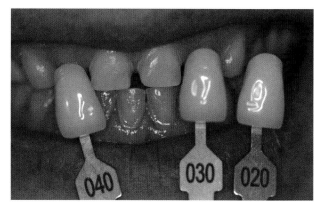

Figure 8-54. Shade selection for the maxillary central incisors.

Vita 3D master shade selection (figs. 8-53, 8-54, and 8-55).

The impressions were sent to the prosthetic laboratory with a detailed laboratory prescription describing exactly what types of incisal effect and surface texture were desired for the final restorations. A custom incisal guide table was created from the duplicate cast of the diagnostic wax-up.

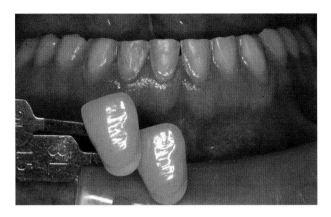

Figure 8-55. Shade selection for the mandibular anterior teeth.

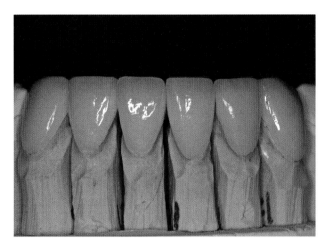

Figure 8-56. Mandibular veneers demonstrating excess bulk of porcelain at the mid facial and line angle areas.

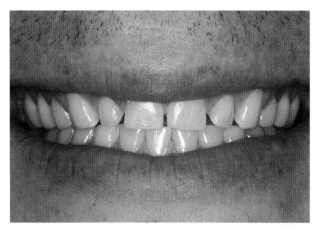

Figure 8-57. Preoperative view of the patient after removal of old direct resin veneers.

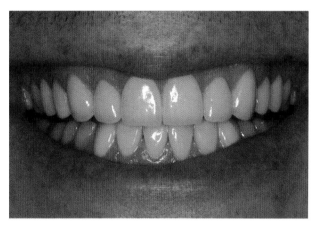

Figure 8-58. Postoperative view of the patient; note improved esthetics and restoration of incisal guidance.

First Delivery Appointment

When the case returned from the laboratory, the veneers were examined for accuracy of fit and esthetics. Upon evaluation, it was determined that the mandibular veneers were too bulky on the mid-facial aspect and the line angles too prominent at the interdental papillae (fig. 8-56). The laboratory was instructed to reduce the mid facial aspect to a thickness of 0.6 mm and to reduce and round the line angles, making them less prominent.

Second Delivery Appointment

After the laboratory corrected the shortcomings, the patient was reappointed for delivery of the restorations. After approval by the patient, the veneers were bonded to place with a light-cured bonding resin (figs. 8-57 and 8-58). Impressions and records were taken to construct a maxillary night guard appliance, and the patient was instructed on the proper care of esthetic restorations.

Cases Involving Fixed and Removable Partial Dentures

The next patient presented with the chief complaints of pain, inability to chew adequately, and the desire to look better. Clinical examination revealed ill-fitting removable partial dentures. The maxillary right first and second premolars and the maxillary right and left canines had failing restorations. The maxillary right central incisor with cantilevered maxillary right lateral incisor was periodontally unsound and deemed unrestorable. The maxillary left first premolar possessed a vertical root fracture, and the mandibular left second premolar was periodontally unsound and unrestorable. The mandibular left second molar was within normal limits. The mandibular left canine, left lateral incisor, right central incisor, and lateral incisor exhibited excessive tooth structure loss

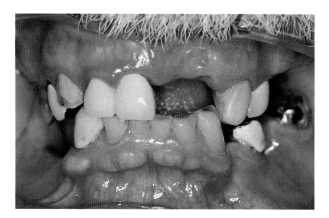

Figure 8-59. Preoperative view of patient requiring reconstruction of fixed and removable partial dentures.

due to attrition. The mandibular right canine had a failing restoration (fig. 8-59).

To design this case properly, complete preoperative records were taken and diagnostic casts were mounted on a semiadjustable articulator. It was determined that the existing vertical dimension of occlusion was within normal limits and did not require modification. The smile analysis demonstrated that an excellent esthetic result was attainable by using a maxillary removable partial denture with semiprecision attachments, and a conventional mandibular partial denture, to restore the edentulous areas.

Treatment Plan

The treatment plan consisted of the following:

Phase 1
1. Prophylaxis and oral hygiene instruction.
2. Extract of all unrestorable teeth: the maxillary right central incisor with its cantilevered lateral incisor, the maxillary left first premolar, and the mandibular left second premolar.
3. Maxillary and mandibular stay plates.

Phase 2
1. Porcelain fused to metal crowns for the remaining teeth, including semiprecision attachments on the distal of the maxillary right second premolar and maxillary left canine teeth. The full gold crown on the mandibular second molar is within normal limits and will remain unchanged.
2. Maxillary semiprecision removable partial denture to replace the missing maxillary teeth.
3. Conventional mandibular removable partial denture to replace the missing mandibular teeth.

First Restorative Appointment

At the first restorative appointment definitive impressions, interocclusal records, face bow transfer, and tooth shade selection (based on the patient's desire) were obtained. These diagnostic aides were obtained for the fabrication of maxillary and mandibular stay plate appliances and custom impression trays for the maxillary and mandibular removable partial dentures. The casts were mounted on a semiadjustable articulator and the teeth to be extracted were removed from the casts. The case was delivered to the prosthetic laboratory for stay plate fabrication. The denture teeth were set on the casts in their most favorable esthetic position while optimizing function and maintaining the existing vertical dimension of occlusion. The stay plates were used to maintain vertical dimension and gauge reduction during the preparation of the remaining teeth.

Second Restorative Appointment

At the second restorative appointment the maxillary right central with lateral incisor pontic, maxillary left first, and mandibular left second premolars were extracted. Additionally, the maxillary and mandibular stay plates were delivered to the patient. The stay plates served to maintain the vertical dimension of occlusion while facilitating healing. They also allowed the patient to adequately function while maintaining his social self-esteem during the healing process.

Third Restorative Appointment

At the third restorative appointment the teeth on the maxillary arch were prepared to receive porcelain-fused-to-metal (PFM) crowns. The abutment teeth for the semiprecision attachments required standard PFM crown preparations, as the attachments that were selected are extracoronal in design (figs. 8-60 and 8-61). A definitive impression of the maxillary arch was made after the preparations were completed. Custom provisional crowns were constructed using a silicone putty matrix, contoured to fit the interim stay plate appliances, and cemented with a provisional cement.

Fourth Restorative Appointment

At the fourth restorative appointment the mandibular teeth, with the exception of the mandibular left second molar, were prepared to receive PFM crowns. Additional reduction was necessary on the lingual surface of the mandibular canine preparations to accommodate the removable partial denture's indirect retainers (fig. 8-62). The definitive impression, interocclusal records, facebow

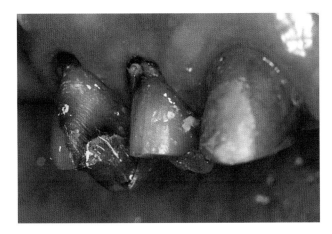

Figure 8-60. Porcelain-fused-to-metal (PFM) preparations for the maxillary right canine and first and second premolars.

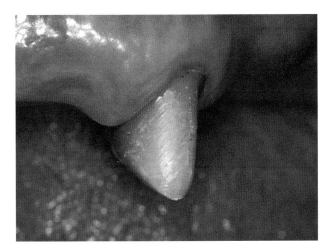

Figure 8-61. PFM preparation for the maxillary left canine.

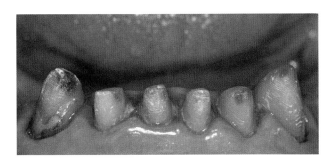

Figure 8-62. PFM preparations for the mandibular anterior teeth.

transfer, shade, and tooth selection were then obtained. The casts were mounted on a semiadjustable articulator and delivered to the prosthetic laboratory for fabrication of the PFM crowns.

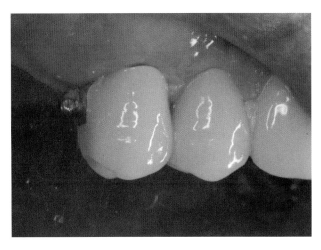

Figure 8-63. PFM restorations, postcementation, for the maxillary right canine and first and second premolars. Note the semiprecision attachment on the distal of the maxillary second premolar crown.

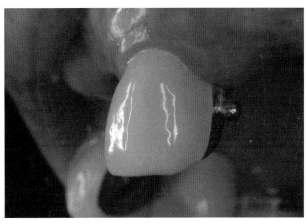

Figure 8-64. PFM restoration, postcementation, for the maxillary left canine.

Fifth Restorative Appointment

At the fifth restorative appointment the PFM crowns were delivered. Resin-modified glass ionomer cement was used to cement the PFM restorations (figs. 8-63, 8-64, and 8-65). The photographs displayed here were taken at the one-year recall appointment. It is important to note the build-up of plaque around the semiprecision attachments on the distal surfaces of the maxillary abutment teeth. For long-term success of this esthetic rehabilitation, it is imperative the patient understands that the proximal surfaces of teeth adjacent to removable partial dentures are often neglected during their regular oral hygiene regimen, and as a result may lead to a catastrophic failure of the reconstruction. Therefore, thorough oral hygiene instruction must be given at the time of prosthetic delivery and reinforced at each recall appointment.

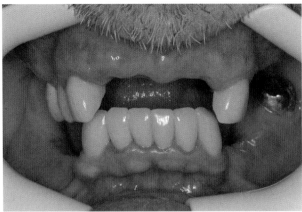

Figure 8-65. PFM restorations, postcementation, for the mandibular anterior teeth.

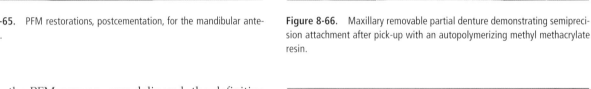

Figure 8-66. Maxillary removable partial denture demonstrating semiprecision attachment after pick-up with an autopolymerizing methyl methacrylate resin.

After the PFM crowns were delivered, the definitive impressions were made for the semiprecision maxillary and conventional mandibular removable partial denture appliances, using the custom impression trays that were previously constructed. The teeth and shade previously selected for the PFM crowns were used for the denture teeth on both removable partial dentures.

Sixth Restorative Appointment

At the sixth restorative appointment the removable partial denture frameworks with the denture teeth set in wax were tried in to verify accuracy of fit of the partial denture castings. Since the female portions of the attachments are not incorporated in the maxillary removable partial denture at this stage, denture adhesive was used to stabilize the maxillary removable partial denture to verify the esthetic arrangement and phonetics of the new prosthesis. The mandibular removable partial denture should exhibit good retention as it uses conventional reciprocal Akers clasps. After patient and doctor approval, the prostheses were returned to the prosthetic laboratory for final processing.

Seventh Restorative Appointment

At the seventh restorative appointment the removable partial dentures were tried in to verify fit function and esthetics. The maxillary semiprecision removable partial denture provides greatly improved esthetics by showing no metal clasps in this patient's full smile. The male portion of the attachment is located on the crown; the female portion is located on the anterior portion of the denture base and is usually constructed of an easily replaceable polyvinyl material. The female portions of

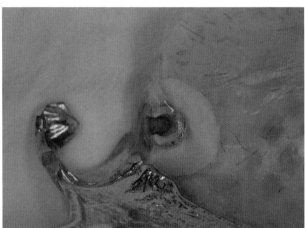

Figure 8-67. Maxillary removable partial denture, demonstrating the semiprecision attachment in the position of the maxillary right second premolar, after trimming and polishing.

the attachments were placed on the male portions, located on the distal of the abutment crowns. Cold cure acrylic was then placed into the female keeper depressions on the anterior portion of the denture base and the partial was fully seated intraorally, held in place until the acrylic fully set, then removed. The excess acrylic was trimmed using rotary acrylic burs and polished with acrylic polishing points (figs. 8-66, 8-67, and 8-68). The mandibular and maxillary removable partials were then inserted and occlusion verified (fig. 8-69).

Conclusion

The preceding case illustrates what can be accomplished when treatment plans are well thought out and devel-

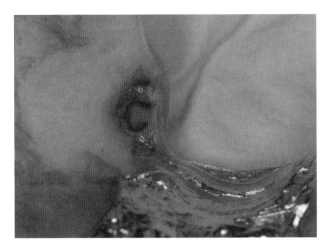

Figure 8-68. Maxillary removable partial denture, demonstrating the semi-precision attachment in the position of the maxillary left canine, after trimming and polishing.

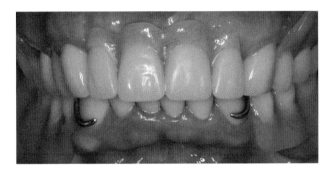

Figure 8-69. Postoperative view of the completed reconstruction with all prostheses in place.

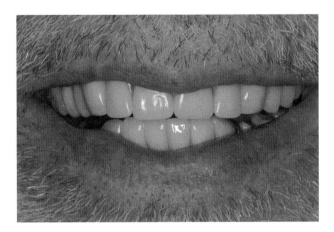

Figure 8-70. Two-to-one view of the completed case. Note that none of the mandibular removable partial denture clasps are visible.

oped. The use of sound esthetic and restorative concepts coupled with solid case design will provide the patient with lasting, esthetically pleasing results. The use of a smile analysis and design led to the choice of a tradi-

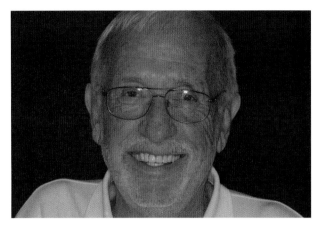

Figure 8-71. Full facial view of the patient, postoperatively.

tional removable partial denture for this patient. During full smile this patient does not display any portion of the mandibular partial denture (figs. 8-70 and 8-71).

Acknowledgements

The authors wish to thank the following individuals for help in providing clinical cases highlighted throughout this chapter:

Gerard Lemongello Jr. DMD, Palm Beach Gardens, Florida. "Immediate Custom Implant Provisionalization: A Prosthetic Technique."

Steven Glassman DDS, New York City, New York. "Smile Correction Using Orthodontics, All Porcelain Crowns and Veneers."

Works Cited

Adell R, Eriksson B, Lekholm U, Branemark P-I, Jent T. 1990. Long term follow up study of osseointegrated implants in the treatment of totally edentulous jaws. *J Oral Maxillofac Implants* 5:347–59.

Anderson B, Odman P, Lindvall AM, Lithmer B. 1995. Single tooth restorations supported by osseointegrated implants: Results and experiences from a prospective study after 2 to 3 years. *Int J Oral Maxillofac Impl* 10(6):702–11.

Baumgarten H, Cocchetto R, Testori T, et al. 2005. A new implant design for crestal bone preservation: Initial observations and case report. *Pract Proced Aesthet Dent* 17(10):735–40.

Bloom DR, Padayachy JN. 2006. Aesthetic changes with four anterior units. *Br Dent J* 200(10):542.

Bollen AM, Huang G, King G, Hujoel P, Ma T. 2004. Activation time and material stiffness of sequential removable orthodontic appliances: Part 1. *Am J Orthod Dentofacial Orthop* 125(3):19A.

Griffith AA. 1924. The phenomenon of rupture and flaw in solids. *Philos Trans R Soc* 221:163–89.

Heymann H. 1997. Nonrestorative treatment of discolored teeth: Reports from an international symposium. *J Am Dent Assoc* Suppl. no. 128: intro.

Kois JC, Kan JY. 2001. Predictable peri-implant gingival aesthetics: Surgical and prosthetic rationales. *Pract Proced Asthet Dent* 13(9):691–98.

Magne P. 2000. Perspectives in esthetic dentistry. *Quintessence Dent Technol* 23:86–89.

Malament KA, Socransky SS. 1999. Survival of Dicor glass ceramic dental restorations over 14 years: Part II. Effects of thickness of Dicor material and design of tooth preparation. *J Prosthet Dent* 81:662–67.

Manns A, Chan C, Miralles R. 1987. Influence of group function and canine guidance on electromyographic activity of elevator muscles. *J Prosthetic Dent* 57(4):494–501.

Mayer TM, Hawley CE, Gunsolley JC, Feldman S. 2002. The single tooth implant: A viable alternative for single tooth replacement. *J Periodontics* 73:687–93.

Meier B, Wiemer KB, Meithke RR. 2003. Invisalign patient profiling: Analysis of a prospective survey. *J Orofac Orthop* 64(5):352–58.

Miller M. 2000. Cosmetic mock-ups. *Reality* 14:3203–7.

Munz D, Fett T. 1999. *Ceramics: Mechanical Properties, Failure Behavior, Material Selection* 1st ed. Berlin: Springer.

Naert I, Koutsikakis G, Duyck J, Quirymen M, Jacobs R, van Steenberghe D. 2000. Biologic outcome of single implant restorations as tooth replacements. A long term follow up study. *Clin Implant Dent Relat Res* 2:209–18.

Nedwed V, Miethke RR. 2005. Motivation, acceptance, and problems of Invisalign patients. *J Orofac Orothop* 66(2):162–73.

Nikaido T, Kunzelmann KH, Chen H, et al. 2002. Evaluation of thermal cycling and mechanical loading on the bond strength of a self-etching primer system to dentine. *Dent Mater* 18:269–75.

Romero E, Chiapasco M, Ghisolfim, Vogel G. 2002. Long term clinical effectiveness of oral implants in the treatment of partial edentulatism: Seven year life table analysis of a prospective study with ITI dental implants system used for single tooth restorations. *Clin Oral Implants Res* 13: 133–43.

Saadoun AP, LeGall M. 1992. Implant positioning for periodontal, functional, and aesthetic results. *Practical Periodontics Aesthet Dent* 4:43–54.

Saadoun AP, Sullivan DY, Krischek, M, LeGall M. 1994. Single tooth implant: Management for success. *Pract Periodontics Assethet Dent* 6:73–82.

Samorodnitzky-Naveh GR, Geiger SB, Levin L. 2007. Patients' satisfaction with dental esthetics. *J Am Dent Assoc* 51(2): 507–24.

Schwartz-Arad D, Hertsberg R, Levin L. 2005. Evaluation of long–term implant success. *J of Periodontology* 10:1623.

Sorensen JA, Munksgaard EC. 1996. Relative gap formation adjacent to ceramic inlays with combination of resin cements and dentin bonding agents. *J Prosthet Dent* 76:472–76.

Swift, E. 1997. Restorative considerations with vital tooth bleaching. *J Am Dent Assoc* Suppl. no. 128:60S.

Touati, B. 1997. Double guidance approach for the improvement of the single tooth replacement. *Dent Implantol Update* 8:89–93.

Touati B, Guez G, Saadoun AP. 1999. Aesthetic soft tissue integration and optimized emergence profile: Provisionalization and customized impression coping. *Pract Periodontics Aesthet Dent* 11:305–14.

Touati B, Nathanson D. 1999. *Esthetic Dentistry and Ceramic Restorations*. Singapore: Martin Duntz.

Vlaskic V, Boyd RL. 2002. Clinical evolution of the Invisalign appliance. *J Calif Dent Assoc* 30(10):769–76.

Suggested Additional Reading

Paul SJ, Pieterobon N. 1998. Aesthetic evolution of anterior maxillary crowns: A literature review. *Pract Periodontics Aesthet Dent* 10(1):87–94.

Suttor D. 2004. Lava zirconia crowns and bridges. *Int J Comput Dent* 7(1):67–76.

Chapter 9

Considerations for Treating the Complex Esthetic Case

James B. Morris DDS

Warden Noble DDS, MS, BS

When planning complex esthetic restorations, it is necessary to evaluate, diagnose, and often treat occlusal factors.

Patients may present with numerous problems, including missing, tipped, or migrated teeth, teeth with increased mobility due to trauma from occlusion and loss of periodontal support, irregular or asymmetrical planes of occlusion, and teeth with extensive loss of enamel and dentin. Additionally, there is often a loss of occlusal vertical dimension, changes in lower face height, and dysfunction of the temporomandibular joints, muscles, and neuromuscular apparatus.

Goals of Occlusal Therapy

A primary goal of occlusal therapy is to reduce and control the forces on teeth, restorations, periodontal structures, and temporomandibular joints (Spear 1997). Ideally, during function forces should be distributed between teeth, periodontium, and temporomandibular joints such that there is no trauma that results in pathology within the stomatognathic system. To achieve control of forces, the following factors are under control of the restorative dentist: (1) position of condyles in the glenoid fossae, (2) vertical dimension of occlusion, (3) plane of occlusion, and (4) interocclusal contact of teeth during centric and eccentric mandibular movements. Additional information on occlusion can be found in chapter 5, dedicated to occlusion. Condylar position and vertical dimension of occlusion will be emphasized in this section.

Positions of Condyles

Centric relation position is generally defined as the maxillomandibular relationship in which the condyles articulate with their respective discs in an anterior-superior position in the fossa (Academy of Prosthodontics 2005). Most patients, however, close into an intercuspal contact position, which is normally located 0.1–1.5 mm anterior to their centric relation position (Rieder 1978).

Centric relation is most valuable as a reference position. In dentitions with missing teeth and worn or mutilated occlusions, the existing habitual intercuspal position may be unstable or nonexistent and may result in a malposition of the condyles. This potentially pathologic interocclusal position should not be propagated in a new occlusal scheme. Therefore, before starting treatment diagnostic casts must be mounted on an adjustable articulator using a face bow transfer with the condyles in a centric relation position. Using centric relation as a reference position, an analysis of the occlusion can be made and treatment decisions can be formulated. For example, as shown in figures 9-1 through 9-4, when this patient closes into his intercuspal contact position, the mandible moves anteriorly and a class III malocclusion appears to be present. However, when the centric relation position is used, the teeth are more edge to edge and the mouth can be restored in a more normal and functional jaw relationship. It would be improper to propagate his existing malocclusion with new restorations. As stated above, diagnostic casts should be mounted in centric relation, appropriate changes should be made in the vertical dimension of occlusion (VDO), and a diagnostic wax-up should be completed. Only at this point can final decisions regarding complex restorative care be finalized.

Treatment planning should be based on the type and extent of treatment to be performed. A practitioner must then decide whether to maintain, modify, or reestablish the existing occlusion (Braly, 1972). Clinical implications are listed in table 9-1. In general, if reestablishment of the existing occlusion is needed, centric relation should be used as a treatment position. Changes in vertical dimension should then be made from centric relation position. It should be emphasized, however, that extensive restorative dentistry can be planned without the need to change the VDO. For example, as shown in the case in figures 9-5 through 9-10, the patient presented with multiple missing and decayed teeth and was seeking improvements in his appearance. Treatment goals of improving comfort, function, and esthetics were attained

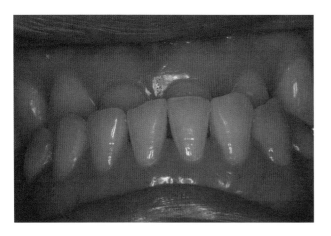

Figure 9-1. Anterior view of patient in maximum intercuspal position.

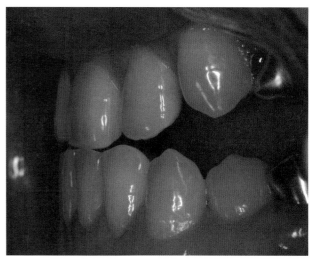

Figure 9-4. Lateral view with patient in centric relation.

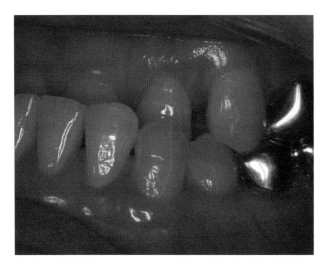

Figure 9-2. Lateral view of patient in maximum interproximal position.

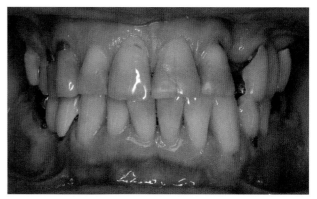

Figure 9-5. Pretreatment anterior view.

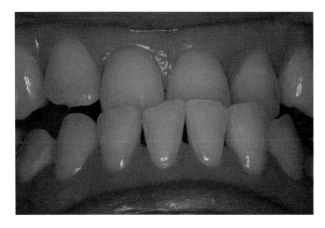

Figure 9-3. Anterior view with patient in centric relation.

Table 9-1. Treatment planning decisions.

Maintain Existing Occlusion	Modify Existing Occlusion	Reestablish Existing Occlusion
• Functional balance exists • Acceptable occlusal plane • Acceptable vertical dimension • No TMJ or muscle pain • Maximum intercuspal position is acceptable	• No change in maximum intercuspal position • No change in vertical dimension • Change individual tooth position or alignment • Minor occlusal adjustment	• Need to establish new intercuspal position • May change vertical dimension • Should use centric relation as treatment position

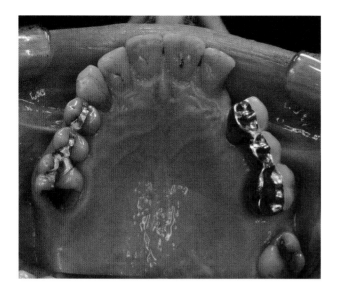

Figure 9-6.   Pretreatment maxillary view.

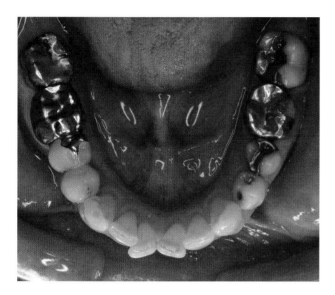

Figure 9-7.   Pretreatment mandibular view.

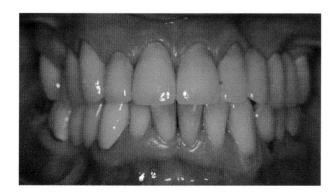

Figure 9-8.   Anterior view of finished case.

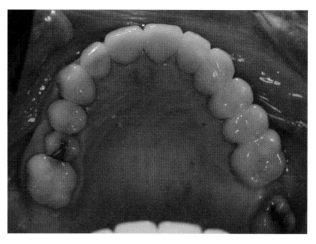

Figure 9-9.   Upper view of finished case.

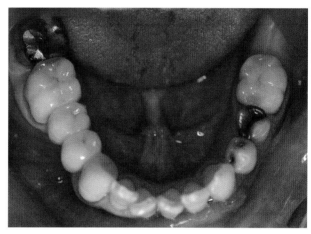

Figure 9-10.   Lower view of finished case.

without altering the VDO. Despite the missing teeth, the maximum intercuspal position was stable and it was not necessary to modify the VDO. Based on the experience and comfort level of the restorative dentist, this case could be treated in segments or could be managed as a "full-mouth reconstruction." However, care must be taken to maintain the existing occlusal relationship.

Maintenance of Vertical Dimension

One of the most important aspects of dental treatment is control of your procedures and treatment plan. Changes in VDO can be a life-altering benefit or misery; therefore, changes in VDO must be undertaken with meticulous diagnostics and documentation. Controlling VDO is most easily facilitated with hard tissue occlusal stops. Without tooth to opposing tooth references, vertical dimension must be approximated until confirmed by patient acceptance. Acceptable VDO requires comfort, function, and proficient speech. The techniques for determining VDO originated with removable prosthodontic therapies and can be quite challenging. Therefore, if a patient presents with an acceptable VDO, occlusal plane, and hard tissue (occlusal stops), maintenance of this position is paramount.

Diagnosing a Loss of VDO

If a change in VDO is necessary, the preliminary diagnostic wax-up and the resulting provisional templates must be recognized as only a proposed position and shape due to the necessity of intraoral refinement, verification, and acceptance by the patient. A common error among practitioners is expectation that the original diagnostic wax-up will be the final template for restorations guiding excursive movements of the mandible. In actuality, the wax-up is a starting point. The provisional restorations fabricated from the primary templates should be evaluated and refined for proper occlusion, guidance in all excursive movements, speech, and finally esthetics. Keep in mind the best esthetics will be compromised with an unacceptable occlusal/functional scheme.

Determining the need to increase VDO may be accomplished with the following techniques:

Excessive freeway space exists (interarch space while the patient's mandible is in a position of rest). Note the average freeway space has been documented by several authors to be 2–4 mm (Zarb 1978). Occasionally, tooth wear proceeds so rapidly that excessive freeway space develops. Examples are congenitally defective enamel and dentin cases, or enamel loss subsequent to acidic/chemical erosion.

Excessive air leakage during speech exists. Patient exhibits lack of slight occlusal contact on posterior teeth while pronouncing words beginning with "ch," "sh," or "z." The desired contact is easily identified with wax tape applied to occlusal surfaces of posterior teeth, keeping the patient from occluding into intercuspation and having the patient pronounce words identifying the closest speaking space as noted previously.

Lack of interarch restorative space exists. Freeway space and the closest speaking space may appear acceptable. In some instances, periodontal surgery and/or orthodontic intrusion is not indicated to provide enough space for your restorations. An increase in the VDO is the only apparent method in which adequate room for the restorative material of choice will be gained. Case selection is critical. Orthodontic and prosthodontic literature support the position of patients with a low or shallow Frankfort-mandibular plane angle being poor

candidates for increases in VDO (Kokich 1996). The most accurate diagnosis is made with the aid of lateral cephalometric radiograph (Dawson 2007). Clinically, the patient is evaluated from a lateral perspective for the intersection of the Frankfort versus the mandibular plane. If the intersection is below or even with the occipital region of the skull, this patient qualifies as having a low or shallow Frankfort-mandibular plane angle. This type of patient frequently presents with a very square mandible and may be angle class III, occasionally angle class I. Better candidates for increases in VDO are frequently angle class II patients with a steeper Frankfort-mandibular plane angle (planes intersecting above the occipital region). Literature supporting changes in the VDO of less than 3 mm at the anteriors is abundant (Dawson 2007).

Vertical Dimension Changes

In order to reestablish stable occlusal contacts, it is often necessary to increase the VDO. However, a careful diagnosis is needed before making clinical decisions. The following are factors that may make vertical dimension of occlusion changes necessary:

- To allow control of function and esthetics
- To restore vertical dimension of occlusion after posterior bite collapse
- To create room for restorations
- To obviate the need for surgical crown lengthening

As the anterior teeth are shortened due to wear and erosion there is often compensatory eruption of the worn teeth that keep the teeth in contact (Murphy 1959). As shown with the patient in figures 9-11 through 9-15, there are short anterior teeth that would provide poor retention for restorations and do not have adequate length to achieve satisfactory esthetic results. There is

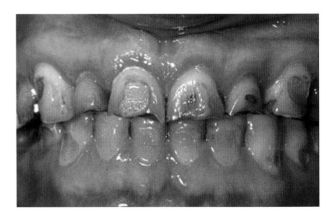

Figure 9-11. Loss of vertical dimension of occlusion, pretreatment anterior view.

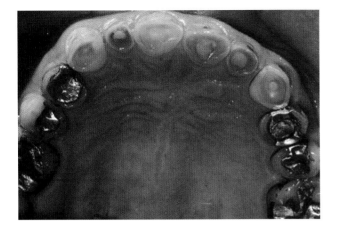

Figure 9-12.   Anterior and posterior wear maxilla.

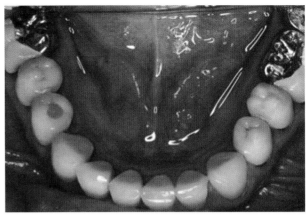

Figure 9-15.   Eighteen years posttreatment, view of mandible.

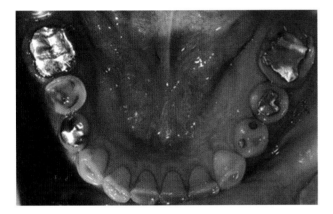

Figure 9-13.   Anterior and posterior wear mandible.

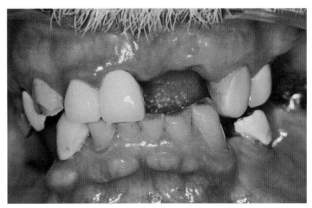

Figure 9-16.   Pretreatment view of posterior bite collapse.

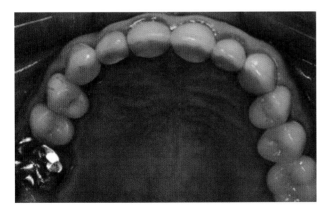

Figure 9-14.   Eighteen years posttreatment, view of maxilla.

also wear of occlusal surfaces on the posterior teeth. When the patient occludes, there is no room for restorations, and it is impossible to achieve anterior guidance. In this situation the teeth were restored at an increased VDO to satisfy both functional and esthetic goals

(Keough, 1992). The postoperative photos (figs. 9-14 and 9-15) show that there has been minimal additional wear after eighteen years of function.

It is also necessary to restore VDO after posterior bite collapse, which includes loss of posterior support due to missing and migrated teeth, caries, and periodontal disease (Rosenberg, Simons, and Gualini 1987). This loss of posterior occlusal support can also result in wear and may lead to periodontal breakdown of anterior teeth. In addition to an increase in VDO, extensive fixed, removable, or implant restorations are often needed.

As shown in figures 9-16 through 9-19, the patient was missing multiple posterior teeth, and teeth numbers 7 and 8 had periodontal bone loss. There was a lack of posterior occlusal support with wear and trauma to lower anterior teeth. Fixed and removable restorations were placed at an increased VDO and treatment goals were achieved. Upper and lower removable partial dentures were used.

Where there has been loss of posterior occlusal support due to dental erosion, it may be necessary to

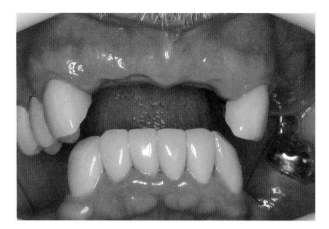

Figure 9-17. Porcelain restorations after extractions.

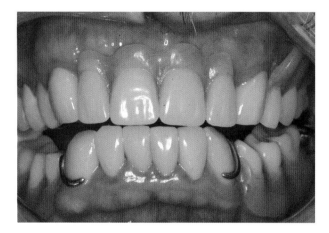

Figure 9-18. Posttreatment with maxillary and mandibular removable partial dentures.

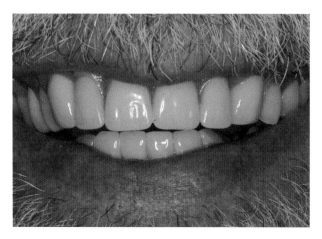

Figure 9-19. Posttreatment smile.

increase VDO to allow room for restorations. In these complete arch restorative cases where there is an absence of adequate room for occlusal reduction for restorations, it may be necessary to do periodontal crown lengthening and perhaps elective endodontic treatment (Keough 2003). Therefore, an increase in vertical dimension may be considered in order to avoid invasive procedures such as crown lengthening or propylactic endodontic treatment.

Various techniques have been proposed for determining the ideal VDO, but there is a lack of scientific evidence to validate their use (Rivera-Morales and Mohl 1991a). So-called physiologic rest position has been used with edentulous patients (Tallgren, 1951). After a resting position for the mandible is determined, the vertical height of the occlusal contact position is placed 2.0–3.0 mm below the resting point. While helpful with edentulous patients, with dentulous patients rest position has been found to be highly variable and not stable (Hickey, Williams, and Woelfel 1961). It has been shown that muscle length is quite adaptable and that patients, particularly those with angle class II occlusions, can usually tolerate changes in VDO of up to 2.0–3.0 mm (Carlsson, Ingervaall, and Kocak 1979). Changes in excess of this amount should be accomplished in gradual steps so muscles can accommodate increases in length.

The use of speech, especially the sibilant sounds or "s" sounds, may be useful to determine if the vertical dimension has been excessively increased (Rivera-Morales and Mohl, 1991b). While a patient is making sibilant sounds, a small space should exist between the teeth. If teeth touch, the vertical dimension may be overopened.

Electronic instrumentation has been advocated to clinically determine the VDO (Jankelson et al. 1995). However, due to a lack of well-controlled clinical trials, clinicians should be cautious and recognize the limitations of these instruments (Rugh and Drago 1981; Clark et al. 1997; Baba, Tsukiyama, and Clark 2000).

In summary, muscles of mastication can adjust and adapt to changes in VDO, but care must be taken to not exceed the adaptive capacity of our patients. If the guidelines below are followed, complex occlusal reconstructions can be completed.

- Always open VDO from a stable centric relation position.
- Open VDO as little as possible to achieve desired goals.
- Consider a period of provisionalization (preferably a removable splint) to allow muscles to adapt to an increase in vertical length.
- Do not increase VDO based on electromyographic recordings.

Periodontal Plastic Surgery

Periodontal tissue management is an important adjunct to complex esthetic restorative dentistry. So-called periodontal plastic surgery involves the cosmetic reconstruction, reshaping, or removal of dento-alveolar tissues (Miller and Allen 1996). Periodontal services are needed to perform root coverage, crown lengthening, alveolar ridge augmentation, and tissue recontouring.

Root Coverage

Many patients are concerned with root exposure due to the apical migration of the dento-alveolar tissues. In addition to esthetic problems, gingival recession can also result in increased susceptibility to root caries and sensitivity.

The prevalence of root recession increases with age and is significant in 90% of patients over eighty years of age (Tjan and Miller 1984). It is related to thin buccal or lingual bone and thin gingival tissue and seen with buccally positioned teeth, periodontal disease, minimal attached gingival, toothbrush abrasion, acid erosion with cervical notching, and subgingival restorations (Kao and Pasquinelli 2002).

After removal or control of various etiologic factors, root coverage treatment is often done using connective tissue–free grafts or so-called pedicle grafts, where periodontal tissues are removed from adjacent areas resulting in an apically or laterally repositioned flap (Allen and Miller 1989). Occasionally, minor gingivalplasty procedures are needed after healing to achieve an ideal result (Hwang and Wang 2006).

As shown in figures 9-20 through 9-23, the use of various grafting procedures should always be considered as a preferred solution to esthetic problems prior to proceeding with more invasive restorations such as porcelain veneers or full-coverage crowns. With this patient, the only necessary restorative procedures were small class V composites on teeth numbers 6 and 11. The use of crowns or veneers would not be justified.

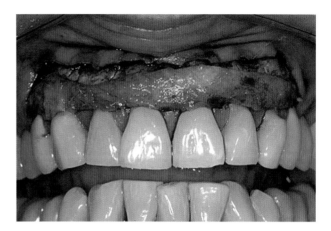

Figure 9-21.   Placement of a connective tissue graft.

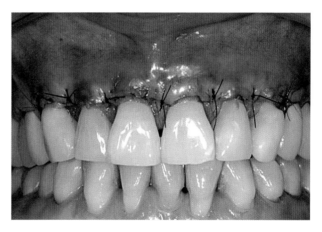

Figure 9-22.   Graft is covered with sutured tissues.

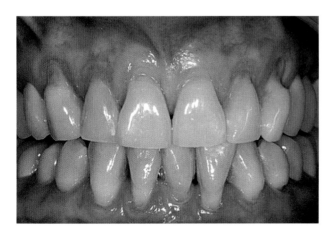

Figure 9-20.   Pretreatment view. Note extensive recession of upper anteriors.

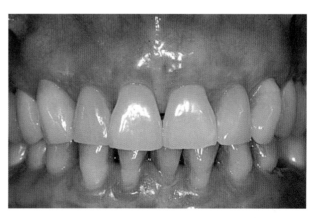

Figure 9-23.   After healing, only small class V restorations were needed (Surgery by Dr. Kirk Pasquinelli).

Crown Lengthening

Crown lengthening is used to improve the position and shape of gingival tissues in an attempt to improve the esthetic outcome and to allow access to healthy root structure to provide adequate retention and support for restorations. The following are general guidelines for crown lengthening surgery:

- Assess restorability: completely remove all caries and restorative material
- Assess endodontic status: treatment needed, prognosis
- Assess periodontal status: overall prognosis of teeth
- Consider electrosurgery or laser surgery: remove excess tissue above the dentogingival complex
- Consider effect of periodontal surgery on adjacent teeth
- Consider orthodontic extrusion: single-rooted teeth (especially with cosmetic concerns)
- Assess cosmetic affects
- Evaluate strategic value of involved teeth

It is important to carefully assess the restorability, endodontic status, and periodontal prognosis before beginning treatment. Small amounts of tissue recontouring can be done using electrosurgery or laser surgery, but more involved procedures involving surgical flaps and bone contouring should be approached cautiously, as the outcome may also affect the esthetics of adjacent teeth. The loss of interproximal papillae can also cause an esthetic problem. It is also important to evaluate the strategic value of the teeth before considering crown lengthening. It may be better to extract teeth with a poor long-term prognosis and to replace them with either an implant or a fixed or removable prosthesis.

As shown in figures 9-24 through 9-26, prior to placement of porcelain veneers on teeth numbers 8 and 9, gingiva has been removed to obtain an even, more esthetic appearance. A different situation is shown in

figures 9-27 and 9-28. In this case, teeth numbers 9 and 10 could be deemed hopeless and be scheduled for extraction. However, by repositioning the gingival tissues apically, healthy root structure is exposed and restorations can be placed on the teeth. Retention of these teeth results in a much better esthetic and functional outcome.

Before considering crown lengthening surgery to correct display of excess gingival tissue, a differential

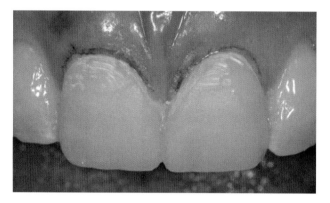

Figure 9-25. Smile design with bis-acrylic.

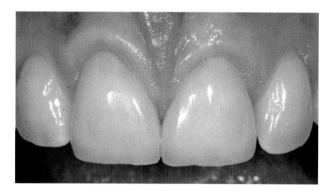

Figure 9-26. Completed veneers (Work by Dr. Lambert Stumpel).

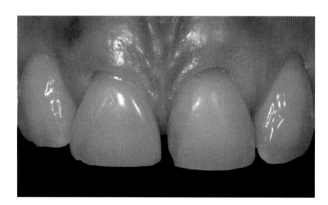

Figure 9-24. Pretreatment tissue asymmetry.

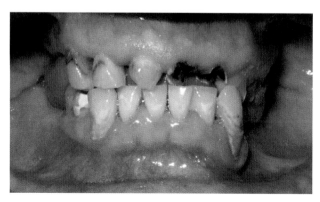

Figure 9-27. Pretreatment view showing caries and fractured teeth.

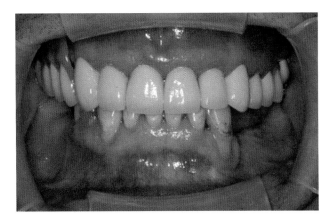

Figure 9-28. Postsurgery showing completed restoration.

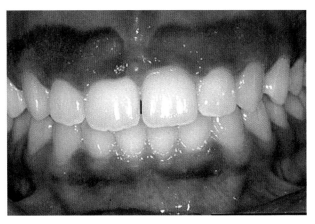

Figure 9-30. Details of irregular gingival tissues.

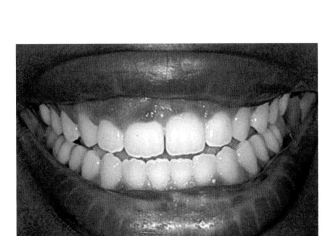

Figure 9-29. Full smile displaying excessive/irregular gingiva.

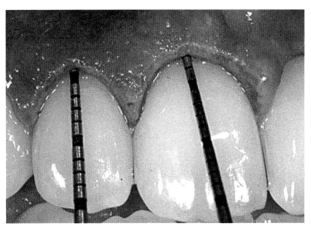

Figure 9-31. After trimming tissue, probe to determine bone position.

diagnosis of the excess gingival display must be made. Etiologic factors that result in excess gingival display include insufficient lip length, hyperactivity of the upper lip, extrusion of the alveolar process, and vertical maxillary excess (Robbins 1999).

If a short or hyperactive upper lip is the cause of the excess gingival display ("gummy smile"), the patient should be informed that no dental restorative treatment currently exists to correct this problem. However, as shown in figures 9-29 through 9-33, selective crown lengthening can improve the esthetics without the need for restorative dentistry. As shown in figures 9-31 and 9-32, it is important to determine the position of the underlying bone before proceeding with surgery. Note also that there is adequate attached gingiva to allow for tissue reduction. In figure 9-32, after exposing the bone, it is clear that bone must be recontoured to achieve an even gingival level. The entire dento-gingival complex has been repositioned apically. The final result is a sig-

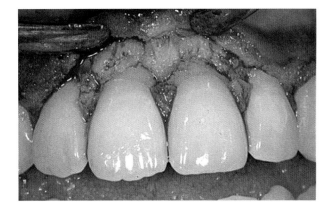

Figure 9-32. Retracted tissue shows irregular bone.

nificant improvement over the pretreatment appearance. Other approaches such as orthodontics or surgery should be considered to help manage excess gingival display (Kokich 1996).

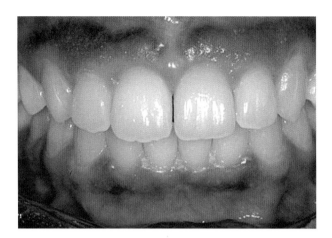

Figure 9-33. Completed case after bone recontouring and healing (Surgery by Dr. Kirk Paquinelli).

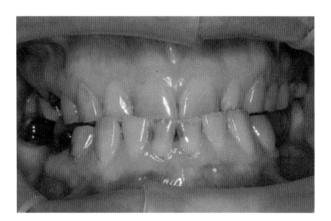

Figure 9-34. Example of altered passive eruption.

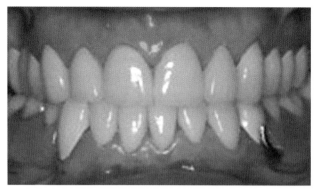

Figure 9-35. Completed case after crown lengthening.

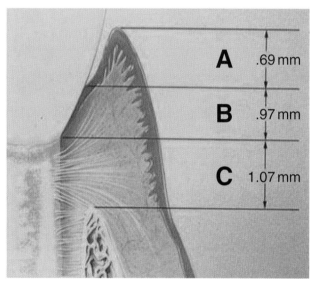

Figure 9-36. Diagram of dento-gingival complex. Do not place crown margins in areas B and C.

Altered passive eruption also results in short maxillary incisor teeth. Teeth that have had loss of incisal length due to wear will tend to continue to erupt to maintain incisal contact. As teeth erupt, the cemento-enamel junction moves incisally, bringing the dento-gingival complex, including the alveolar bone, with it. In this instance surgical crown lengthening with osseous reduction would be indicated (Dolt 1997). As shown in figures 9-34 and 9-35, crown lengthening followed by porcelain-fused-to-metal crowns resulted in an excellent esthetic result. It should be noted that in this clinical situation there is usually no need to increase the VDO.

There are many clinical situations where crown lengthening can improve the prognosis of a questionable tooth and render it restorable. In particular, teeth with loss of coronal tooth structure due to caries, fractures, or endodontic treatment may be saved if tissue is removed and restoration margins can be placed more apically. The following is a list of indications for crown lengthening:

- Short teeth due to wear
- Inadequate tooth structure for retention due to subgingival fracture or caries
- Uneven gingival levels
- Altered passive eruption
- Hyperplastic tissue due to drug systemic reactions

Great care must be taken when crown lengthening is done in the esthetic zone. To achieve a satisfactory result it is necessary to understand the relationship between clinical crown length, the biologic width of attachment, the dento-gingival complex, and the alveolar crest (Gunay et al. 2000; Becker, Oshenbein, and Becker 1998). The biologic width refers to the space in the dento-gingival complex occupied by the junctional epithelium (epithelial attachment) and supracrestal connective tissue fibers, as indicated by areas B and C in figure 9-36. If crown margins are placed into the epithelial attachment or supracrestal fibers, an unsightly and pathologic chronic inflammation may persist. Therefore, this "biologic width" must not be violated, and the dento-gingival complex should be repositioned apically to allow for placement of the margin of the restoration coronal to the epithelial attachment (Gargiulo, Wentz, and Orban 1961).

It is important to also evaluate the characteristics of the gingival tissue if crown lengthening procedures are being considered. As noted in table 9-2, tissues can be grouped into those with a thick or thin "biotype" (Pasquinelli 2005). These differences are illustrated in figures 9-37 and 9-38. If there is inadequate attached ginigva or if the tissue biotype is very thin, it is difficult to achieve

Table 9-2. Characteristics of gingival tissue.

Thick Gingival Tissue	Thin Gingival Tissue
• Dense, fibrotic soft tissue	• Delicate, friable soft tissue
• Large amounts of attached gingiva	• Minimal attached gingiva
• Thick underlying osseous form	• Thin underlying bone
• Reacts to disease with pocket formation and intrabony defects	• Reacts to insults and disease with gingival recession

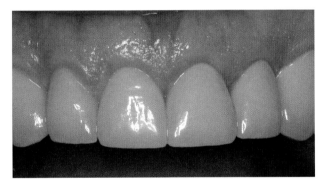

Figure 9-37. Thick gingiva. Note stippling, flatness, and attached gingiva.

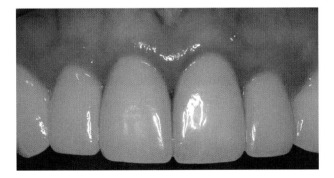

Figure 9-38. Thin gingiva. Note minimal texture and reduced attached gingiva.

reattachment, and crown lengthening may not be indicated. Surgically, thin tissues are very difficult to manipulate and the underlying bone is very thin. Thick gingival tissues are more easily manipulated and healing is more predictable.

The amount of osseous material to be removed depends in large part on the proposed location of the planned restorative margin. Usually, the osseous crest should be at least 3.0 mm apical to the crown margin, which allows for formation of a new and healthy biologic width. The actual placement of the final restorative margin depends on the esthetic requirements of the patient. For example, margins in all-ceramic crowns do not have to be placed as far subgingivally as metal collars on porcelain-fused-to-metal crowns. Other factors such as contour of the final restoration, thickness and width of the attached gingival, dimension of the biologic width, and quality of oral hygiene should be considered (Nevins and Skurow 1984). After crown lengthening, remodeling and maturation of the attachment apparatus can take more than three months, although it should be noted that there is the possibility of future changes in the volume of tissue covering root surface (Waal and Castellucci 1994; Ramfjord, Engler, and Hiniker 1966). Before final restorations are completed, minor gingivoplasty may be needed to create ideal gingival contours.

Restoratively, there are limits to what can be accomplished with crown lengthening. As alveolar bone is surgically removed, teeth have less support. With less bone there are less favorable crown-root ratios, and the long-term prognosis of restorations may be compromised. There can also be problems with poor emergence profiles of restorations after surgery.

Ridge Augmentation

After removal of a tooth or implant there is usually less alveolar bone in both apical and lingual directions (Carlsson, Thilander, and Hedegard 1967; Schropp et al. 2003). The final bone contour after extraction can be influenced by the pre-extraction position of the tooth, form and biotype of the periodontium, tooth shape, and position of the osseous crest (Kois 1998; Kois 2001). This collapse of bone and soft tissue results in esthetic problems with implants and pontics and often requires reconstruction and augmentation of the edentulous area.

Various techniques are available to rebuild collapsed ridges. Soft tissue grafts, bone block grafts, guided bone regeneration, and alveolar distraction osteogenesis have been used alone or in combination to enhance the functional and esthetic result when treating the edentulous spaces (Pasquinelli 2005; Langer and Calagna 1980; Buser et al. 1995; Seibert 1983; Tolman 1995; Chin 1998).

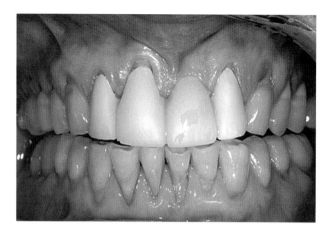

Figure 9-39. Pretreatment view showing extensive recession.

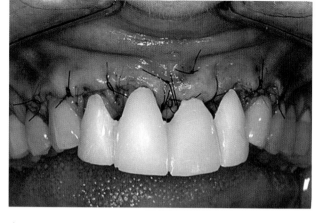

Figure 9-42. Sutured tissue with original provisional restoration.

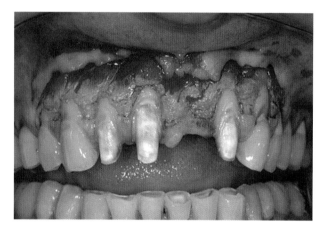

Figure 9-40. View of retracted tissue showing edentulous ridge defect.

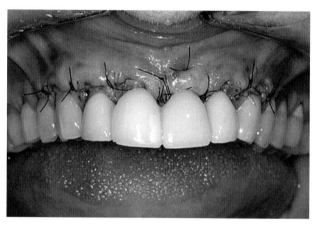

Figure 9-43. Modified provisional restoration in place.

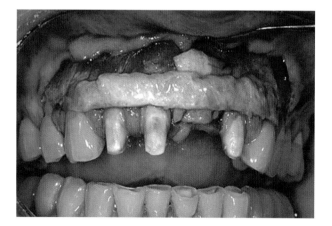

Figure 9-41. View of connective tissue grafts in place.

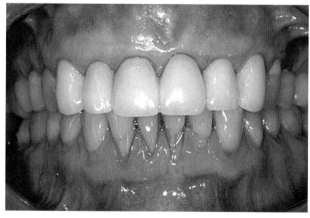

Figure 9-44. Final all-ceramic restorations in place (Surgery by Dr. Kirk Pasquinelli).

As shown in figures 9-39 through 9-44, when a fixed partial denture is being used, connective tissue grafts are an effective way to restore missing tissue volume. In this case, a combination of ridge augmentation and gingival repositioning was needed to prepare the tissue for the final all-ceramic restorations. Figure 9-39 shows a patient with extensive recession. During periodontal surgery, connective tissue grafts were used to both augment the extraction site and to provide a support for the repositioned tissue. The provisional restoration was readapted and a satisfactory esthetic result was obtained. It should be noted that construction of the final prosthesis should be delayed at least three months to allow for tissue maturation and shrinkage.

For implant site preparation, a combination of bone grafts and connective tissue grafts is often needed (Pasquinelli 2005). As shown in figures 9-45 through 9-55, a large postextraction soft-tissue defect was allowed to heal and minor orthodontic treatment was done to create ideal spacing and root angulations between the teeth. An implant was placed and graft materials were used to rebuild the lost edentulous bone. Finally, all-ceramic restorations were placed on the anterior teeth.

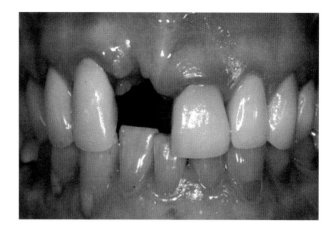

Figure 9-45. Pretreatment view showing extensive ridge defect.

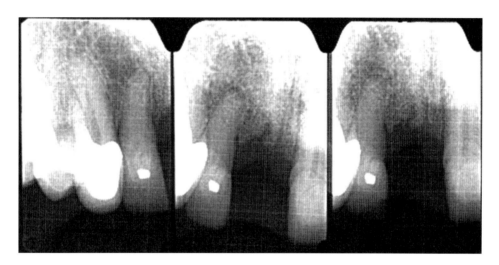

Figure 9-46. Pretreatment radiographs showing ridge defect.

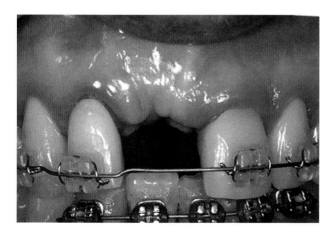

Figure 9-47. Minor orthodontic treatment completed to optimize spacing.

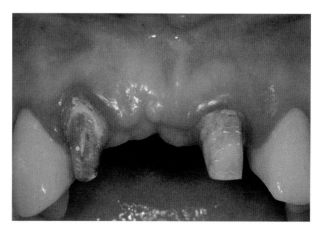

Figure 9-48. Ridge healed and prepared for implant.

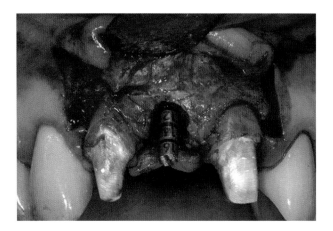

Figure 9-49. Implant pilot hole drilled.

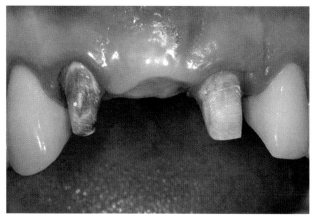

Figure 9-52. Implant site healed.

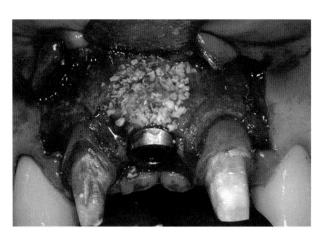

Figure 9-50. Implant placed with bone graft material.

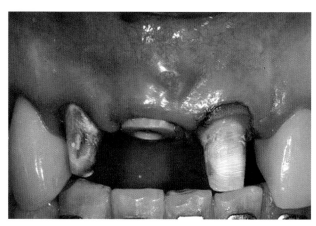

Figure 9-53. Implant healing cap in place.

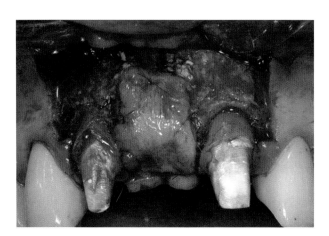

Figure 9-51. Implant covered with connective tissue graft.

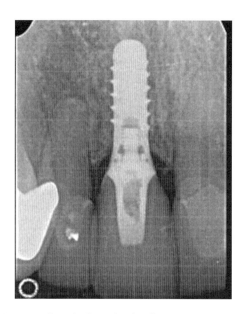

Figure 9-54. Radiograph of completed implant/restoration.

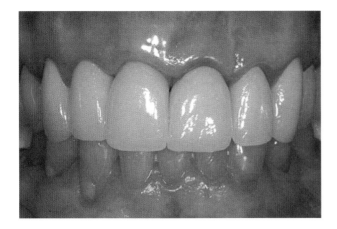

Figure 9-55. Final all-ceramic crowns in place.

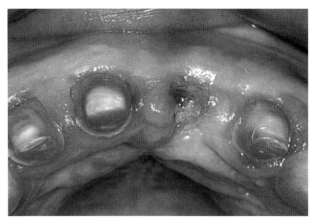

Figure 9-57. Completed depression in tissue for ovate pontic.

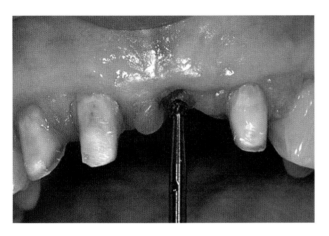

Figure 9-56. Ovate pontic site preparation.

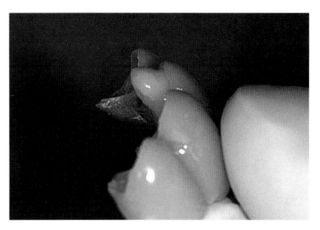

Figure 9-58. Provisional restoration is modified.

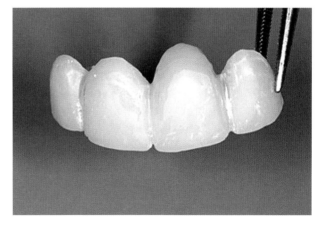

Figure 9-59. Modified provisional ready for seating. Tissue heals around acrylic addition.

Pontic site preparation is another useful adjunct for esthetic reconstruction. A scalloping of convex surfaces of the edentulous area can enhance the contour and cleansibility of a modified ridge-lap or ovoid pontic (Eissmann, Radke, and Noble 1971; Shillingberg et al. 1997). This can be easily accomplished using rotary instruments, laser, electrosurgery, or a scalpel. In recent years the use of ovate pontics has been increasing. For optimal results the buccal aspect of the ridge and the interproximal papillae must be preserved. To achieve excellent esthetic results with an ovate pontic, note that as the extraction site heals an ovoid depression can be developed using a bur, as shown in figures 9-56 and 9-57. Figures 9-58 through 9-60 show that with the addition of acrylic to a temporary removable partial, a removable partial denture, or a fixed provisional restoration, an ovoid depression is made into which the apical aspect of the pontic is placed. The tissue heals around the acrylic extension and the new pontic fits into the depression.

In summary, the esthetic-oriented restorative dentist must be well educated in and aware of the adjunctive therapies which can be provided by other dental specialties. Interdisciplinary diagnosis and treatment planning are an integral part of esthetic dentistry.

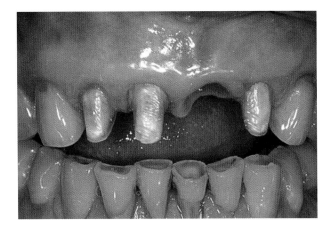

Figure 9-60. Pontic site prepared for final restoration.

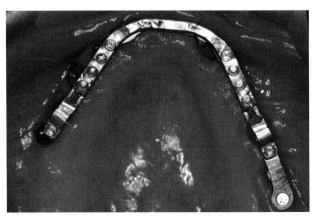

Figure 9-61. View of implant-supported bar to retain overdenture.

Esthetics with Fixed-Removable Restorations

It is impossible to prescribe comprehensive restorative dentistry without the use of removable prostheses. Despite the fact that the number of edentulous adults in the United States is decreasing, it is estimated that approximately 23% of adults aged 65 and older are completely edentulous (Mojon 2003). The number of partially edentulous patients is difficult to estimate, but it is clear that the partially edentulous population is far greater than the edentulous population, and therefore a significant component of restorative dentistry must involve treatment of this population.

Regarding esthetic dentistry, there are unique challenges found when making fixed and removable combination restorations. It is often difficult to obtain a satisfactory shape and shade match when using various esthetic restorative dental materials adjacent to stock denture teeth. When there is loss of alveolar structures, it can be difficult to blend denture base materials with a patient's gingival tissues. It is also understandable that many patients object to a display of metal when clasps or attachments are used to support and retain a removable prosthesis. Finally, many patients experience compromised comfort and function with removable appliances (Feine and Heydicke 2003; Zarb 1997).

Due in part to the problems noted above, dentists have sought treatment alternatives to negate the use of removable prostheses, including the concept of shortening the dental arch, sometimes called a "bicuspidized occlusion" (Armellinini and von Fraunhofer 2004; Frias, Toothaker, and Wright 2004), and the increasingly popular use of dental implants to support fixed and removable restorations. In particular, dental implants have been associated with increased longevity, better

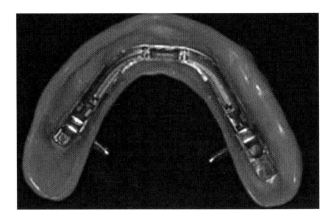

Figure 9-62. Overdenture with cast housing to fit over implant-retained bar.

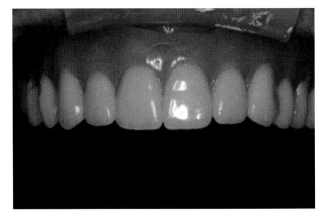

Figure 9-63. Maxillary implant/bar-retained overdenture.

patient satisfaction, and improved function (Weber and Sukotjo 2007). The prosthesis shown in figures 9-61, 9-62, and 9-63 is an example of an appliance that can be removed by the patient for cleaning but is fixed in the mouth during periods of functional use. The overdenture is held in place by small pins that can be engaged by the patient. It fits accurately over a milled, implant-supported bar.

Implant-supported fixed and removable restorations are considered the standard of care in modern dental practices (Cho 2004; Sadowsky 2001; Weber and Sukotjo 2007). However, as shown in the following list, there are situations where dental implants are not an option, and a removable prosthesis must be used (Wostman et al. 2005):

- Extensive loss of alveolar bone due to trauma, pathology, or periodontal disease
- Anatomical restrictions, such as proximity of the alveolar nerve or minimal bone below the maxillary sinuses
- Financial limitations of patients
- Certain medical or behavioral considerations

A large segment of the population cannot afford the high cost of fixed restorations and must accept removable alternatives rather than implant-supported fixed restorations. Medical problems such as uncontrolled diabetes, autoimmune problems, or certain chemotherapy regimes may affect the osseointegration process. Also, behavioral or patient management issues can be problematic. Therefore, the use of removal appliances in esthetic restorative dentistry must be discussed.

The display of metal is a major esthetic problem with removable partial dentures. To overcome this problem, there are four basic solutions. These are listed below:

- Use of "I" bar or "RPI" removable partial denture design
- Use of rotational path design removable partial dentures
- Use of precision or semiprecision attachments
- Use of "shortened dental arch" concepts

One method of minimizing display of metal is with the use of so-called RPI clasps, especially in patients who do not display their teeth during smiling or speech (Krol, Jacobson, and Finzen 1999; Carr, McGivney, and Brown 2005). The contour of the fixed restoration used as support for the partial denture can be modified to place the small I-bar clasp as far apically on the tooth as possible. The use of circumferential or "Akers" clasps should be avoided as these are often not esthetically acceptable. The example shown in figure 9-64 illustrates how the RPI design minimizes coverage of the tooth with metal and approaches the retentive undercut from under the lip.

Rotational path removable partial dentures are another excellent esthetic solution (Krol, Jacobsen, and Finzen 1999). The teeth adjacent to the edentulous space are contoured with an undercut into which the anterior

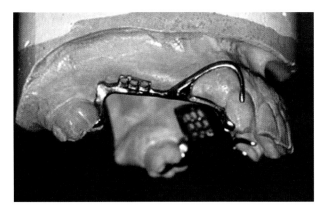

Figure 9-64. "RPI" clasp design showing minimal coverage of tooth.

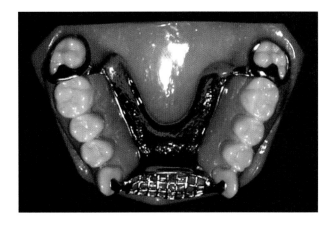

Figure 9-65. Rotational path design framework on cast.

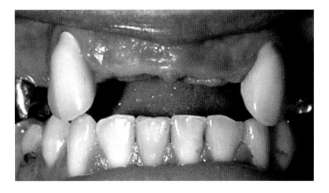

Figure 9-66. Removable partial denture will engage undercuts on the mesial of teeth 6 and 11 for retention.

segment of the removable partial denture seats. The prosthesis is then rotated around this point until the rigid posterior segments are fully seated in place. Conventional circumferential clasps placed in posterior areas retain the appliance. As shown in figures 9-65, 9-66, and 9-67, by engaging the undercut, the appliance

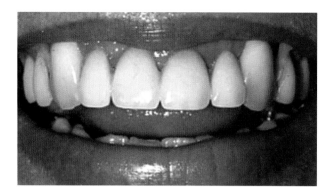

Figure 9-67. Rotational path removable partial denture in place. Note no display of clasps.

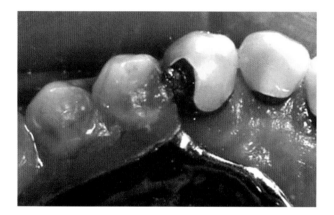

Figure 9-68. View of rigid precision attachment in place.

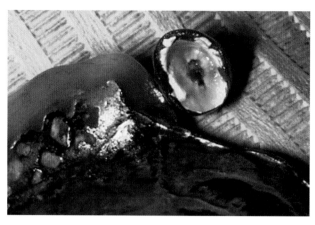

Figure 9-69. Abutment tooth fracture caused by leveraged stress from attachment.

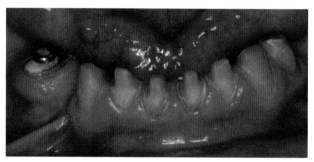

Figure 9-70. Locator attachment is shown on tooth 29.

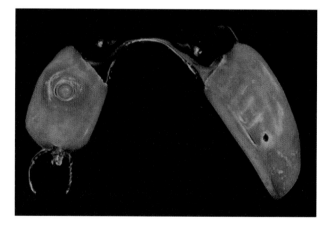

Figure 9-71. Nylon-retentive element shown in removable partial denture.

is held firmly in place. No clasps are needed in the anterior area.

Various precision attachments can be used to preclude the use of clasps in the esthetic zone. Attachment systems have been classified as rigid and resilient (Staubli 1996). Rigid systems should not be used when a distal extension base is supported by soft tissue only, as movement of the base can generate pathologic forces in the abutment teeth resulting in trauma to periodontal tissues or fracture of crowns and roots of teeth. Figures 9-68 and 9-69 illustrate a failed rigid attachment assembly where heavy occlusal forces have fractured the tooth, retaining the removable partial denture. Thus, the use of rigid precision attachment systems should usually be limited to class III-type tooth-supported removable partial dentures.

Various resilient attachment systems are available and may be used with either tooth- or tissue-supported cases. One system is the Locator (Zest Anchors, Inc., Escondido, CA) attachment system, wherein the removable framework is retained and supported by a friction-fitting nylon housing. As shown in figures 9-70 through

9-72, the nylon attachment can be changed to increase retention or can be replaced after excessive wear. The ERA (APM-Sterngold, Attleboro, MA) attachment system can also be useful for free-end distal extension cases where there has been excessive loss of bone in edentulous areas adjacent to natural teeth. This extra-

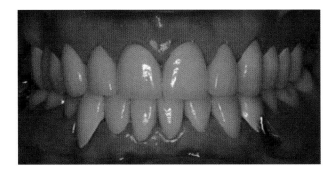

Figure 9-72. Mandibular removable partial denture in mouth. Note lack of clasp on right side.

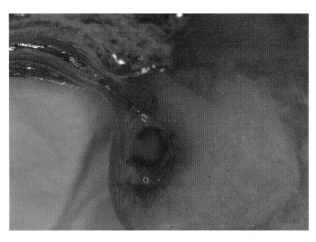

Figure 9-74. Extracoronal attachment-matrix.

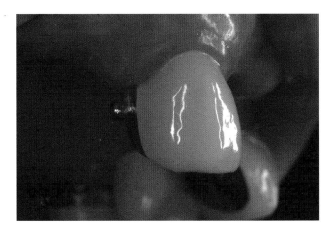

Figure 9-73. Extracoronal attachment-patrix.

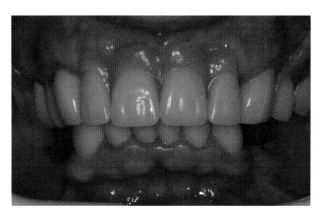

Figure 9-75. Removable partial denture in mouth.

coronal attachment can be placed lower in the edentulous area, thus providing more interocclusal room for the attachment housing and possibly decreasing the torque on the tooth by lowering the fulcrum point. The long-term retention with both of these attachment systems has been found to be very satisfactory (Petropoulos, Smith, and Kousvelari 1997; Kampen et al. 2003).

Another extracoronal attachment utilizing a replaceable nylon matrix is the Bredent VKS-SG system (Bredent GmbH and Co. KG, Sending, Germany). As shown in figures 9-73 through 9-75, this system is highly versatile regarding position and spacing requirements while also satisfying cosmetic demands.

The concept of the shortened dental arch has gained acceptance in recent years. A shortened dental arch is defined as a dentition where most of the posterior teeth are missing (Frias, Toothaker, and Wright 2004). For clinical situations when implants cannot be placed, many patients can function with bicuspid occlusion only, without the use of a removable partial denture (Budtz-Jorgensen, Bochet, Grundman, and Borgis 2000). Since there is no significant loss in masticatory function

or nutritional status and there is improvement in patient satisfaction, a shortened dental arch approach is a viable treatment planning option (Wostmann et al. 2005; Jepson et al. 2003).

Correct anatomical contouring and custom characterization of denture base materials can result in a much-improved esthetic result. As shown in figures 9-76 and 9-77, contours on removable appliances should mimic underlying bony contours, resulting in a very natural appearance (Brigante 1981). As is obvious when comparing the dentures in figures 9-78 and 9-79, custom characterization of denture base materials and the use of "restorations" in denture teeth can result in a very realistic prosthesis. These are somewhat specialized procedures, and the services of a high-quality dental laboratory should be sought.

Finally, techniques can be employed to create a satisfactory color match and tooth contour at the interface of denture teeth and teeth made from various restorative

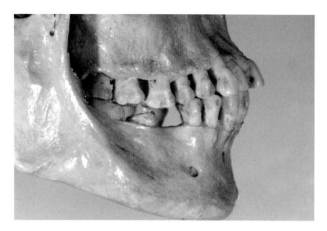

Figure 9-76. Underlying bone contours should be replicated in acrylic.

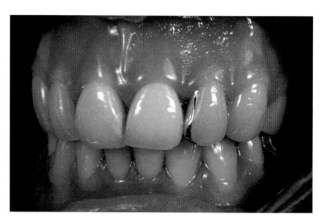

Figure 9-79. Characterization results in a very natural-looking denture (Courtesy of Dr. Robert Brigante).

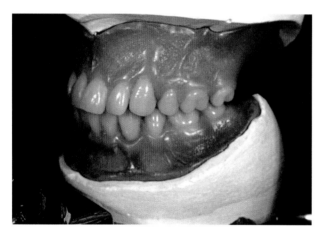

Figure 9-77. Creating natural contours on dentures enhances esthetic results.

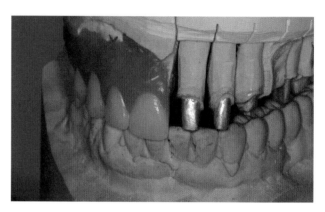

Figure 9-80. Denture teeth set on master cast.

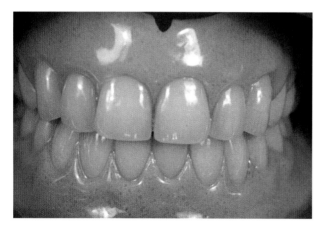

Figure 9-78. An example of a poor esthetic result.

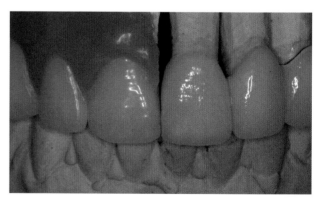

Figure 9-81. Porcelain-metal crowns matched to denture teeth.

materials. It is suggested that the denture teeth be selected prior to completion of restorative procedures. Denture teeth should be set on the master cast and sent to the dental laboratory at the time ceramic restorations are made, as shown in figures 9-80 through 9-82. This will allow the technician to copy the color and shape of the denture teeth and achieve an excellent esthetic result.

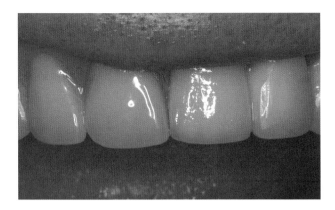

Figure 9-82. Completed fixed-removable restoration.

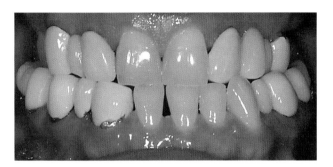

Figure 9-83. Pretreatment restorations.

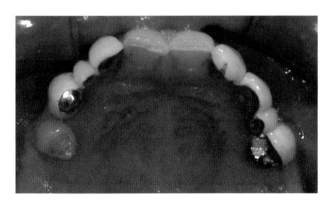

Figure 9-84. Pretreatment maxillary view.

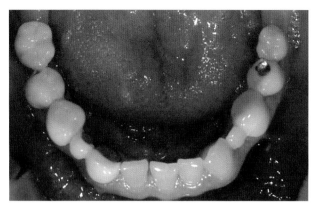

Figure 9-85. Pretreatment mandibular view.

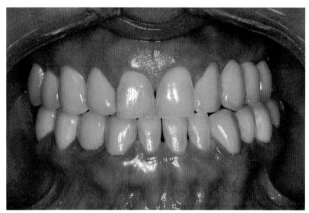

Figure 9-86. Posttreatment restorations.

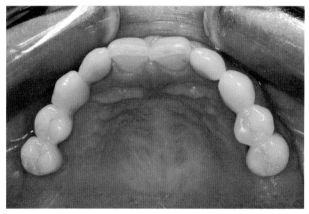

Figure 9-87. Posttreatment maxillary view.

Orthodontic Treatment in Preparation for Restoration

Frequently, dentitions present with inadequate spacing to allow anatomic restoration with correct symmetry. Orthodontic movement of the teeth is the most conservative way to provide correct anatomic space for pontics and alignment of potential abutments. Additionally, deep impinging occlusions require orthodontic correction to provide correct anterior guidance (Kokich 1996). The case presented in figures 9-83 through 9-88 repre-

sents an example of prosthetic restoration of congenitally missing teeth without preprosthetic orthodontic treatment, compared with the same patient being retreated prosthetically following orthodontic correction of the inadequate pontic space and alignment of the abutment teeth.

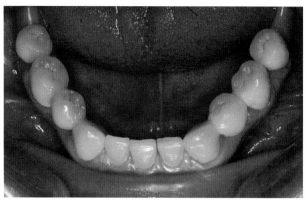

Figure 9-88. Posttreatment mandibular view.

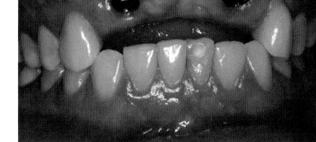

Figure 9-89. Pretreatment implant position.

Implants in the Esthetic Zone

Precise treatment planning and coordination are required for implant placement and restoration to be esthetically successful. Less-than-ideal implant sites are the most common cause of increased complexity of the case. Inadequate bone height, width, and density or inadequate amounts of attached gingiva all affect the implant esthetic success (Zarb 1997; Taylor 2005). Implant manufacturers are evolving at very competitive rates, and thus the choice of materials for the abutment and prosthesis have greatly improved the restorative dentist's ability to meet patient expectations in the esthetic zone. The implant treatment plan should be supervised by the restorative dentist from the initial planning of the case. The restorative doctor is (especially in the eyes of the patient) ultimately responsible for the esthetic outcome and satisfaction of the patient. Considerations for implant treatment planning include the following items.

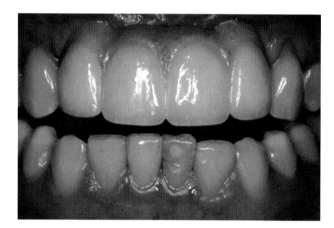

Figure 9-90. Posttreatment restoration.

Site Development

The potential implant site must duplicate the healthy periodontium supporting a natural tooth (Pasquinelli 2005). Frequently, hard and/or soft tissue grafting is required to provide adequate bulk of bone and attached gingival at an implant site. More often in cases of previous extraction without grafting of the supporting tissues, retrograde periodontal surgery is indicated to provide adequate bone height and width. When two adjacent implants are planned in the esthetic zone, it is extremely difficult to reproduce the interdental papillae without preprosthetic bone grafting. If there is adequate space for a pontic in the area, gingival-colored ceramics may provide the esthetics necessary and thus avoid the site-development surgery (figs. 9-89 through 9-91).

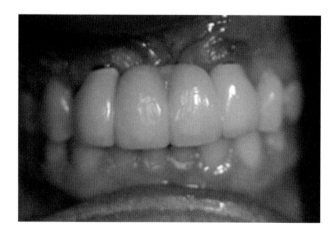

Figure 9-91. Pretreatment restoration.

Grafting surgery may be avoided in cases where a single implant is immediately placed following extraction of patient's natural tooth, thus preserving the adjacent interdental papillae. In some cases of planned extraction, orthodontic extrusion of the terminal root has been shown to provide the adequate bone height and gingival frame to improve the prognosis of esthetic success (Tarnow 1994).

Abutment Selection

The choice is either metallic or nonmetallic. The nonmetallic choice is zirconium oxide due to the impressive strength compared to other ceramics. The choice to use zirconium oxide abutments is dictated by the contours of the final restoration and the subsequent strength of the prepared abutment. Due to the shape of teeth and restorative space available, metallic abutments may be utilized in the esthetic zone without sacrificing excellent esthetic results.

Additionally, thin biotype tissues will be complimented esthetically with a ceramic abutment emerging through the marginal gingival compared to a metallic abutment showing through the gingival transparency. Thin, spire-shaped abutments are at a higher risk of fracture and will not resist the lateral forces placed on the final restoration. The decision to use the nonmetallic abutments should be made at the initial stages of treatment planning and confirmed at the diagnostic waxing stage of the treatment plan. Good candidates for nonmetallic abutments are areas in the esthetic zone where there is room for the abutment to have opposing walls circumferentially while the prosthetic room for the restoration is of adequate esthetic thickness buccal-lingually (see figures 9-92 through 9-94). Thick- and thin-biotype patients are good candidates for nonmetallic abutments as long as the restoration follows margin design/placement as described in the gingival biotype section. When restorative space dictates that the thinnest abutment material must be used, high noble alloy or titanium is the metal of choice. In thin gingival areas such as thin

biotypes, a gold hue will provide better esthetics than a silver or gray alloy. An advantage of the metallic abutments is the resistance to fracture when preparation requires very thin walls on the abutment.

Cement-Retained or Screw-Retained Crowns

In the esthetic zone, screw access holes are very difficult to hide, but screw retention allows retrievability. Cement-retained crowns look, feel, and function like natural teeth, but they sacrifice retrievability. A provisional cement could be utilized, but provisional cement use may lead to premature cement failure. Literature continues to document successful use of definitive crown and bridge luting cements on implant restorations (Taylor 2005). All-ceramic crowns should be cemented due to the integrity of the ceramic material being compromised by the sharp angles inherent to the shape of a screw-retained restoration. The conceptual need of retrievability with regard to single crowns is debatable. If a single implant-supported crown fails due

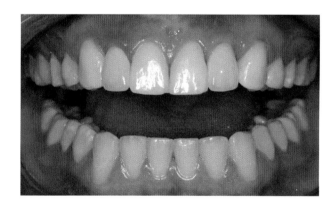

Figure 9-93. Posttreatment restorations.

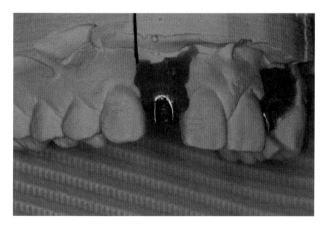

Figure 9-92. Pretreatment abutment position.

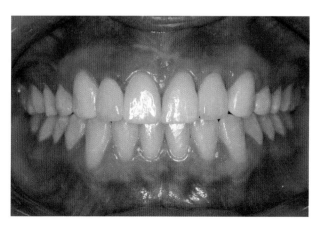

Figure 9-94. Posttreatment restorations in maximum intercuspation.

to fracture, it should be replaced as a crown on a natural tooth would be replaced (Taylor 2005). If resistance and retention of the cement-retained crown are compromised by the shape of the abutment, using a lingual horizontal set screw is an option to provide the resistance and retention.

All-Ceramic or Metal-Ceramic Crowns

All-ceramics will look the best by the translucent nature of the restorative material and are the material of choice if the prosthetic space allows. Some occlusal schemes such as deep, impinging occlusions and/or tooth anatomy do not allow the adequate prosthetic room required for the all-ceramic restoration. If the restoration must be screw retained for retention or a deep impinging occlusion precludes the use of all-ceramic crowns, then metal-ceramic crowns must be utilized. Additionally, if a fixed partial denture is treatment planned, a metal framework may be indicated for durability, although the use of zirconium oxide fixed partial denture frameworks is available in limited edentulous spans (Taylor 2005). Finally, if adjacent existing restorations are metal-ceramic, then best matching will be achieved with like materials.

Works Cited

Academy of Prosthodontics. 2005. Glossary of prosthodontic terms, 8th ed. *J Prosthet Dent* 94(1):21–22.

Allen E, Miller P. 1989. Coronal positioning of existing gingiva: Short-term results in the treatment of shallow marginal tissue recession. *J Periodont* 60(6):316–319.

Armellini D, von Fraunhofer, Anthony. 2004. The shortened dental arch: A review of the literature. *J Prosthodont* 92(6):531–35.

Baba K, Tsukiyama Y, Clark G. 2000. Reliability, validity and utility of various occlusal measurement methods and techniques. *J Prosthet Dent* 83:83–89.

Becker W, Oschenbien C, Becker B. 1998. Crown lengthening: The restorative connection. *Compendium* 19:239–254.

Braly B. 1972. Occlusal analysis and treatment planning for restorative dentistry. *J Prosthet Dent* 27:168–171.

Brigante R. 1981. Patient assisted esthetics. *J Prosthet Dent* 46(1):143–147.

Budtz-Jorgensen, Bocht, Grundman, Borgis. 2000. Aesthetic considerations for the treatment of partially edentulous patients with removable dentures. *Pract Periodontics Aesthet Dent* 12(8):765–72.

Buser D, Dula K, Belser U, Hirt H-P, Berthold H. 1995. Localized ridge augmentation using guided bone regeneration: Part II. Surgical procedure in the mandible. *Internat J Periodontics Restorative Dent* 15:11–29.

Carlsson G, Thilander H, Hedegard G. 1967. Histological changes in the upper alveolar process after extractions with or without insertion of an immediate full denture. *Acta Odontol Scand* 25:1–31.

Carlsson G, Ingervall B, Kocak G. 1979. Effect of increasing vertical dimension on the masticatory system in subjects with natural teeth. *J Prosthet Dent* 41:284–289.

Carr A, McGivney G, Brown D. 2005. *Removable Partial Prosthodontics*, 11th ed. St. Louis, MO: Elsevier Mosby.

Chin M. 1998. The role of distraction osseogenesis in oral and maxillofacial surgery. *J Oral Maxillofacial Surg* 56:805–6.

Cho G. 2004. Evidence-based approach for treatment planning options for extensively damaged dentitions. *J Calif Dent Assoc* 32(12):983–90.

Clark G, Tsukiyama Y, Baba K, Simmons M. 1997. The validity and utility of disease detecting methods and of occlusal therapy for temporomandibular disorders. *Oral Surg Oral Med Oral Path* 83:101–6.

Dawson PE. 2007. *Functional Occlusion: From TMJ to Smile Design*. St. Louis, MO: Mosby.

Dolt A. 1997. Altered passive eruption: An etiology of short clinical crowns. *Quintessence Internat* 28:363–72.

Eissmann H, Radke R, Noble W. 1971. Physiologic design criteria for fixed dental restorations. *Dent Clinics North America* 15(3):543–68.

Feine JS, Heydicke G. 2003. Implant overdentures versus conventional dentures. In *Implant Overdentures: The Standard of Care*, Feine JS, Carlsson G, eds., 37–45. Carol Stream, IL: Quintessence.

Frias VS, Toothaker R, Wright R. 2004. Shortened dental arch: A review of the current treatment concepts. *J Prosthodont* 13(2):104–10.

Gargiulo A, Wentz F, Orban B. 1961. Dimensions and relations of the dento-gingival junction in humans. *J Periodont* 32:261–67.

Gunay H, Seeger A, Tschernitschek H, Geurtsen, W. 2000. Placement of the preparation line and periodontal health: A prospective 2-year clinical study. *Internat J Periodontal Restorative Dent* 20(2):173–81.

Hickey J, Williams B, Woelfel J. 1961. Stability of mandibular rest position. *J Prosthet Dent* 11:566–72.

Hwang D, Wang H-L. 2006. Flap thickness as a predictor of root coverage: A systemic review. *J Periodontol* 77(10):1625–34.

Jankelson B, Sparks S, Crane P, Radke J. 1995. Neural conduction of the Myomonitor stimulus: A quantitative analysis. *J Prosthet Dent* 34:245–53.

Jepson N, Allen F, Moynihan P, Kelly F. 2003. Patient satisfaction following restoration of shortened dental arches in a randomized controlled trial. *Internat J Prosthodon.* 16:409–14.

Kampen F van, Cune M, Vanderbilt A, Bosman F. 2003. Retention and post- insertion maintenance of bar-clip, ball and magnet attachments in mandibular overdenture treatment: An in vivo comparison after 3 months of function. *Clin Oral Implants Res* 14(6):720–26.

Kao R, Pasquinelli Kirk. 2002. Thick vs. thin gingival tissue: A key determinant in tissue response to disease and restorative treatment. *J Calif Dent Assoc* 30:521–26.

Keough B. 1992. Occlusal considerations in periodontal prosthetics. *Int J Periodontics Restorative Dent* 12:359–71.

Keough B. 2003. Occlusion-based treatment planning for complex dental restorations: Part I. *Int J Periodontics Restorative Dent* 23:237–47.

Kois J. 1998. Esthetic extraction site development: The biologic variables. *Contemp Esthetics Restorative Practice* 2:10–18.

Kois J. 2001. Predictable single tooth peri-implant esthetics: Five diagnostic keys. *Compendium* 22:199–206.

Kokich V. 1996. Esthetics: the orthodontic-periodontic-restorative connection. *Semin Orthodont* 2:21–30.

Krol A, Jacobsen T, Finzen F. 1999. *Removable Partial Denture Design Outline Syllabus*, 5ᵗʰ ed. San Rafael, CA: Indent.

Langer B, Calagna L. 1980. Subepithelial grafts to correct ridge concavities. *J Prosthet Dent* 44:363–70.

Miller PD, Allen EP. 1996. The development of periodontal plastic surgery, *Periodont 2000* 11:7–17.

Mojon P. 2003. The world without teeth: Demographic trends. In *Implant Overdentures: The Standard of Care*, Feine JS, Carlsson GE, eds., 3–14. Carol Stream, IL: Quintessence.

Murphy T. 1959. Compensating mechanisms in facial height adjustment to functional tooth attrition. *Aust Dent J* 4:312.

Nevins M, Skuro H. 1984. The intra-cervicular restorative margin, the biologic width and the maintenance of the gingival margin. *Internat J Periodontics Restorative Dentistry* 4(3):30–49.

Pasquinelli K. 2005. Periodontal plastic surgery as an adjunctive therapeutic modality for esthetic restorative dentistry. *J Calif Dent Assoc.* 35(3):217–21.

Petropoulos V, Smith W, Kousvelari E. 1997. Comparison of retention and release periods for implant overdenture attachments. *Internat J Oral Maxillofacial Implants* 12(2):176–85.

Ramfjord S, Engler W, Hiniker J. 1966. A radioautographic study of healing following simple gingivectomy: Part II. The connective tissue. *J Periodont* 37:179–89.

Rieder C. 1978. The prevalence and magnitude of mandibular displacement in a survey population. *J Prosthet Dent* 39:324–29.

Rivera-Morales W, Mohl N. 1991a. Relationship of vertical dimension to the health of the masticatory system. *J Prosthet Dent* 65:547–53.

Rivera-Morales W, Mohl N. 1991b. Variables in closest speaking space compared with interocclusal distance in dentulous subjects. *J Prosthet Dent* 65:228–32.

Robbins W. 1999. Differential diagnosis and treatment of excess gingival display. *Prac Periodontal Aesthetic Dent* 11:265–72.

Rosenberg ES, Simons J, Gualini F. 1987. Clinical aspects and treatment of posterior bite collapse due to accelerated wear. *Int J Periodontics Restorative Dent* 17:67–82.

Rugh J, Drago C. 1981. Vertical dimension: A study of clinical rest position and jaw muscle activity. *J Prosthet Dent* 45:670–75.

Sadowsky S. 2001. Mandibular implant-retained overdentures: A literature review, *J Prosthet Dent* 86(5):468–473.

Schropp L, Wenzel A, Kostopoulos L, Karring T. 2003. Bone healing and soft tissue uniform changes following single-tooth extraction: A clinical and radiographic 12-month prospective study. *Internat J Periodontics Restorative Dent* 23:313–23.

Seibert J. 1983. Reconstruction of deformed partially edentulous ridges using full thickness onlay grafts: Part I. Technique and wound healing. *Compend Contin Educ Dent* 4:437–53.

Shillingburg H, Hobo S, Whitsett L, Jacobi R, Brackett S. 1997. *Fundamentals of Fixed Prosthodontics*, 3ʳᵈ ed. Chicago: Quintessence.

Spear FM. 1997. Fundamentals of occlusal therapy considerations. In *Science and Practice of Occlusion*, McNeill C, ed., 421–434. Chicago: Quintessence.

Staubli P. 1996. *Attachments and Implants Reference Manual*, 6ᵗʰ ed. San Mateo, CA: Attachments International.

Tallgren A. 1951. Changes in adult face height due to aging, wear and loss of teeth and prosthetic treatment. *Acta Odontol Scand* 15(Suppl. 24):1–122.

Tarnow. 1994. Solving restorative esthetic dilemmas with semilunar coronally positioned flap. *J Esthet Dent* 6(2):61–64.

Taylor TD. 2005. Evidence based considerations for removable prosthodontic and dental implant occlusion: A literature review. *Journal of Prosthetic Dentistry* no. 15:20–24.

Tjan AH, Miller GD. 1984. The esthetic factors in a smile. *Journal of Prosthet Dent* 51(1):24–28.

Tolman D. 1995. Reconstrutive procedures with endosseous implants in grafted bone: A review of the literature. *Internat J Oral Maxillofacial Implant* 10:275–94.

Waal H de, Castellucci G. 1994. The importance of restorative margin placement to the biologic width and periodontal health: Part II. *Internat J Periodontics Restorative Dent* 14(1):70–83.

Weber HP, Sukotjo C. 2007. Does the type of implant prosthesis affect outcomes in the partially edentulous patient? *Internat J Oral Maxillofacial Implants* 22(Suppl):140–70.

Wostmann B, Jorgensen E-B, Jepson N, Mushimoto E, Palmqvist S, Sofou A, Owall B. 2005. Indications for removable partial dentures: A literature review. *Internat J Prosthodont* 6.

Zarb GA. 1978. *Prosthodontic Treatment for the Partially Edentulous Patient*. St. Louis, MO: Mosby.

Zarb G. 1997. Biomechanics of the edentulous state. In *Prosthodontics: Treatment for Edentulous Patients*, 11ᵗʰ ed., Zarb G, Bolender C, Carlsson G, eds., 8–29, St. Louis, MO; Mosby.

Suggested Additional Reading

Aghaloo T, Moy P. 2007. Which hard tissue augmentation techniques are the most successful in furnis hing bony support for implant placement. *Internat J Oral Maxillofacial Implant* 22(Suppl):49–70.

Camargo P, Melnick P, Camargo L. 2007. Clinical crown lengthening in the esthetic zone. *J Calif Dent Assoc* 35(7): 487–98.

Pasquinelli K. 1999. Periodontal plastic surgery. *J Calif Dent Assoc* 27:597–610.

Chapter 10
Direct Restorative Materials

Karen A. Schulze DDS, PhD

Mark Macaoay DDS, BS

Jeffrey P. Miles DDS

The growing demand for esthetic results has changed the way dentistry is practiced in the twenty-first century. While amalgam is still an economically and clinically adequate restorative material, concerns over esthetics, alleged toxicity, environmental concerns, lack of bonding, and the need for aggressive tooth preparation have made composites a popular alternative for restoring missing tooth structure.

Dental composites have advantages as a restorative material in terms of esthetics, conservation of tooth structure, adhesion to tooth structure, and low thermal conductivity. However, modern composites have failed to completely replace amalgam due to decreased wear resistance, a tendency for water sorption, inconsistent dentin adhesion, variable conversion, and most important, polymerization shrinkage. These negative factors can lead to recurrent caries, postoperative sensitivity, and staining at the margins. Controlled studies have shown that most of these drawbacks can be overcome with meticulous isolation and placement technique (Leinfelder 1995; Lutz 1995).

A variety of materials are available for use as direct dental restorative material: resin composites, glass-ionomers, and hybrid materials that combine substances from both resin composites as well as glass-ionomers. Among these materials, composite resins occupy a paramount position. This chapter will describe the dental hard tissue and its ability to form a bond with restorative materials. Adhesive systems, a variety of restorative materials, and light-curing devices will be discussed as well.

Fundamental Concepts of Enamel and Dentin Adhesion

To understand the goals and difficulties of adhering esthetic materials to tooth structure, one must have a general knowledge of the composition of dental hard tissues.

Characteristics of Enamel, Dentin, and Cementum

Enamel, dentin, and cementum possess very different organic and inorganic components. Enamel has the highest density (2.8–3.0 g/cc) and the highest percentage (93–98%) of inorganic material by weight. Enamel mainly consists of calcium, phosphorus, carbon, magnesium, and sodium. Enamel contains between 1.5% and 4% water and between 0.5% and 3% organic material by weight, including proteins, lipids, citrate, lactate, and carbohydrates (figs. 10-1a and 10-1b; Provenza and Seibel 1986; Kinney, Marshall, and Marshall 2003). Dentin, in contrast, is a living but less mineralized tissue, containing only 60%–70% inorganic materials by weight. The organic substrate (20%–30% by weight) is primarily composed of collagen (fig. 10-2). Dentin also contains approximately 10% water (Marshall et al. 1997).

Enamel resists occlusal forces but is brittle and easily fractured, while dentin is flexible but not wear resistant. Together they form a "composite" structure unique to teeth (Kraus, Jordan, and Abrams 1969; Habelitz et al. 2001).

Cementum covers the anatomic root and partially covers the apical walls of the root canal. The structure and hardness are similar to human bone, but it lacks vascularity (30–50 KHN). It is the least mineralized dental hard tissue. The inorganic content is about 65% by weight. The organic matrix is about 23% by weight, and the remaining 10% is water. The organic matrix is composed of approximately 90% collagen by weight. The coronal portion of the root is layered with noncellular cementum while the apical region is covered with cellular cementum. It is continually rebuilt throughout life, being applied in layers (Ho et al. 2007).

Enamel Conditioning and Bonding

The first step of the bonding procedure is conditioning the enamel with phosphoric acid. This results in a frosty-looking surface. Conditioning increases the enamel's

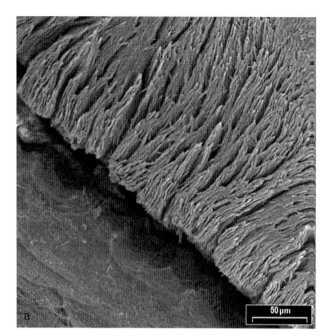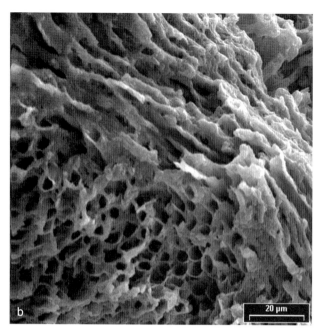

Figure 10-1.   a. Scanning electron microscope (SEM) image showing enamel rods etched with 10% phosphoric acid running from the dentin enamel junction to the outer surface of the tooth. Because of the acid treatment, a gap is formed at the dentin enamel junction, exposing the dentin with a scalloped surface. b. Hunter-Schreger bands after etching enamel with 10% phosphoric acid. They represent areas of enamel rods cut in cross-sections dispersed between areas of rods cut longitudinally (Courtesy of Dr. Stefan Habelitz).

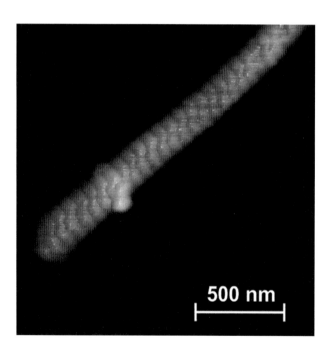

Figure 10-2.   Atomic force microscopy image of a single dentinal collagen fibril in air after 10% citric acid etching. Note the unique periodicity pattern and an attachment of organic or inorganic nature.

surface energy ("wetability") and the surface area by creating microretentive zones. The amount of inorganic material removed depends on acid concentration, duration of the etching process, and the chemical composi-

tion of the etchant (Buonocore 1955; Brudevold, Buonocore, and Wileman 1956). Low-viscosity bonding materials penetrate the microporosities and result in micromechanical retention. Basically, the main bonding mechanism of current resin adhesives can be regarded as an exchange process involving substitution of inorganic tooth material by resin monomers that, upon setting, become micromechanically interlocked in the enamel surface (Van Meerbeek, Vargas, and Inoue 2001). This bond to enamel not only effectively seals the restoration margin, it also protects the more vulnerable bond to dentin against degradation (De Munck et al. 2003).

Dentin Conditioning and Bonding

Opening the dentin tubules by conditioning results in direct contact with the pulp through liquid in the dentinal tubules (figs. 10-3a, 10-3b, 10-3c, and 10-3d). The primary purpose of dentin bonding is to seal the dentinal tubules and establish as tenacious a bond as possible between the restorative materials and dentin. Secondarily, the pulp should not be irritated by the bonding material and microleakage—including bacterial invasion—should not occur. The bonding zone should resist occlusal forces and chemical attacks in the oral cavity. The bonding procedure should not be technique sensitive. The materials should be easy to handle,

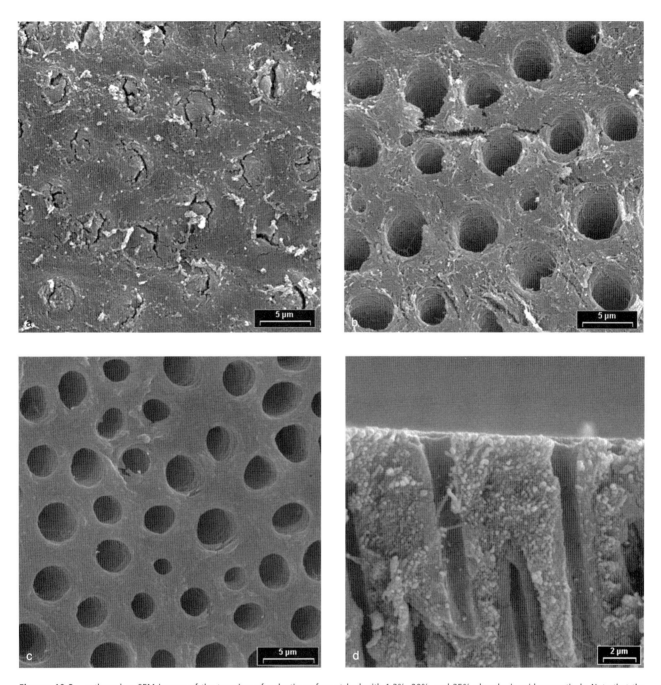

Figures 10-3. a through c. SEM images of the top view of a dentin surface etched with 1.3%, 20%, and 35% phosphoric acid, respectively. Note that the dentin tubules are opened completely when etched with 35% phosphoric acid (Courtesy of Dr. Sofia Oliveira). d. Side view of etched dentin. The smear layer has been removed using 35% phosphoric acid.

require little time to apply, and provide consistent results (Schulze et al. 2005).

Instrumentation of the dentin and removal of decay creates a smear layer, which can be a barrier to dentin bonding. Historically, any attempt to bond onto or through the smear layer has resulted in lower average bond strengths compared to "conditioned" dentin sur-

faces. Therefore, acids were introduced as a simple method of removing the smear layer (Buonocore 1955). In the "total-etch" technique, acid is applied to dentin and enamel for the same amount of time. Due to varying amounts of solubility between enamel and dentin, ideal etching with 35% phosphoric acid requires approximately 30 seconds of contact time for enamel and 20

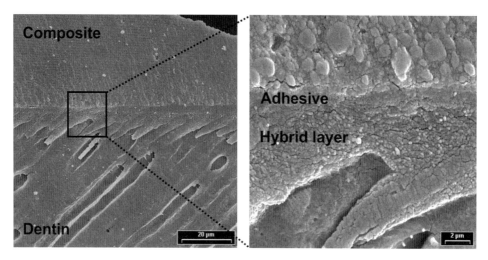

Figure 10-4. Cross-sectional SEM image of a dentin-composite bonding interface. Single Bond (3M ESPE) was the bonding material and Z100 (3M ESPE) the composite. The enlarged area illustrates the bonding interface with a hybrid layer formation.

seconds for dentin. Manufacturers of bonding systems are aware of this and make every attempt to manufacture materials that work well with both enamel and dentin.

The etching process removes the smear layer and some hydroxylapatite, uncovering a collagen network. Since the dentin tubules contain liquid (primarily water), a hydrophilic monomer is more likely to penetrate into the tubules and the collagen network. This action creates a hybrid layer, first described by Nakabayashi, Kojima, and Masuhara in 1982 (fig. 10-4). About 5 to 10 μm of the dentin surface are demineralized, and up to 30 μm of the collagen network is exposed after acid etching. The goal is to penetrate the entire etched surface with adhesive monomers.

The application of a hydrophilic primer prepares the dentin and the collagen network for the adhesive (Roulet and Degrange 2000). It keeps the dentin surface moist and prevents the collagen fibers from collapsing. The application of the methacrylate-containing adhesive creates the chemical link to the hydrophobic composite. The low viscosity of the adhesive coupled with the application pressure forces the adhesive into the tubules. After light curing, resin tags are formed. Neither the thickness of the hybrid layer nor the length of the resin tags seems to play an important role in bond strength (Yoshiyama et al. 1995).

Adhesive Systems

The first-generation adhesive systems, introduced in the early 1960s, were composed of polyurethanes, cyanoacrylates, glycerophosphoric acid dimethacrylate, N-phenyl glycine, and glycidylmethacrylate. Due to very low bond strengths (2 megapascals [MPa] on average), these systems were not clinically successful. Twenty years later the second-generation adhesives were introduced, containing bis-GMA esters designed to adhere to the phosphate-calcium bonds in the minerals of dentin. Although the initial bond strength increased to approximately 9 MPa on average, the bond hydrolyzed over time and the composite restorations failed. In 1982, Bowen, Cobb, and Rapson introduced the third-generation dentin bonding systems containing oxalates, which achieved an average bond to dentin of 21 MPa (near that of the bond between enamel and composite). Although these systems represented a significant improvement over their predecessors, their clinical performance was not satisfactory (Bowen et al. 1982).

Fourth-generation dentin bonding agents showed promising results. Clinical procedures were simplified by etching the enamel and dentin simultaneously with the total-etch technique. These three component systems required the separate application of a primer and an adhesive following the etching process. These systems improved dentin bond strengths and reduced pulpal irritation (fig. 10-5; Summitt et al. 2006).

The fifth-generation bonding systems represent a simplified version of the fourth-generation bonding system. Like all previous systems, conditioning of dentinal surface is accomplished by acid-etching. The main difference with these systems is that the primer and the adhesives are combined into a single component. Generally, these systems use two layers of a combined primer and adhesive, the first layer acting as a primer on the etched surface and the second layer bringing the adhesive monomers into the tubules (fig. 10-6). Some fifth-generation materials require only one layer of this

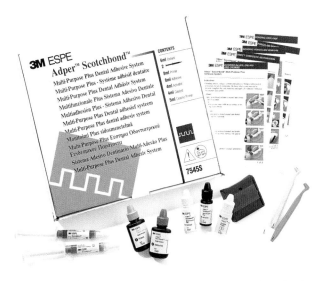

Figure 10-5. Three-step etch-and-rinse adhesive: Adper Scotchbond Multi-Purpose, 3M ESPE (fourth-generation bonding agent).

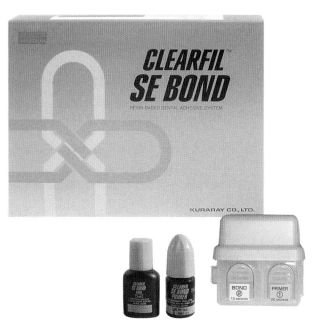

Figure 10-7. Two-step etch adhesive: Clearfil SE Bond, Kuraray America (sixth-generation bonding agent).

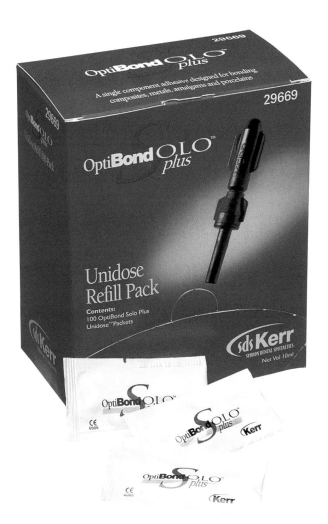

Figure 10-6. Two-step etch-and-rinse adhesive: Optibond Solo Plus, Kerr Corporation (fifth-generation bonding agent).

combined primer and adhesive. These systems require that the dentinal surface remains moist after conditioning to ensure good bonding and reduce the potential for postoperative sensitivity.

The sixth generation consists of a self-etching primer and an adhesive. These systems combine the etching and priming process with the application of their first component. No separate acid-etching is necessary. The self-etching primer conditions and primes the dentin through the use of an acidic monomer (pH 2). After application, the first component is not rinsed off, allowing the clinician to continue with the application of the adhesive to establish a hybrid layer (fig. 10-7).

The seventh-generation dentin bonding can be described as all-in-one systems. These products usually consist of packages with two compartments that must be combined, mixed, and immediately applied to the dentin surface. With these materials, conditioning, priming, and adhesion are accomplished in one step (fig. 10-8). Generally, these bonding systems have a higher film thickness than their predecessors, which may present a problem for bonding indirect restorations. Because these systems are so new and lack long-term research, caution is recommended until studies have established long-term clinical efficacy.

Although one-step adhesives are the simplest to use, their adhesive performance is less than that of multistep adhesives, exhibiting lower bond strength and durability, phase separation, enhanced water sorption, and reduced shelf life. (Van Landuyt et al. 2007)

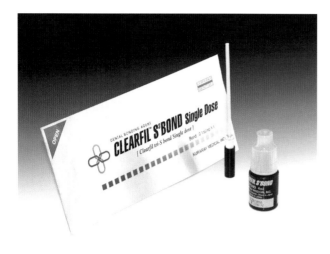

Figure 10-8. One-step self-etch adhesive: Clearfil S3 Bond, Kuraray America (seventh-generation bonding agent).

After aging, three-step total-etch adhesives maintain the best bonding integrity, and they remain the gold standard among adhesives, despite the rather elaborate and lengthy procedures required (Shirai et al. 2005). Table 10-1 displays the recent classification of adhesive systems adapted from Van Meerbeek (2008). To establish a bond with the underlying intact dentin, there are basically two options: (1) removal of the smear layer prior to bonding with an etch-and-rinse procedure, or (2) use of an adhesive system that can penetrate beyond the smear layer while incorporating it following a self-etch approach. Diffusion is the primary mechanism to obtain such micromechanical retention. However, no matter how splendid the shape and color, a satisfactory composite filling does not last long without a solid bond to the remaining tooth structure.

Composites

Modern dental composites consist of three major components modified with other compounds that aid or initiate the polymerization process and preserve the shelf life of the product. The three major components are filler, matrix, and coupler. Each composite system uses different formulations of these individual components to achieve various characteristics. This allows the clinician to choose specific products indicated for each specific lesion location, lesion size, occlusal load, and individual caries risk. The correct combination of filler, matrix, and coupler will have appropriate flow characteristics and optimum physical, thermal, and optical properties.

The filler is manufactured to an appropriate size for each intended application. The primary purpose of filler particles is to strengthen the composite and to reduce the amount of matrix material. Though not taking part in the polymerization reaction, the filler acts to increase hardness and wear resistance and to decrease polymerization shrinkage and water sorption while improving optical properties and viscosity. Commonly used fillers have extremely low coefficients of thermal expansion, greatly reducing the stresses between the restoration and tooth structure. Diagnostic sensitivity has improved through the incorporation of radiopaque compounds.

Composite systems contain fillers such as quartz, colloidal silica, or silica glass containing barium, strontium, other radiopaque particles or resin compounds. Filler particles are produced by grinding quartz or glass to particles in the range of 0.1–100 microns. Submicron silica particles are created by a process in which a silicon compound is fired in an oxygenated environment to form large chains of SiO_2 particles. The silica surfaces form bonds with the monomer molecules leading to a thicker resin paste. Because of this effect, the microfilled composites contain a small volume of colloidal silica as the inorganic component. The remainder is pulverized organic filler with particle sizes in the 5–30 micron range (Anusavice 2003).

The matrix of a composite system is a plastic resin material that binds the filler particles. This organic matrix generally includes bis-GMA (bisphenol A glycidylmethacrylate) or UDMA (urethane dimethacrylate), and TEGDMA (triethylene glycol dimethacrylate). While bis-GMA is generally the major component in the matrix phase of a composite system, other components are frequently used to decrease the viscosity of the composites and minimize polymerization shrinkage. The use of EBPADMA (ethoxylated bisphenol A dimethacrylate) has further decreased the water sorption characteristics of dental resins (Dhuru 2004). Consequently, it has been used as a partial or complete substitute for bis-GMA in newer composite systems (Sideridou and Achilias 2005).

Silane is the usual coupling agent linking filler to matrix. The use of silane reduces the gradual loss of the filler particles from the composite surface caused by occlusal wear and abrasion. Inorganic filler particles are coated with layers of liquid silane and blended with resin to create high bond strength and prevent water diffusion through the matrix-filler interface (Dhuru 2004). Chemically, one end of the silane molecule bonds to the filler while the other end couples with the resin. This adhesive bond allows for more durable, longer lasting restorations.

Initiators and accelerators activate and catalyze the polymerization reaction in composite systems. Light-cured composites commonly contain a photoinitiator called camphorquinone, activated by the 460–480 nm wavelength light emitted by visible light-curing units. The camphorquinone reacts with tertiary amines,

Table 10 1. Currently available dental adhesive systems.

4th Generation	5th Generation	6th Generation	7th Generation
3 steps	2 steps	2 steps	1 step
Etch+Prime+Bond	Etch+Bond (Priming incl.)	Prime (Etching incl.)+Bond	Bond (Etching+Priming incl.)
Adper™ Scotchbond™ Multi-Purpose (Plus)[a]	Adper™ Scotchbond™ 1 XT Adhesive (Single Bond Plus)[a]	AdheSE®[n]	Absolute2[k]
ALL-BOND 2®[b]	Bond-1®[c]	Adper™ Scotchbond™ SE[a]	AdheSE® One[n]
ALL-BOND 3™[b]	Clearfil® Photo Bond[d]	ALL-BOND SE™ (including ALL-BOND SE™ Liner)[b]	Admira® Bond[m]
Bond-It®[c]	Clearfil® New Bond[d]	Clearfil™ Liner Bond 2[d]	Adper™ Easy Bond[a]
Clearfil® Liner Bond[d]	Excite®[n]	Clearfil™ Liner Bond 2V[d]	Adper™ Prompt™ L-Pop™[a]
cmf adhesive system[e]	Excite® DSC[n]	Clearfil™ Protect Bond[d]	ALL-BOND SE™[b]
Ecusit®-Primer/Mono[f]	Gluma® Comfort Bond[g]	Clearfil™ SE Bond[d]	AQ Bond[p]
Gluma® Solid Bond[g]	Gluma® One Bond[g]	Contax®[f]	Tokuyama® Bond Force[s]
OptiBond®[h]	Go![i]	FL-Bond[r]	Clearfil® S3 Bond[d]
OptiBond FL®[h]	Heliobond[n]	Frog[i]	Futurabond NR[m]
Paama 2[i]	One Coat® Bond[o]	Microbond/Microbond Duo[e]	G-BOND[t]
PermaQuick[j]	ONE-STEP®[b]	Nano-Bond®[c]	Hybrid Bond[p]
ProBOND®[k]	ONE-STEP® PLUS[b]	One Coat Self Etching Bond[o]	iBond®[g]
Quadrant UniBond[l]	OptiBond® Solo Plus[h]	ONE-STEP PLUS®/TYRIAN™ SPE[b]	James-2[e]
Solobond Plus[m]	OptiBond® Solo Plus™/Dual Cure[h]	Peak™ Self-Etch[i]	OptiBond® All-In-One[h]
Syntac®[n]	Peak LC Bond[i]	Tokuso® Mac Bond II[s]	One-Up® Bond F[s]
	Polibond[m]	Unifil® Bond[t]	One-Up® Bond F Plus[s]
	Prime & Bond® NT™[k]		Reactmer Bond[r]
	Prime & Bond® NT™ Dual Cure[k]		Tyrian™ SPE[b]
	PQ1[i]		Xeno® III[k]
	Quadrant Uni-1-Bond[l]		Xeno® IV[k]
	Solist®[f]		Xeno® V[k]
	Solobond M[m]		
	Stae[i]		
	Super-Bond C&B[p]		
	TECO™[q]		
	XP BOND™[k]		

[a] 3M ESPE, St. Paul, MN

[b] BISCO Inc, Schaumburg, IL

[c] Pentron Clinical Technologies, Wallingford, CT

[d] Kuraray America, Inc, New York, NY

[e] Saremco, Rebstein, Switzerland

[f] DMG, Hamburg, Germany

[g] Heraeus Kulzer, Armonk, NY

[h] Kerr Corporation, Orange, CA

[i] SDI Limited, Bensenville, IL

[j] Ultradent Products, Inc., South Jordan, UT

[k] DENTSPLY International, York, PA

[l] Cavex Holland BV, Haarlem, Holland

[m] VOCO America, Sunnyside, NY

[n] Ivoclar Vivadent, Amherst, NY

[o] Coltène/Whaledent, Cuyahoga Falls, OH

[p] Sun Medical Co, Shiga, Japan

[q] Zenith/DMG, Englewood, NJ

[r] Shofu Dental Corporation, San Marcos, CA

[s] Tokuyama Dental Corp., Tokyo, Japan

[t] GC America, Alsip, IL

Reprinted from Van Meerbeek, B. 2008. With permission from AEGIS Publications, LLC.

Note: This list represents a sampling of available products.

leading to a free radical reaction that continues until the resin is fully polymerized.

Chemically activated (self-curing) composites contain a benzoyl peroxide (BP) initiator in one component and an aromatic tertiary amine activator in the other component. The amine reacts with the BP to form free radicals initiating polymerization.

Polymerization inhibitors and stabilizers are commonly added to composite systems for extended shelf life. Ultraviolet light–absorbing compounds provide increased working time for chemically activated resins.

Macrofilled Composites

Macrofilled (traditional) composites were some of the first composite systems produced. Their inorganic quartz or glass fillers consist of large particle sizes ranging from 15 to 100 μm at the first generation. These systems are difficult to polish, due to scattering of light from the relatively large surface particles. Over time, mastication and brushing wears away the resin matrix, exposing the more wear-resistant filler particles. These are then easily dislodged from the surface, leaving resin-lined pits to further scatter light and wear away in turn. Macrofilled composite restorations also tend toward discoloration and staining, caused in part by the rough-textured surface (Leinfelder 1993). The smaller particle size of modern products ranges between 1 and 10 μm. Macrofills are now used mainly for large buildups underneath extracoronal restorations due to their relatively high strength.

Microfilled Composites

Microfilled composites have low filler content with inorganic particles of submicron size. Problems of surface roughening and low translucency associated with macrofilled and small particle composites are overcome by the incorporation of sintered colloidal silica particles. Sintering helps to produce particles that are small enough for good polishability. Because of the small size of fillers, there is a large surface area of the filler in contact with the resin. This high surface area means that it is very difficult to obtain a high filler loading, as a large amount of resin is required to wet the surfaces of the fillers. To ensure adequate filler loading, additional pre-polymerized resin particles of 10–40 μm in size containing small colloidal silica particles are often incorporated (approx. 40% vol.). The main characteristics of these composites are the high polish that can be achieved and maintained over time and excellent enamel-like translucency. Unfortunately, these composites have a lower strength relative to other composites and are contraindicated for use in areas exposed to high occlusal or incisal forces. Inferior physical and mechanical properties are due to the fact that a higher percentage of the

composite is made up of resin. The larger amount of resin compared with inorganic filler also results in greater water sorption, a higher coefficient of thermal expansion, and decreased elastic modulus. Therefore, they are indicated for restorations of anterior teeth and cervical lesions. With the trend toward simplification, together with the search for universal materials and the evolution of hybrid materials, the use of microfilled composites will become more restricted.

Hybrid Composites

Hybrid composites, often called microhybrids, contain a blend of submicron (0.04 μm) and small particle fillers in micrometer range (0.2–5 μm). They are successfully used as universal composite since they combine not only different sizes of fillers but also different types of fillers: glass particles for good physical properties and SiO_2 particles for good polishability (fig. 10-9a,b; Gedik and

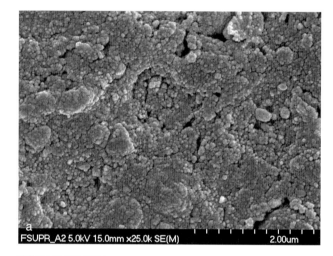

FSUPR_A2 5.0kV 15.0mm x25.0k SE(M)   2.00um

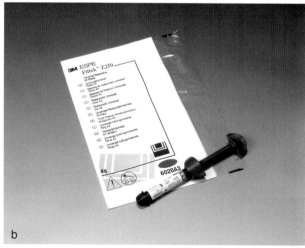

Figure 10-9. a. SEM image of the topographic surface from a hybrid composite: Filtec Supreme; note the different sizes of filler particles (Courtesy of 3M ESPE). b. Microhybrid composite Filtek Z250, 3M ESPE.

Hurmuzlu 2005). Regrettably, one problem with hybrid composite resins is their inability to maintain their gloss. Given the need for a highly polishable composite resin with optimal physical properties for use in the anterior and posterior region, manufacturers developed micro-hybid composites. Microhybrid composites have a reduced particle size ranging from 0.04 μm to 1 μm and a high filler loading (more than 60% vol.). They polish and handle better than their hybrid counterparts and they are better universal or all-purpose composites. Physical and mechanical properties for these systems generally fall between those of the macrofilled and SPF composites.

A more modern material is the *nanofilled composite*, but the fact that microfiller and submicron filler are combined is not new (Tian and Gao 2007). The monomer matrix usually contains filler 3 to 10 micrometers in size to resist occlusal loading in molar regions and nano-sized fillers for improved surface quality. The nanofilled composites, recommended mostly for universal applications, provide excellent esthetic results (fig. 10-10).

Specialized Composites

Packable and flowable composites were developed in response to requests from dental practitioners for composites with special handling properties.

Packable Composites
Packable composites (once inaccurately called condensables) have characteristics that are derived from alteration of the filler loading or the resin matrix. The increased viscosity can be accomplished in a number of ways:

- By increasing the filler particle size range
- By modification of the filler particle shape such that the particles have a tendency to interlock
- By modification of the resin matrix such that stronger intermolecular attractions are created
- By the addition of dispersants, which lower the viscosity and allow an increase in filler loading

Packable composites have not met expectations as far as improved wear resistance, nor ease of placement in posterior preparations (Yip and Poon 2003). They continue to exhibit the unwanted composite characteristics of polymerization shrinkage and a fairly shallow depth of cure (Petersen 2005).

Flowable Composites
Flowable composites have reduced filler content providing a consistency that allows the material to intimately adapt to a preparation form (fig. 10-11). The shortcomings of these materials, such as decreased wear resistance and higher polymerization shrinkage, should not affect the results when used only for selected treatments. However, the resulting lower viscosity makes the material extremely useful in tight marginal areas or cavities with an undercut that is difficult to fill with composites. They can also be used to close an endodontic access and for class V restorations. Another useful application is for preventive restorations in areas too large to be restored with fissure sealants.

Polymerization Shrinkage

Polymerization shrinkage, which can be as much as 7%, is a major hurdle in composite systems. Volumetric shrinkage in adhesive restorations causes stress that may lead to cracking and crazing of tooth structure or warping of the restoration, potentially leading to gap formation, microleakage, sensitivity, margin staining, and recurrent caries. While enamel bevels, incremental

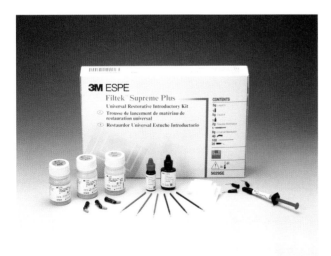

Figure 10-10.   Universal nanocomposite Filtek Supreme Plus, 3M ESPE.

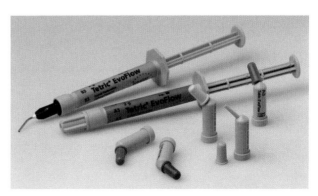

Figure 10-11.   Flowable composite Tetric EvoFlow, Ivoclar Vivadent.

curing techniques, and ramped light curing have been suggested to minimize shrinkage, most tests have shown them to have no significant effect on overall shrinkage or stress within the tooth and restoration (Kuijs and Fennis 2003; Giachetti and Russo 2006). Since filler particles do not contribute to polymerization shrinkage, the higher the filler loading, the less shrinkage occurs (Fortin and Vargas 2000). Although increasing the molecular weight of a monomer reduces curing shrinkage and improves mechanical properties, it also increases viscosity. Thus it is necessary to use lower molecular weight monomers to dilute bis-GMA. This allows a sufficiently high filler level while producing resin pastes with consistencies suitable for clinical manipulation. Balancing polymerization shrinkage, wear resistance, and manipulation properties remains a challenge for composite manufacturers.

Forces developed by polymerization contraction create stress in the dental structure as well as the restoration. The interruption of the adhesive bond takes place in the zones where the bond is weakest, and the contraction forces tend to destroy the adhesive interface, creating conditions for recurrent caries, postoperative sensitivity, and pulpal pathology (Albers 2001).

Composite activated by a light source initiates a chemical reaction that does not terminate with the elimination of light but continues for over twenty-four hours. Elimination of the polymerization stresses cannot be achieved completely but can be minimized. The larger the cavity, the larger the stress, and even with a layering technique using numerous increments of material, part of the forces generated remain beyond our control.

Biocompatibility

For the present, it is believed that the safety of composite resins should not be of concern to the general public. Composites are believed to release some components and breakdown products to the oral environment including uncured resins, diluents, additives, plasticizers, and initiators, amounts depending on the degree of cure. Cytotoxicity has been demonstrated in vitro. Delayed hypersensitivity reactions have been reported but are very rare, probably due to the small amount of chemicals released.

Water Sorption and Solubility

The water sorption, occurring mainly by direct absorption into the resin component of the composite, depends on the resin content and the quality of the bond between the resin and the filler (table 10-2). Excessive water sorption has a detrimental effect on color stability and wear resistance. A composite that absorbs water will also absorb other fluids from the oral cavity, resulting in discoloration.

Mechanical Properties

Polishability is improved by the incorporation of softer glass fillers of a smaller size. Microfilled composites have the best esthetics due to their excellent polishability and their ability to retain surface smoothness over time.

Glass filler can be attacked over time by acidulated fluoride solutions or gels, gradually becoming more susceptible to abrasive wear and shortening its functional lifetime compared to silica-reinforced resins. See more properties in table 10-2.

Optical Properties

The translucency of a composite restoration is dependent on the index of refraction of all materials incorporated within it. A natural translucency results from a close match of index of refractions among the filler,

Table 10-2. Properties of composite restorative materials.

Characteristic/Property	Macrofilled (Traditional)	Hybrid	Microfilled	Flowable Hybrid	Packable Hybrid	Enamel	Dentin
Compressive strength (MPa)	250–300	300–400	250–350	—	—	384	297
Tensile strength (MPa)	50–65	40–90	30–50	—	40–45	10	52
Elastic modulus (GPa)	8–15	11–20	3–6	4–8	3–13	84	18
Thermal expansion coefficient (ppm/°C)	25–35	19–40	50–60	—	—	—	—
Water sorption (mg/cm^2)	0.5–0.7	0.5–0.7	1.4–1.7	—	—	—	—
Knoop hardness (KHN)	55	50–60	25–35	—	—	350–430	68
Curing shrinkage (vol%)	—	2–3	2–3	3–5	2–3	—	—
Radiopacity (mm Al)	2–3	2–4	0.5–2	1–4	2–3	2	1

Adapted with permission from Anusavice 2003.

resin, and tooth. Most bis-GMA and TEGDMA mixtures have been manufactured to exhibit similar refractive indices to glass and quartz fillers for optimal optical properties.

Discoloration of composites can manifest itself in one of three ways:

- Marginal discoloration is due to debris penetrating a marginal gap between the restoration and the tooth.
- Surface discoloration, related to the surface roughness, is more likely to occur with composites employing large filler particles.
- Bulk discoloration is a particular problem with chemically cured composites containing amines.

Radiopacity

To allow for accurate diagnosis of recurrent caries at the gingival margins of posterior composites, these restorative materials need to exhibit radiopacity at least equal to that of enamel.

Thermal Properties

Important thermal properties of composites include thermal expansion and thermal conductivity. Ideally, the thermal dimensional changes of restorative materials should approximate those of tooth structure to control marginal leakage and maintain enamel bonding. Modern composites have a coefficient of thermal expansion four to six times that of natural tooth structure, but because of their low thermal conductivity, deleterious

effects are not as great as previously expected (Powers and Hostetler 1979). While composite manufacturers have created materials with decreased filler content in an attempt to reduce viscosity, this also increases the coefficient of thermal expansion.

Polyacid-Modified Resin Composites (Compomers)

Compomers are essentially composite materials that have been modified to release fluoride over an extended period of time. In order to achieve this, some elements of glass-ionomer cements have been incorporated into composite resin. Compomers set mainly with a free radical polymerization reaction activated by blue light. However, they contain glass fillers, which are similar to the composition of the fluoride-containing glasses used in glass-ionomer cements (fig. 10-12). They are susceptible to acid attack and provide the source of fluoride ions. Water is absorbed into the material from the oral environment and allows an acid-base reaction between the glass and carboxyl groups on resin monomers. This provides for a slow but continuous release of fluoride, not previously possible with composite resin.

Properties of Polyacid-Modified Resin Composites

Compomers have a lower fluoride release profile than glass-ionomer cements and resin-modified glass-ionomer cements (Itota et al. 2004). Similar to resin composite materials, compomers have good handling

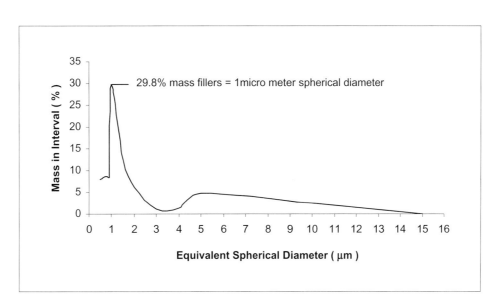

Figure 10-12.   Filler size versus the filler mass distribution of compomer filler particles from Dyract, Dentsply Caulk. Note: two main particle sizes, 1 μm and 5 μm, are present, with 0.5 μm the smallest and 15 μm the largest filler size.

characteristics, easily adapt to cavity walls without sticking to the placement instruments, are easy to shape, and do not slump. The polymerization shrinkage and water sorption tendencies are similar to that of composites. Where the compomer differs from the composite is the rate of water uptake. The hydrophilic resin matrix in a compomer provides a more rapid pathway for the absorption of water, with equilibrium being reached in a matter of days rather than weeks, months, or years for composites. The mechanical properties are inferior to that of the composite resin, with a reduced compressive,

diametral, and flexural strength (Schulze, Soederholm, and Zaman 2003). Therefore, compomers do not have the same range of applications as composite resins; in fact, the range of applications is similar to that of glass-ionomer cements and resin-modified glass-ionomer cements. Their use is limited to low-stress-bearing situations such as class V lesions, permanent restorations in the primary dentition, and long-term temporaries in the permanent dentition (see table 10-3; Krämer et al. 2006; Pascon et al. 2006; Gallo et al. 2005; Duggal, Toumba, and Sharma 2002).

Table 10-3. Examples of currently available restorative materials.

Resin Composites	Polyacid-Modified Resin Composites (Compomers)	Resin-Modified Glass-Ionomers	Glass-Ionomers
Microfilled	Dyract[®f]	Fuji™ II LC[l]	Ketac™ Molar[i]
Durafill® VS[a]	F-2000[i]	Fuji Filling™ LC[l]	Fuji IX GP[l]
Renamel® Microfill[b]	Compoglass[®e]	Photac™ Fil[i]	Ketac™ Fil[i]
Matrixx™ Anterior[c]		Vitremer™[i]	Ketac™ Silver[i]
EPIC®-TMPT[d]		Ketac™ Nano[i]	Fuji II™[i]
Helio Progress[®e]			Miracle Mix[®l]
Heliomolar[®e]			
Hybrid			
Spectrum® TPH[®f]			
Charisma[®a]			
Herculite XRV™[g]			
Renamel® Microhybrid[b]			
Tetric® Ceram[e]			
Venus[®a]			
Point 4™[g]			
Synergy® D6[h]			
Filtek™ Z250[i]			
Nanofilled			
Filtek™ Supreme Plus[i]			
Nanohybrid			
Premise[g]			
Aelite Aesthetic Enamel[j]			
Clearfil Majesty™ Esthetic[k]			

Note: List is not complete.

[a] Heraeus Kulzer Inc, Armonk, NY.

[b] Cosmedent, Inc, Chicago, IL.

[c] Discus Dental, Culver City, CA.

[d] Parkell, Inc, Edgewood, NY.

[e] Ivoclar Vivadent, Amherst, NY.

[f] DENTSPLY Caulk, Milford, DE.

[g] Kerr Corporation, Orange, CA.

[h] Coltène/Whaledent Inc, Cuyahoga Falls, OH.

[i] 3M ESPE, St. Paul, MN.

[j] BISCO Inc, Schaumburg, IL.

[k] Kuraray America, Inc, New York, NY.

[l] GC America Inc, Alsip, IL.

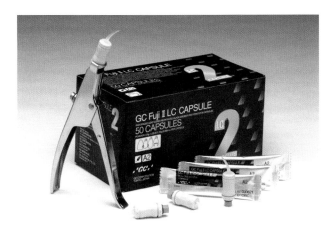

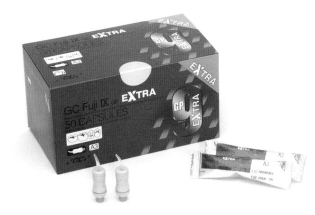

Figure 10-14. Glass-ionomer cement GC Fuji IX (GC America).

Figure 10-13. Resin-modified glass-ionomer GC Fuji II LC (GC America).

Resin-Modified Glass-Ionomer Cements

Resin-modified glass-ionomer cements (RMGIs) are a result of the manufacturer's attempt to improve the handling characteristics of regular glass-ionomer cements by incorporating visible light-curing resin (fig. 10-13).

The material is dispensed either in capsule form or as a powder-liquid system, the powder consisting of a radiopaque fluoro-alumino-silicate glass and the photoactive liquid kept in a dark bottle. The acid-base setting reaction, the same as for the glass-ionomer cements, is initiated when the powder and liquid are mixed. The material differs from other glass-ionomer cements in that this reaction is much slower, giving a considerably longer working time. A rapid set is initiated by ultraviolet light. Once mixed, the material polymerizes after 30 seconds of exposure to light. If not exposed to light, the material will eventually set in 15 to 20 minutes. It should be noted that these materials will continue to set via the acid-base reaction for some time after the polymerization process has been completed. Some RMGIs contain a chemical curing process, providing an activator and initiator in their two component systems. This has the advantage that if the light is not penetrating to the full depth of the restoration, the chemical reaction ensures full depth of cure of the resin component without the need for incremental placement.

Properties of RMGIs

RMGIs have the ability to release fluoride and bond to dentin and enamel (Forsten 1990; Forsten and Karjalainen 1990; Forsten 1995). In addition, they have prolonged working time and a rapid set once exposed to visible light. The restoration can be polished immedi-

ately. Their strength and resistance to desiccation and acid attack is believed to be better than glass-ionomer cements. RMGIs have been specifically designed as bases or liners for use under composites, amalgams, and ceramic restorations as well as direct restorative material for class V lesions (Burgess, Norling, and Summitt 1994; Uno, Finger, and Fritz 1996; McComb et al. 2002).

Glass-Ionomer Cements

Glass-ionomer cements (GICs) are valued as dental materials for their ability to bond to enamel and dentin and their ability to release fluoride. The main components of glass-ionomer cements are glass, poly-acid, tartaric acid, and water.

The glass can be made from a wide variety of materials allowing for a range of properties. The glasses contain three major components: silica (SiO_2), alumina (Al_2O_3), and a flux of calcium fluoride (CaF_2). This mixture together with other variable ingredients is fused at a high temperature, shock cooled, and finely ground to a powder. For restorative materials, the particle size ranges between 3 and 50 μm, while for the luting and lining materials it is reduced to less than 20 μm. The rate of release of ions from glass, which determines the setting, the solubility, and the release of fluoride, is a function of the type of glass employed.

Tartaric acid is an important component of the GIC, as it has a significant influence on the working and setting time. Many GICs consist of a glass powder and an aqueous solution of polyacrylic or poly-maleic acid and tartaric acid. More modern GICs are of the water-hardening type: the glass powder is blended with freeze-dried polyacid and tartaric acid and is mixed with a specified amount of distilled water. The difficulty of dispensing and mixing the correct amount of powder and liquid means that preproportioned capsules are preferable for consistency of performance (fig. 10-14).

The setting reaction of the GIC is via an acid-base reaction. The reaction involves three overlapping stages:

1. Dissolution
2. Gelation
3. Hardening

Dissolution starts when the liquid is mixed with the powder. The acids go into solution and react with the outer layer of the glass. The gelation phase—the initial setting—begins with the rapid action of the calcium ions, which, being divalent and more abundant initially, react more readily with the carboxyl groups of the acid than do the trivalent aluminum ions. Although the material appears hard at its initial setting time (3–7 minutes), it will continue to set for up to one month.

Properties of GICs

What makes the GICs most attractive is their ability to bond directly to dentin and enamel, even when placed in bulk. To obtain a good bond, the surface must first be treated with a conditioner to remove debris and to produce a clean, smooth surface. The best conditioner appears to be polyacrylic acid. The major limitation on the bond strength of GICs is their low tensile strength and low toughness.

The esthetic appearance of GIC has always been considered inferior to that of composite resin because of its greater opacity. The cements appear dull and lifeless, limiting their application in esthetic areas to class V and noncritical class III cavities (Abdalla, Alhadainy, and García-Godoy 1997; Loher, Kunzelman, and Hickel 1997). A loss of esthetic quality can also arise from staining, which, if excessive, could cause a restoration to be considered a clinical failure necessitating replacement. Staining around the margins has been found to be far less pronounced in GIC than in composite resin. Nevertheless, for those patients who are known to have a high caries risk, it may be better to forsake some of the esthetic qualities of composites in return for the fluoride protection provided by the GIC. It is believed that this significantly increases the caries resistance of enamel adjacent to the restoration (Diaz-Arnold et al. 1995; Forsten 1998). GICs are available in powder-liquid systems or in capsule form. Their clinical applications are presented in table 10-4.

After placement of the glass-ionomer cement into the cavity, the use of a varnish is often recommended by the manufacturer. Solutions of natural and synthetic resins dissolved in an organic solvent such as acetone are generally used. Contamination of the filling materials with saliva or blood should be avoided during insertion, setting, and finishing. The cavity and surrounding area

Table 10-4.   Clinical applications of glass-ionomer cements.

Direct Restorative Material	Cavity Base or Liner
— Class V lesions involving abfractions, abrasions, or erosion lesions	— Base under composites, amalgams, and ceramics
— Class III lesions involving exposed root dentin	— Blocking out undercuts
— Class I and II lesions on deciduous dentition	
— Temporary anterior and posterior restorations	
— Repair of crown margins	

should be dry, although excessive desiccation must not occur.

Future Trends

Polymerization shrinkage of composite resin during light curing remains the main problem for practitioners. While in the past this problem was approached by optimizing filler particle sizes, researchers are currently working to improve the resin matrix. A new material group, called ormocers, contain larger monomers in the methacrylate resin, which may reduce the shrinkage but not solve the problem altogether (Efes, Dörter, and Gömeç 2006; Al-Harbi and Farsi 2007; Rosin et al. 2007; Bottenberg, Alaerts, and Keulemans 2007). The latest approach is the "silorane" composite with a new resin using cationic ring-opening polymerization (Weinmann, Thalacker, and Guggenberger 2005). These composites are recommended for posterior use only because of low opacity, limited shade selection, and incompatibility with methacrylate-based composites and bonding systems (Eick et al. 2006; Eick et al. 2007). The manufacturer claims less than 1% shrinkage with silorane, which would help to reduce marginal gap formation, microleakage, and secondary caries.

Light-Curing Units (LCUs)

Dental curing lights have continually evolved since the UV-emitting lights of the 1970s. Currently, there are a variety of light-curing units on the market with special features that give clinicians the ability to adjust intensity and cure time characteristics depending on the technique employed and the specific material being used. The degree to which these materials cure is dependent on the intensity, duration, and quality of light to which they are exposed. Other factors affecting polymerization are the type, shade, and thickness of the composite, and the distance, orientation, and diameter of the light tip. Exposure time is the easiest factor to control among these variables. However, surveys have shown that dentists tend to cure for inadequate periods of time. This may stem from a lack of awareness of the importance of adequate light intensity and of the importance of the other factors mentioned above that can affect light intensity and degree of polymerization (Strydom 2002). Therefore, it is important to fully understand the type of light and the type of material being used and determine its optimum settings before applying it in clinical practice.

The following terms describe the functional properties of curing lights that are important to understand in purchasing and using a light-curing unit.

Power density is the intensity of light per unit area measured in mW/cm^2. Both power density and spectral distribution are important factors in the effectiveness of a curing light. Curing light output must be monitored to ensure that it functions adequately for curing composite in the time allotted.

Spectral distribution is a measure of light intensity at each component wavelength. Ideally, a light should have the same peak spectral distribution as the photo-initiator being used. LCU spectral emissions beyond that needed for photo-initiation are wasted energy, dissipated as heat and visual glare. Camphorquinone, the most common photo-initiator, is most efficiently activated or converted by light energy in the 460–480 nm spectra, with maximum absorption occurring between 465 and 470 nm (Owens and Rodriguez 2007).

Depth of cure is a description of how deep the composite is cured beneath the surface. It is related to the ability of light to penetrate through material. Darker composites require longer curing times to reach that same depth of cure compared with lighter composites.

Temperature rise is a concern when treating vital teeth. In addition to the exothermic reaction exhibited by composite conversion, the light from LCUs will also cause a temperature rise. Many of the units tested had no adverse pulpal reactions at the time and intensity tested under manufacturers' instructions. Significantly, halogen bulbs tend to produce higher pulpal temperatures than other curing units (up to 2°C), while lasers and plasma-arc lights produce the highest heat increases on the surface (up to 21°C) and within the resin restorations (up to 14°C) (Dunne, Davies, and Millar 1996).

Types of Light-Curing Units

Plasma Arc Curing Devices

Plasma Arc Curing (PAC) sources contain a gaseous mixture of ionized molecules and electrons emitting high intensity light upon electrical discharge (fig. 10-15).

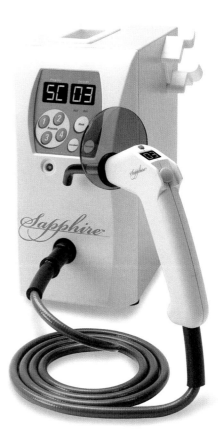

Figure 10-15. Sapphire Supreme plasma arc curing and whitening light (Denmat, Santa Maria CA).

PAC lights generally have a higher light intensity than standard halogen units. They claim to produce a deeper cure in a shorter amount of time. This accelerated cure—along with the heat produced by PAC units—has sparked controversy over whether these lights can cause damage to the dental pulp, to the composite resin, or to the margins of the restoration. While some claim that there is no difference in polymerization quality following the manufacturers' instructions, a study found that the Knoop hardness of specimens cured by a PAC light was significantly lower than those cured by a quartz-tungsten-halogen curing light (Yazici, Kugel, and Gül 2007). Curing time is the most significant advantage of the plasma arc curing light. About three seconds is required for a typical shade A2 composite restoration. Short curing time reduces chair time and the risk of moisture contamination during the curing process. The disadvantages of PAC lights include high heat production, high initial cost, high maintenance costs, and large physical size. Temperature during curing must be controlled by accurate timing of cure and air-cooling. The relative cost is high compared with that of other light-curing units. Replacement of the lamps is costly. Most of the devices are large, heavy, and bulky. The Sapphire Plasma Arc light was the only light tested that was able to maintain over 80% of its maximum intensity at a distance of 10 mm. Other lights lost over 90% of their curing power at 10 mm, with most falling below the International Organization of Standardization's suggested minimum intensity of 300 mW/cm² (Price 2004).

Laser

Laser sources are also used as curing devices. They emit light at a few distinct frequencies within the desired region, eliminating the need for filtering of undesired wavelengths. Argon laser units have the ability to produce an increased initial depth and degree of cure in less time than halogen LCUs. The narrow range of wavelength consistent with the activation wavelength of camphorquinone allows the laser to cure faster and at a lower power than current halogen LCUs. One manufacturer claims that the argon laser needs only one-fourth of the exposure time of other LCUs: 10 seconds for 2 mm depth of cure compared with the 40 seconds recommended for other LCU systems (Fleming and Maillet 1999). However, faster curing times have been correlated with increased shrinkage, brittleness, and marginal leakage. Argon laser units are relatively expensive, ranging from US$12,000 to US$20,000. At approximately twenty pounds, the unit is still fairly cumbersome and occupies considerably more space than a conventional LCU. The laser can generate a substantial amount of heat, the cooling fans tend to be noisy, and there is a 30-second time lag between turning the unit on and actual light emission. These shortcomings can be overcome, in part, with units now available that can be centrally installed, with curing wands radiating into individual operatories (Fleming and Maillet 1999). However, when a laser is used in the oral cavity, the dentist must determine the risk to surrounding tissues, including periodontal and pulp tissues. It is also important to know that laser lights require proper warning signs in the operatory and are subject to increased government regulation. The combination of cost, size of equipment, and concerns over microleakage argue against lasers as LCUs for a general dental office.

Quartz-Tungsten-Halogen Light Curing Units

Quartz-tungsten-halogen (QTH) light-curing units continue to be very popular devices due to their more reasonable size and cost (fig. 10-16). The light source consists of a halogen bulb with a filament. As a current passes through the filament, it heats up and emits electromagnetic radiation. QTH bulbs emit a significant amount of light energy outside the peak range of camphorquinone. Some would argue that this energy is wasted since light emitted outside of the range of the photo-initiator has

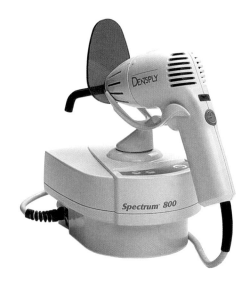

Figure 10-16. Spectrum 800 quartz-tungsten-halogen light-curing unit (Dentsply Caulk, York, PA).

little or no effect on the polymerization of the light-cured resin. Instead, it produces heat, which may be detrimental to pulpal health and the health of surrounding tissues, depending on the duration and intensity of the light. Additionally, the performance of the QTH bulb progressively diminishes, eventually leaving composite materials incompletely cured.

Light-Emitting Diode Curing Units

Light-emitting diode (LED) curing units convert electronic energy into light energy more efficiently, producing less heat than QTH lights (fig. 10-17). The first-generation LEDs did not meet manufacturers' claims and required exposure times twice as long as conventional QTH curing lights (Leonard and Swift 2007). However, the latest generation of LED curing lights shows significant improvement over their predecessors. Advantages associated with LED curing lights include ergonomic handling capabilities, less heat generation, and minimal maintenance concerns (Owens and Rodriguez 2007). Less heat means no need for cooling fans and less need for large, heavy heat sinks. LED LCUs are also inexpensive and the diodes used in this technology are known to have long life expectancy, while exhibiting low voltage requirements. They are designed to emit specific light waves, avoiding wasted energy. The units have better resistance to shock and vibration and are portable and safe. They are quiet in operation. LEDs have some disadvantages as well. Their technology is new to dentistry, and the concept is still evolving. Their curing times are longer than those of PAC lights and some enhanced halogen lights. Their batteries must be recharged, and they cost more than conventional halogen lights.

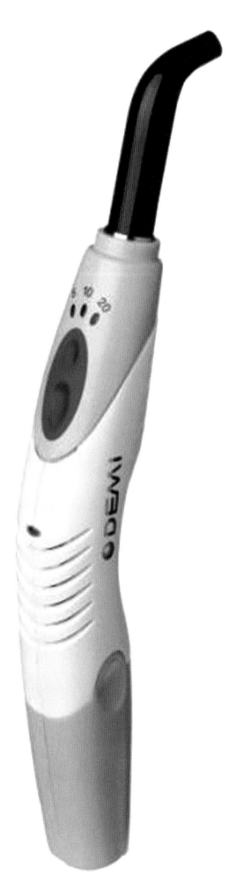

Figure 10-17. Demi, cordless light-emitting diode curing light (Kerr/Sybron, Orange CA).

Works Cited

Abdalla AI, Alhadainy HA, García-Godoy F. 1997. Clinical evaluation of glass ionomers and compomers in class V carious lesions. *Am J Dent* 10(1):18–20.

Albers HF. 2001. *Tooth-Colored Restoratives: Principles and Techniques*. Philadelphia: BC Decker.

Al-Harbi SD, Farsi N. 2007. Microleakage of Ormocer-based restorative material in primary teeth: An in vivo study. *J Clin Pediatr Dent* 32(1):13–7.

Anusavice Ken. 2003. *Phillips' Science of Dental Materials*. 11th ed., Philadelphia: Saunders.

Bottenberg P, Alaerts M, Keulemans FA. 2007. Prospective randomised clinical trial of one bis-GMA-based and two ormocer-based composite restorative systems in class II cavities: Three-year results. *J Dent* 35(2):163–71.

Bowen RL, Cobb EN, Rapson JE. 1982. Adhesive bonding of various materials to hard tooth tissues: Improvement in bond strength to dentin. *J Dent Res* 8(4):278–82.

Brudevold F, Buonocore M, Wileman W. 1956. A report on a resin composition capable of bonding to human dentin surfaces. *J Dent Res* 35(6):846–51.

Buonocore MG. 1955. A simple method of increasing the adhesion of acrylic filling materials to enamel surfaces. *J Dent Res* 34(6):849–53.

Burgess J, Norling B, Summitt J. 1994. Resin ionomer restorative materials: The new generation. *J Esthet Dent* 6(5): 207–15.

De Munck J, Van Meerbeek B, Yoshida Y, Inoue S, Vargas M, Suzuki K, Lambrechts P, Vanherle G. 2003. Four-year water degradation of total-etch adhesives bonded to dentin. *J Dent Res* 82(2):136–40.

Dhuru VB. 2004. *Contemporary Dental Materials*. Textbook Series in Dentistry. Oxford University Press.

Diaz-Arnold AM, Holmes DC, Wistrom DW, Swift EJ. 1995. Short-term fluoride release/uptake of glass ionomer restoratives. *Dent Mater* 11(2):96–101.

Duggal MS, Toumba KJ, Sharma NK. 2002. Clinical performance of a compomer and amalgam for the interproximal restoration of primary molars: A 24-month evaluation. *Br Dent J* 193(6):339–42.

Dunne SM, Davies BR, Millar BJ. 1996. A survey of the effectiveness of dental light-curing units and a comparison of light testing devices. *Br Dent J* 180(11):411–6.

Efes BG, Dörter C, Gömeç Y. 2006. Clinical evaluation of an ormocer, a nanofill composite and a hybrid composite at 2 years. *Am J Dent* 19(4):236–40.

Eick JD, Kotha SP, Chappelow CC, Kilway KV, Giese GJ, Glaros AG, Pinzino CS. 2007. Properties of silorane-based dental resins and composites containing a stress-reducing monomer. *Dent Mater* 23(8):1011–7.

Eick JD, Smith RE, Pinzino CS, Kostoryz EL. 2006. Stability of silorane dental monomers in aqueous systems. *J Dent* 34(6):405–10.

Fleming MG, Maillet WA. 1999. Photopolymerization of composite using the argon laser. *J Can Dent Assoc* 65(8):447–50.

Forsten L. 1990. Short- and long-term fluoride release from glass ionomers and other fluoride-containing filling materials in vitro. *Scand J Dent Res* 98(2):179–85.

Forsten L. 1995. Resin-modified glass ionomer cements: Fluoride release and uptake. *Acta Odontol Scand* 53(4):222–5.

Forsten L. 1998. Fluoride release and uptake by glass-ionomers and related materials and its clinical effect. *Biomaterials* 19(6):503–8.

Forsten L, Karjalainen S. 1990. Glass ionomers in proximal cavities of primary molars. *Scand J Dent Res* 98(1):70–3.

Fortin D, Vargas MA. 2000. The spectrum of composites: New techniques and materials. *J Am Dent Assoc* 131(Suppl): 26S–30S.

Gallo JR, Burgess JO, Ripps AH, Walker RS, Ireland EJ, Mercante DE, Davidson JM. 2005. Three-year clinical evaluation of a compomer and a resin composite as class V filling materials. *Oper Dent* 30(3):275–81.

Gedik R, Hurmuzlu F. 2005. Surface roughness of new microhybrid resin-based composites. *J Am Dent Assoc* 136(8): 1106–12.

Giachetti L, Scaminaci Russo D. 2006. A review of polymerization shrinkage stress: Current techniques for posterior direct resin restorations. *J Contemp Dent Pract* 7(4):79–88.

Habelitz S, Marshall SJ, Marshall GW, Balooch M. 2001. Mechanical properties of human dental enamel on the nanometer scale. *Arch Oral Biol* 46(2):173–83.

Ho SP, Marshall SJ, Ryder MI, Marshall GW. 2007. The tooth attachment mechanism defined by structure, chemical composition and mechanical properties of collagen fibers in the periodontium. *Biomaterials* 28(35):5238–45.

Itota T, Carrick TE, Yoshiyama M, McCabe JF. 2004. Fluoride release and recharge in giomer, compomer and resin composite. *Dent Mater* 20(9):789–95.

Kinney JH, Marshall SJ, Marshall GW. 2003. The mechanical properties of human dentin: A critical review and re-evaluation of the dental literature. *Crit Rev Oral Biol Med* 14(1):13–29.

Krämer N, García-Godoy F, Reinelt C, Frankenberger R. 2006. Clinical performance of posterior compomer restorations over 4 years. *Am J Dent* 19(1):61–6.

Kraus BS, Jordan RE, and Abrams L. 1969. Histology of the teeth and their investing structures. In *Dental Anatomy and Occlusion: A Study of the Masticatory System*, 135. Baltimore: Williams and Wilkins.

Kuijs RH, Fennis WM. 2003. Does layering minimize shrinkage stresses in composite restorations? *J Dent Res* 82(12):967–71.

Leinfelder KF. 1993. Posterior composites state-of-the art application. *Dent Clin North Am* 3(37):411–8.

Leinfelder KF. 1995. Posterior composite resins. *J Am Dent Assoc* 126(5):663–4, 667–8, 671–2.

Leonard D, Swift EJ. 2007. Light emitting diode curing lights-revisited. *Journal of Esthetic and Restorative Dentistry* 19(1): 56–62.

Loher C, Kunzelman RH, Hickel R. 1997. Clinical evaluation of glass-ionomer cements (LC), compomer and composite restorations in class V cavities: Two years results. *J Dent Res* 76(Spec Iss):1190.

Lutz F. 1995. The postamalgam age. *Oper Dent* 20(6):218–22.

Marshall GW, Marshall SJ, Kinney JH, Balooch M. 1997. The dentin substrate: Structure and properties related to bonding. *J Dent* 25(6):441–58.

McComb D, Erickson RL, Maxymiw WG, Wood RE. 2002. A clinical comparison of glass ionomer, resin-modified glass ionomer and resin composite restorations in the treatment of cervical caries in xerostomic head and neck radiation patients. *Oper Dent* 27(5):430–7.

Nakabayashi N, Kojima K, Masuhara E. 1982. The promotion of adhesion by the infiltration of monomers into tooth substrates. *J Biomed Mater Res* 16(3):265–73.

Owens BM, Rodriguez KH. 2007. Radiometric and spectrophotometric analysis of third generation light-emitting diode (led) light-curing units. *J Contemp Dent Pract* 8(2): 43–51.

Pascon FM, Kantovitz KR, Caldo-Teixeira AS, Borges AF, Silva TN, Puppin-Rontani RM, Garcia-Godoy F. 2006. Clinical evaluation of composite and compomer restorations in primary teeth: 24-month results. *J Dent* 34(6):381–8.

Petersen RC. 2005. Discontinuous fiber-reinforced composites above critical length. *J Dent Res* 84(4):365–70.

Powers JM, Hostetler RW. 1979. Thermal expansion of composite resins and sealants. *J Dent Res* 58(2):584–7.

Price RB, Felix CA, Andreou P. 2004. Effects of resin composite composition and irradiation distance on the performance of curing lights. *Biomaterials* 25(18):4465–77.

Provenza DV, Seibel W. 1986. *Oral Histology: Inheritance and Development*, 2nd ed. Philadelphia: Lea & Febiger.

Rosin M, Schwahn C, Kordass B, Konschake C, Greese U, Teichmann D, Hartmann A, Meyer G. 2007. A multipractice clinical evaluation of an ORMOCER restorative: 2-year results. *Quintessence Int* 38(6):306–15.

Roulet J-F, Michel D. 2000. *Adhesion: The Silent Revolution in Dentistry*. Chicago: Quintessence.

Schulze KA, Oliveira SA, Wilson RS, Gansky SA, Marshall GW, Marshall SJ. 2005 Effect of hydration variability on hybrid layer properties of a self-etching versus an acid-etching system. *Biomaterials* 26(9):1011–8.

Schulze KA, Soederholm KJ, Zaman AA. Aug 2003. Assessment of rheological and compressive properties in experimental compomer materials. *J Dent* 31(6):373–82.

Shirai K, De Munck J, Yoshida Y, Inoue S, Lambrechts P, Suzuki K, Shintani H, Van Meerbeek B. 2005. Effect of cavity configuration and aging on the bonding effectiveness of six adhesives to dentin. *Dent Mater* 21(2):110–24.

Sideridou ID, Achilias DS. 2005. Elution study of unreacted Bis-GMA TEGDMA, UDMA, and Bis-EMA from light-cured dental resins and resin composites using HPLC. *J Biomed Mater Res B Appl Biomater* 74(1):617–26.

Strydom C. 2002. Curing lights: The effects of clinical factors on intensity and polymerisation. *Sadj* 57(5):181–6.

Summitt JB, Robbins JW, Hilton TJ, Schwartz RS. 2006. *Fundamentals of Operative Dentistry, a Contemporary Approach*. Chicago: Quintessence.

Tian M, Gao Y. 2007. Bis-GMA/TEGDMA dental composites reinforced with electrospun nylon 6 nanocomposite nanofibers containing highly aligned fibrillar silicate single crystals. *Polymer Guildf* 48(9):2720–8.

Uno S, Finger WJ, Fritz U. 1996. Long-term mechanical characteristics of resin-modified glass ionomer restorative materials. *Dent Mater* 12(1):64–9.

Van Landuyt KL, Snauwaert J, De Munck J, Peumans M, Yoshida Y, Poitevin A, Coutinho E, Suzuki K, Lambrechts P,

Van Meerbeek B. Systematic review of the chemical composition of contemporary dental adhesives. 2007. *Biomaterials* 28(26):3757–85.

Van Meerbeek B. 2008. Mechanisms of resin adhesion: Dentin and enamel bonding. *Functional Esthetics and Restorative Dentistry (A Supplement to Compendium)* Serie 2(1):18–25.

Van Meerbeek B, Vargas S, Inoue S. 2001. Adhesives and cements to promote preservation dentistry. *Oper Dent* Suppl. no. 6:119–44.

Weinmann W, Thalacker C, Guggenberger R. 2005. Siloranes in dental composites. *Dent Mater* 21(1):68–74.

Yazici AR, Kugel G, Gül G. 2007. The knoop hardness of a composite resin polymerized with different curing lights and different modes. *J Contemp Dent Pract* 8(2):52–9.

Yip KH, Poon BK. 2003. Clinical evaluation of packable and conventional hybrid resin-based composites for posterior restorations in permanent teeth: Results at 12 months. *J Am Dent Assoc* 134(12):1581–9.

Yoshiyama M, Carvalho R, Sano H, Horner J, Brewer PD, Pashley DH. 1995. Interfacial morphology and strength of bonds made to superficial versus deep dentin. *Am J Dent* 8(6):297–302.

Chapter 11
Direct Composite Restorative Techniques

Brian J. Kenyon DMD, BA

Kenneth G. Louie DDS, BS

Bina Surti DDS

Initial Clinical Procedures

Some of the essential procedures that are completed prior to a direct composite preparation and restoration include diagnosis and treatment planning, shade selection, assessment of occlusion relative to the proposed restoration, and a field of isolation decision.

An important step in esthetic restoration of an anterior tooth is shade selection. A shade guide is only useful for a general determination of color. For underlying tooth color to be taken into account, custom shade tab composite disks of about one millimeter in thickness are fabricated and held facial to the area of the tooth to be restored (see fig. 11-1; Terry 2003). In addition, a test shade of approximate thickness of the restoration is applied and light cured on the tooth to confirm color choice.

A pretreatment assessment of occlusion with articulating paper is done to guide the practitioner in preparation design (Bryant 1992). The objective is to avoid the development of excessive occlusal contacts on the restorative material or margins, which may result in decreased restoration longevity.

Adequate isolation and moisture control is essential for a composite restoration. The most complete method of achieving field isolation is the rubber dam. A comparison of cotton roll and rubber dam isolation found a significant increase in composite bond strength (18.9 to 14.4 megapascals) when the latter was used for isolation (fig. 11-2; Barghi, Knight, and Berry 1991).

Following the rubber dam application, a wedge is placed gingival to the preparation to keep the field dry, protect the rubber dam and gingiva, decrease the risk of adjacent tooth damage, and to separate the teeth slightly to help develop an appropriate interproximal contact (fig. 11-3).

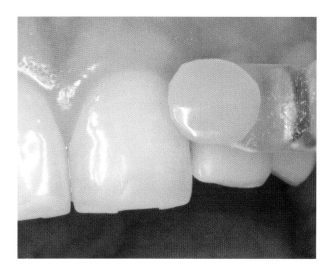

Figure 11-1. Custom shade tab composite disks of about 1 mm in thickness are fabricated.

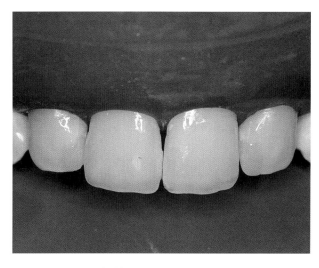

Figure 11-2. Optimal rubber dam isolation increases access, visibility, and bond strength.

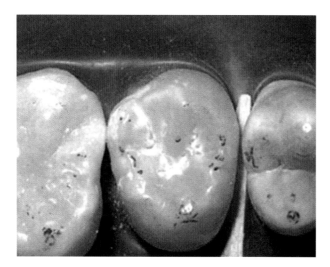

Figure 11-3.   A wedge is placed gingival to the preparation.

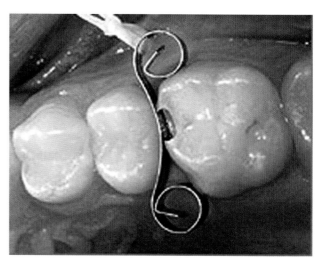

Figure 11-4.   An Interguard (Ultradent, South Jordan, UT) is used to protect adjacent teeth from iatrogenic damage. Courtesy of Ultradent.

Anterior Direct Restorations

This section discusses the restorative treatment of class III and class IV lesions, diastema closure, and facial veneering with light-cured composite. For each class, it delineates preparation design, material placement, finishing, and polishing.

Class III Composite Preparation

The size, depth, and extension of a class III composite preparation are determined by the characteristics of the lesion, the access path for visualization or instrumentation, removal of decalcified tooth structure, and/or the defective restoration (Terry 2004; Terry 2005b). Adjacent tooth structure is protected from iatrogenic damage with a metallic strip such as an Interguard (Ultradent, South Jordan, UT; fig. 11-4).

If the lesion is equidistant between the facial and lingual surfaces (fig. 11-5), a lingual approach is preferable to minimize restorative material showing on facial surfaces. Facial access is used if the caries lesion or an existing restoration extends more to the facial than the lingual. Ideally, the preparation is somewhat rectangular with rounded corners so retention does not entirely depend on adhesion. All or part of the interproximal contact is maintained due to the difficulty restoring the original tightness and anatomical shape. Ideally, there is a 0.5-mm gingival extension. The proximal outline form follows the facial contour. Unsupported enamel is removed with the possible exception of a thin facial wall, and rounded internal line angles are created. A slight bevel (0.5 mm at 45 degrees) is placed on the accessible lingual cavosurface margin to maximize enamel bond

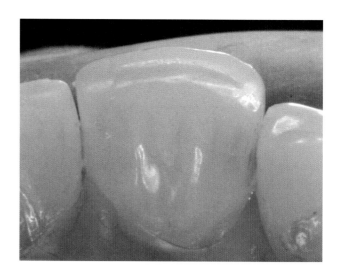

Figure 11-5.   Preoperative lingual view of class III caries lesion on tooth #9-D.

strength, remove friable enamel, make margins smooth, and enhance composite adaptation (Munechika et al. 1984; Dietschi et al. 1995). A facial bevel is added only if the preparation extends prominently to that surface. A retention groove is not utilized unless the preparation walls are overly divergent toward the cavosurface.

Class III Composite Placement Technique

A polyester matrix strip is placed between teeth to confine material within the preparation. A wedge is often used interproximally to hold the matrix in place and tight to tooth structure at the gingival margin (fig. 11-6). Following the cleaning of the tooth with a prophy-

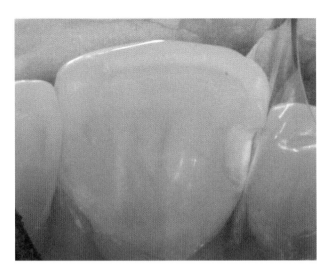

Figure 11-6. Lingual view of class III composite preparation and matrix strip/wedge placement.

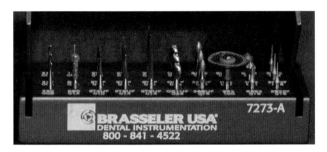

Figure 11-7. Department of Restorative Dentistry, University of the Pacific, Arthur A. Dugoni School of Dentistry Composite Preparation and Finishing System.

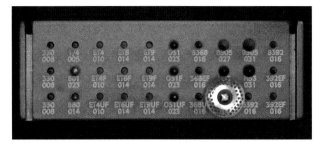

Figure 11-8. Bur numbers for the Department of Restorative Dentistry, University of the Pacific, Arthur A. Dugoni School of Dentistry Composite Preparation and Finishing System.

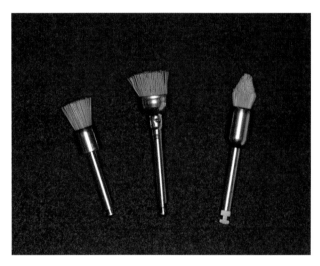

Figure 11-9. Jiffy Composite Polishing Brushes, Ultradent, South Jordan, UT.

laxis cup, pumice, and the adhesive process, composite material is placed and shaped with hand instruments. A small preparation does not require incremental placement and allows matrix wrapping as remaining tooth structure maintains contours. A medium to large preparation necessitates a layering technique to minimize polymerization shrinkage, maximize the quality of cure, and ensure a natural-looking restoration. To hide the show-through of the darkness of the mouth, the composite material is layered with shades that replace the anatomical dentin and enamel portions of the tooth preparation (Araujo et al. 2003). Each layer is light cured after it is added and smoothed. If the insertion of composite is done carefully, very little excess will need to be removed at this stage. The principal purpose of finishing and polishing is to restore a surface similar in smoothness and contour to the adjacent tooth structure. A #12 scalpel blade may be used to remove some of the excess proximal material. Shaping and smoothing is continued with finishing burs of appropriate shape and coarseness (figs. 11-7 and 11-8). Sandpaper strips or diamond strips

are used to polish proximal surfaces and margins gingival to the contact point. A silicon-impregnated brush (fig. 11-9) and a composite polishing point with paste (figs. 11-10 and 11-11) are utilized to impart a shine or luster to the surface. The restoration is treated with a fluoride-releasing composite surface sealant, an unfilled light-cured resin material (fig. 11-12). The material fills in surface irregularities, marginal discrepancies, and may reduce wear of composite restorations (Kawai 1993). The tooth is etched for fifteen seconds, rinsed and dried, surface sealant applied, air thinned, and light cured for twenty seconds. Floss is used to confirm the adequate interproximal contact of the definitive restoration (fig. 11-13).

Class IV Composite Preparation

A class IV restoration replaces incisal tooth structure lost from caries, trauma (fig. 11-14), wear, or a defective

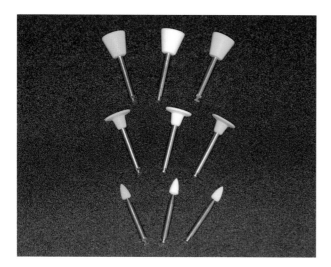

Figure 11-10. Jiffy Composite Polishing Cups, Disks, and Points, Ultradent, South Jordan, UT.

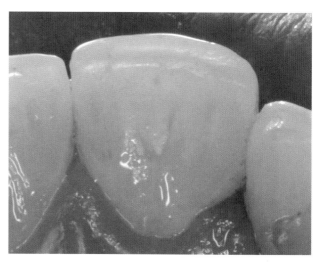

Figure 11-13. Postoperative lingual view of the definitive restoration exhibits the successful esthetic result achieved.

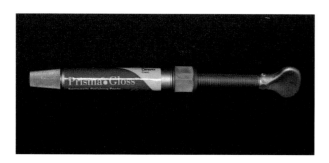

Figure 11-11. Prisma Gloss Composite Polishing Paste, Dentsply Caulk, York, PA.

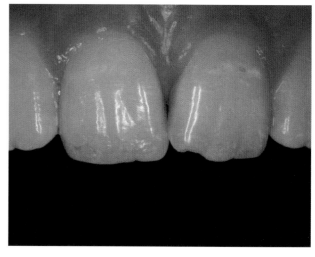

Figure 11-14. Preoperative facial view of class IV lesion on tooth #9.

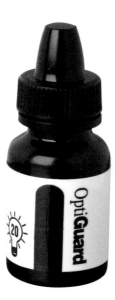

Figure 11-12. The fluoride-releasing surface sealant Optiguard, Kerr Dental, Orange, CA. Courtesy of Kerr Dental.

restoration. If the class IV lesion is significant, a diagnostic cast is prepared to be used for the fabrication of a diagnostic restoration (fig. 11-15) and silicone matrix. The silicone matrix is sectioned and used in the creation of the lingual shell of composite, which will act as a base for subsequent increments (fig. 11-16; Boer 2007a; Terry and Geller 2004). The dentin shade is obtained from the gingival one-third where enamel is thinnest (fig. 11-17). The enamel shade is acquired from the middle one-third where enamel is thickest (fig. 11-18). The incisal region

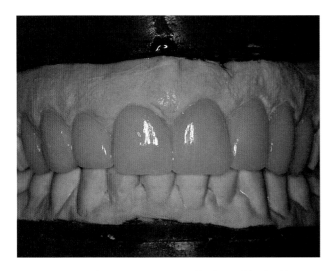

Figure 11-15. A diagnostic cast is prepared to be used for the fabrication of a diagnostic restoration and silicone matrix. Courtesy of Martin B. Goldstein, DMD.

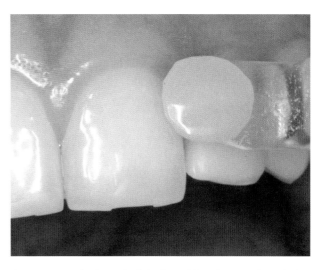

Figure 11-17. The dentin shade is obtained from the gingival one-third.

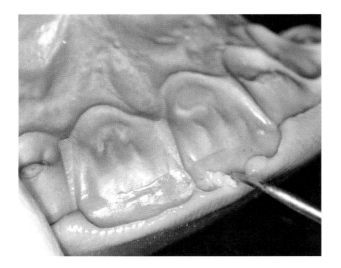

Figure 11-16. The silicone matrix is sectioned and used in the creation of the lingual shell of composite.

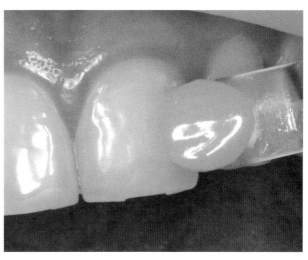

Figure 11-18. The enamel shade is obtained from the middle one-third.

of the tooth is checked for translucency and the shade is chosen accordingly (fig. 11-19; Felippe et al. 2004; Milnar 2004; Felippe et al. 2005).

Beveling at ends of enamel rods increases strength of enamel bonding. A longer bevel or chamfer preparation creates more surface area for strength and provides a long gradual show-through of tooth structure for better color transition and esthetics. A 2-mm knife-edge-type bevel is created facially (fig. 11-20). Clinicians tend to make the bevel of large class IV restorations far too uniform in both depth and width, which will often hinder the chameleon effect and increase the chance of

visible detection of the restoration. Varying the depth and width of the bevel will greatly enhance the ability of the clinician to produce a lifelike result (fig. 11-21). If the preparation is on dentin facially, a butt joint margin is made. Lingually on enamel, a slight bevel (0.5 mm) or narrow chamfer margin is developed—preferably not in the contact zone (LeSage 2007).

Class IV Composite Placement Technique

Following the cleaning of the tooth with a prophylaxis cup and pumice, the preparation is etched (15 seconds

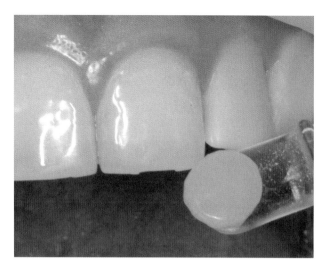

Figure 11-19. The incisal region of the tooth is checked for translucency and the shade is chosen accordingly.

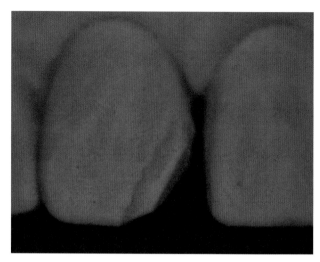

Figure 11-21. The facial bevel is made less uniform in depth and width to disguise the visible detection of the restoration margin.

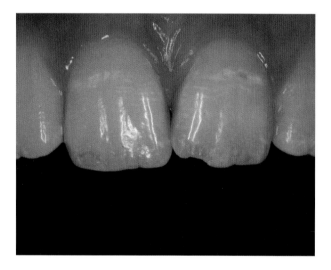

Figure 11-20. A 2-mm knife-edge-type bevel is placed facially.

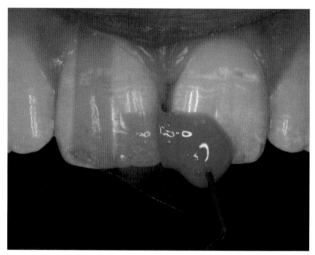

Figure 11-22. The preparation is etched past the end of the bevel.

with 34% phosphoric acid) past the end of the bevel (fig. 11-22). After the completion of the adhesive process (fig. 11-23), the composite material is placed incrementally (fig. 11-24). The material is allowed to go slightly past the bevel (fig. 11-25). This allows for a disappearing margin and leads to an excellent esthetic result (fig. 11-26).

To restore a more significant class IV lesion (fig. 11-27), the first layer of composite is added to the silicone matrix, placed on the tooth, and light cured (figs. 11-28 and 11-29). The lingual shell is made using the enamel shade (semitranslucent shades) and acts as a base for the subsequent increments. The dentin shade is utilized to replace dentin and the incisal shade of composite creates the incisal edge so that it matches the translucency of the

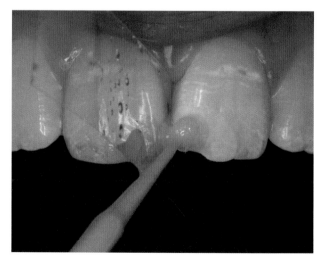

Figure 11-23. Adhesive materials are applied.

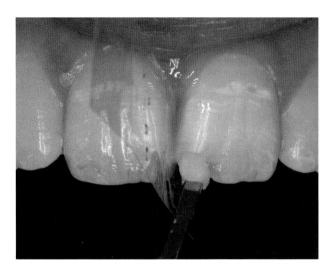

Figure 11-24. The first increment of composite is applied.

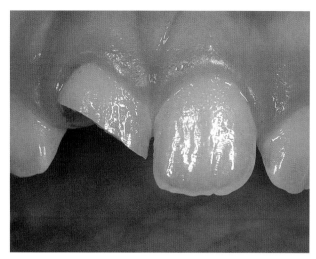

Figure 11-27. Preoperative facial view of a more significant class IV lesion.

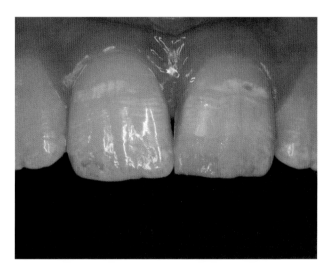

Figure 11-25. The composite material is allowed to go slightly past the bevel.

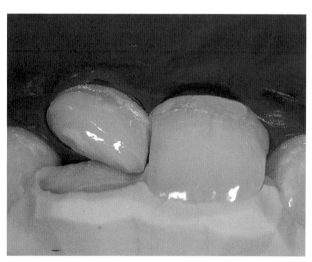

Figure 11-28. Facial view of a silicone matrix placed on the anterior teeth.

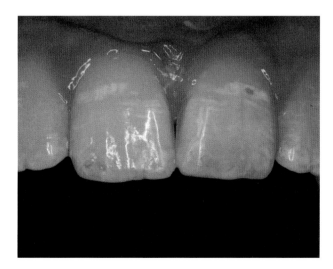

Figure 11-26. Postoperative facial view of the definitive restoration exhibits the successful esthetic result achieved.

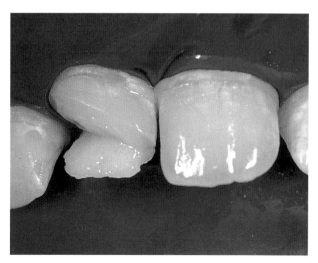

Figure 11-29. The first layer of composite is added to the silicone matrix, placed on the tooth, and light cured.

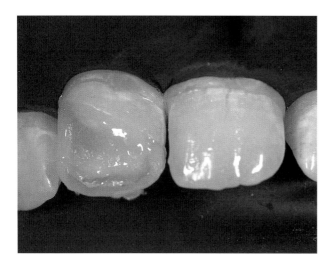

Figure 11-30. The dentin shade replaces dentin and the incisal shade of composite creates the incisal edge.

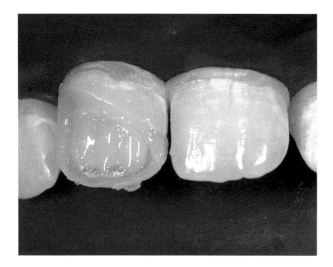

Figure 11-31. The dentin lobes are fabricated with the dentin shade.

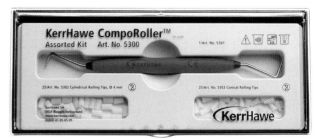

Figure 11-32. The CompoRoller Kerr Dental, Orange, CA, is used to prevent inclusions and voids in the composite material. Courtesy of Kerr Dental.

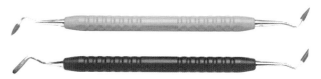

Figure 11-33. Optrasculpt (Ivoclar Vivadent, Amherst, NY) is a double–ended composite placement instrument. Courtesy of Ivoclar Vivadent.

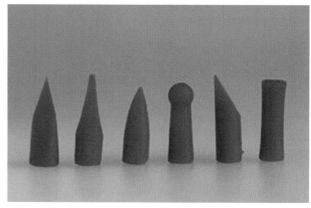

Figure 11-34. Six different tip styles are available for use with the Optrasculpt instrument. Courtesy of Ivoclar Vivadent.

adjacent incisors (fig. 11-30). The dentin lobes are then fabricated with the dentin shade (fig. 11-31). An incisal shade of composite is applied between dentin lobes and is followed by an enamel shade of composite on the facial surface. Internal characterization may be done by creating a notch in the final layer and placing special tints.

An instrument such as the CompoRoller (Kerr Dental, Orange, CA; fig. 11-32) may be used to remove the white edge of composite as it is expressed from the compule, and to avoid an inclusion or void in the material. The composite is placed and thinned or feather-edged past the bevel of the preparation. Optrasculpt (Ivoclar Vivadent, Amherst, NY; fig. 11-33) is a double-ended composite placement instrument that allows easy and

selective modeling as a result of slight elasticity of the disposable tips. It is available in six different tip styles that may be rotated a full 360 degrees on the instrument and snapped into place in the desired position. The six tip styles are (1) a point for creating detailed anatomy, pits, fissures, and a lingual contour; (2) a spatula for a class V restoration and a facial surface; (3) a pyramid for creating detailed anatomy; (4) a ball for the concavity of a lingual surface of an anterior tooth; (5) a chisel for a marginal ridge and a cervical margin of a class V restoration; and (6) a cylinder for the initial increment of a class I or class II composite restoration (fig. 11-34). A sable brush and wetting resin may be used to smooth and shape the outer layer of the class IV restoration prior to light curing (fig. 11-35; LeSage 2007).

To remove excess composite, flame- and football-shaped finishing burs are used. Sandpaper strips or diamond strips are utilized to remove inadvertent interproximal excess. Regular or pointed polishing brushes made of silicon carbide particles may be employed to smooth and polish the restoration, followed by rubber points, disks, and cups with polishing paste (Ferreira, Lopes, and Baratieri 2004). The restoration is completed with a fluoride-releasing composite surface sealant, an unfilled light-cured resin material. The definitive class IV restoration is demonstrated in figure 11-36.

Diastema Closure Preparation

Diagnosis and treatment planning are essential prior to beginning a case of diastema closure or reduction. A diastema may be treated clinically using orthodontics, with direct or indirect restorative materials, or a combination of these treatment modalities. If restorative treatment is chosen, width of the maxillary anterior teeth should not exceed 80% of length. Frequently, two to six teeth require augmentation for an optimal esthetic diastema closure. A diagnostic wax or composite mock-up is done to demonstrate the possible conclusion of the diastema closure. The mock-up is used to construct a silicone matrix and to guide the clinician with the fabrication of temporary diagnostic restorations (figs. 11-37, 11-38,

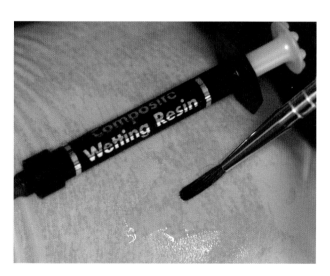

Figure 11-35. A sable brush and wetting resin are used to smooth and shape the outer layer of the class IV restoration prior to light curing.

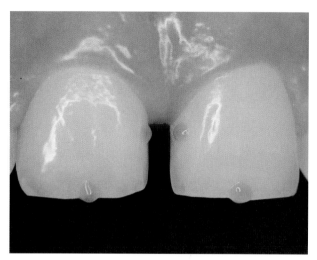

Figure 11-37. Preoperative facial view of the diastema showing the spots to be etched prior to the fabrication of the diagnostic restorations. Courtesy of Adilson Yoshio Furuse.

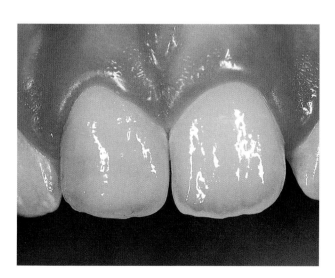

Figure 11-36. Postoperative facial view of the definitive restoration.

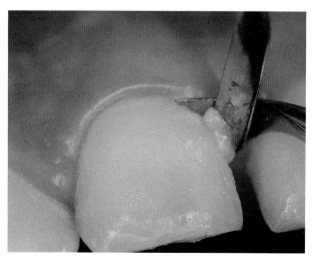

Figure 11-38. Diagnostic restorations are fabricated. Courtesy of Adilson Yoshio Furuse.

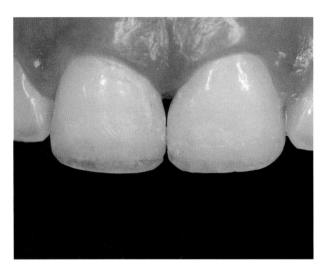

Figure 11-39. Diagnostic restorations completed. Courtesy of Adilson Yoshio Furuse.

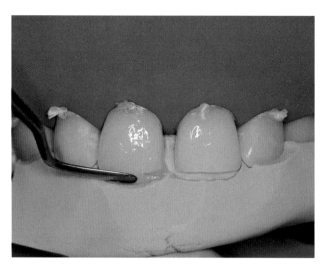

Figure 11-41. A silicone matrix is used to guide the construction of the incisal edge of tooth #8. Courtesy of Adilson Yoshio Furuse.

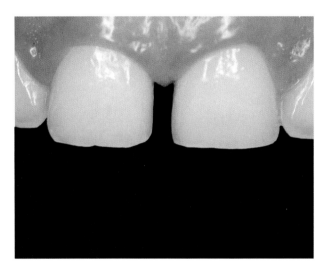

Figure 11-40. After removal of the diagnostic restorations it is evident that the interdental papilla has accommodated to the new tooth contours. Courtesy of Adilson Yoshio Furuse.

and 11-39). The use of diagnostic restorations allows the patient to evaluate proposed esthetic changes and may help to properly form the interdental papilla near the restorations (fig. 11-40). The patient is encouraged to go home with the diagnostic restorations and seek the opinion of family and friends. When the patient returns, the practitioner obtains authorization for treatment.

In the majority of cases, tooth preparation is not required for diastema closure or reduction (Fahl 2006, 2007). Because of the large enamel surface area to be bonded and the minimal amount of potential dentin bonding, it is advised that clinicians consider the use of a total-etch bonding system over a self-etch bonding system for this particular clinical situation. Acid etching of enamel and bonding agent provide adequate retention for the composite. Preparation may be necessary to remove tooth discoloration or to create enough space for the restorative material to mask a dark color. This may be accomplished with a diamond bur, sandpaper strips, or air abrasion.

Diastema Closure Placement Technique

The composite material is layered with shades that replace the anatomical dentin and enamel portions of the tooth preparation to produce a lifelike restoration. As with other large anterior composite restorations, the dentin shade is obtained from the gingival one-third, the enamel shade is taken from the middle one-third, and the incisal region of the tooth is checked for translucency with the shade chosen accordingly. Following dental prophylaxis of the treatment teeth and the adhesive process, the first layer of composite is added to the silicone matrix, placed on the tooth, and light cured (fig. 11-41). The lingual shell (fig. 11-42) is made using the enamel shade and acts as a base for the subsequent light-cured increments of composite (Fahl 2006, 2007). The dentin lobes are then fabricated with a dentin shade. An incisal shade of composite is applied between dentin lobes and is followed by an enamel shade of composite on the facial surface (fig. 11-43). Internal characterization may be done by creating a notch in the final layer and placing special tints.

To remove excess composite, flame and football-shaped finishing burs are used. Sandpaper strips or

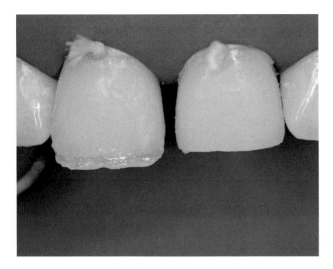

Figure 11-42. The lingual shell of composite acts as a base for the subsequent increments of composite. Courtesy of Adilson Yoshio Furuse.

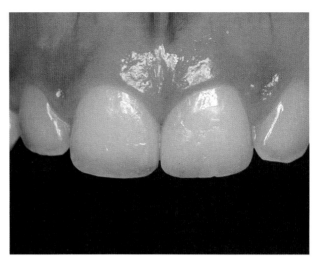

Figure 11-44. Facial view of the definitive diastema closure restorations. Courtesy of Adilson Yoshio Furuse.

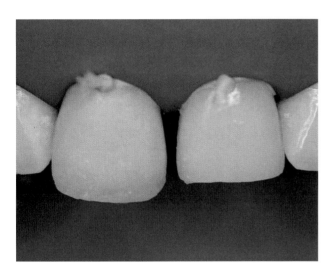

Figure 11-43. The dentin lobes are fabricated with a dentin shade, an incisal shade composite is placed between the lobes, and an enamel shade composite is applied to the facial surface. Courtesy of Adilson Yoshio Furuse.

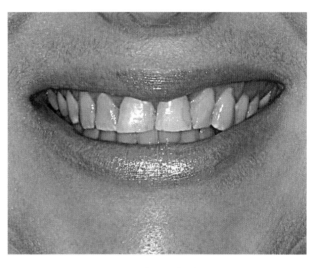

Figure 11-45. Preoperative facial view of a direct composite veneer case. Courtesy of Martin B. Goldstein, DMD.

diamond strips are used to remove inadvertent interproximal excess. Regular or pointed polishing brushes made of silicon carbide particles may be used to smooth and polish the restoration, followed by rubber points, disks, and cups with polishing paste. The restoration is completed with a fluoride-releasing composite surface sealant, an unfilled light-cured resin material (fig. 11-44).

Direct Composite Veneer Preparation

Direct composite veneers may or may not require tooth preparation. With a composite veneer, the tooth base is maintained under the restoration and may influence its

final color (fig. 11-45). This is called the chameleon effect (Helbig et al. 2002). For underlying tooth color to be taken into account, custom shade tab composite disks of about one millimeter in thickness are fabricated and held facial to the area of the tooth to be restored. In addition, a test shade of approximate thickness of the restoration is placed and light cured on the tooth to confirm color choice. The enamel shade is obtained from the middle one-third where enamel is thickest. The incisal region of the tooth is checked for translucency and the shade is chosen accordingly. A diagnostic wax or composite mock-up is done to demonstrate the possible conclusion of the direct composite veneer case (fig. 11-46).

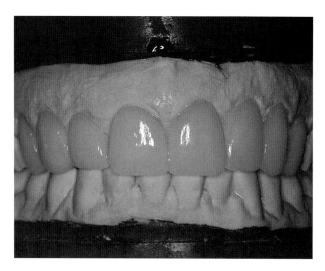

Figure 11-46. A diagnostic wax or composite mock-up of the direct composite veneer case is done. Courtesy of Martin B. Goldstein, DMD.

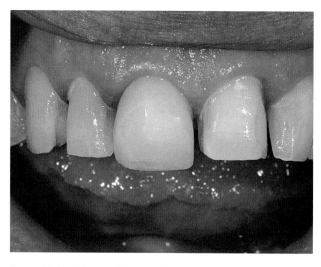

Figure 11-48. The maxillary central incisor is restored first. Courtesy of Martin B. Goldstein, DMD.

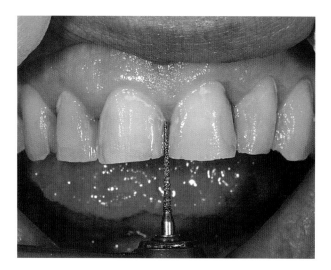

Figure 11-47. Enamel is maintained to achieve the strongest and most durable bond of the direct composite veneer to tooth structure. Courtesy of Martin B. Goldstein, DMD.

Preparation may be necessary to avoid overcontouring of the final restoration or to provide a thickness of composite material to mask tooth discoloration (fig. 11-47). Whenever possible, enamel is maintained to achieve the strongest and most durable bond of the restoration to tooth structure.

Direct Composite Veneer Placement

Following dental prophylaxis of the treatment teeth and the adhesive process, if the tooth has a dark discoloration, an opaque layer or masking agent may be applied over the adhesive and polymerized (Felippe et al. 2003). Caution must be taken when using a masking agent. These materials may increase the likelihood of metamerism of the final restoration due to the increased opacity that is created. Translucency, the appearance of dental lobes, and characterization of the incisal edge may be done in the incisal third of the restoration with appropriate shades of composite. The flat areas of the composite restoration may be modified to give the illusion of a wider or narrower tooth. Horizontal lines accentuate the width of teeth and vertical lines highlight the length of teeth. Labial embrasures may be increased or decreased to make a tooth look narrower or wider. Ideally, width of the maxillary anterior teeth should not exceed 80% of length. If the facial appearance and occlusion allow, the length of the teeth may be increased by adding to the incisal edge. Refer to chapter 2 to assist you in determining which direction to lengthen teeth. However, it may be more appropriate to increase tooth length with laser or surgical procedures. It is recommended that the clinician first restore the central incisors individually (figs. 11-48 and 11-49) and then complete the teeth posterior to the centrals.

Following polymerization of the composite, excess composite is removed and shaping is done with flame-shaped finishing burs. Sandpaper strips or diamond strips are used to remove inadvertent interproximal excess. Regular or pointed polishing brushes made of silicon carbide particles may be used to smooth and polish the restoration, followed by rubber points, disks, and cups with polishing paste. The restoration is completed (fig. 11-50) with a fluoride-releasing composite surface sealant, an unfilled light-cured resin material.

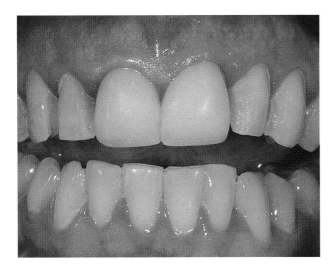

Figure 11-49.   The other maxillary central incisor is restored next. Courtesy of Martin B. Goldstein, DMD.

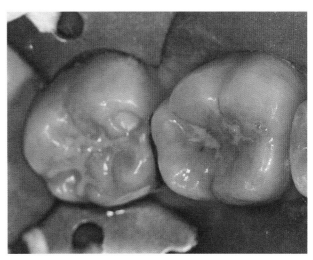

Figure 11-51.   Preoperative occlusal view of class I lesions on teeth #18 and #19.

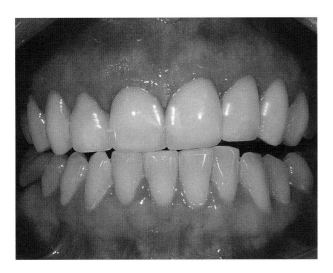

Figure 11-50.   Postoperative facial view of the definitive restorations exhibits the successful esthetic result achieved. Courtesy of Martin B. Goldstein, DMD.

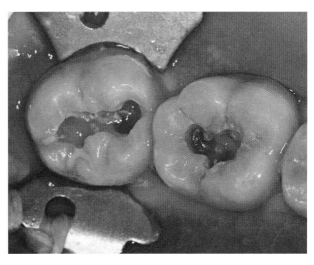

Figure 11-52.   Initial tooth preparation with an access path for removal of remaining decay.

Posterior Direct Restorations

This section discusses the restorative treatment of class I, class II, and class V lesions with light-cured composite. For each class, it delineates preparation design, material placement, finishing, and polishing.

Class I Composite Preparation

The size, depth, and extension of a class I preparation are dictated by the characteristics of the caries lesion and/or a defective restoration (fig. 11-51). The primary goal of a direct composite tooth preparation is the conservation of tooth structure. The preparation removes defective tooth structure, ideally remains small, shallow, narrow, out of occlusion, and has rounded internal line angles. A small tooth defect with light occlusion requires minimal tooth preparation because only bond strength is required to provide retention and resistance. With a larger tooth defect where increased forces are applied, mechanical retention and resistance with increased bond area may be required to provide adequate strength for the restoration. An isthmus width of less than one-third the intercuspal distance is ideal for direct composite. Tooth preparation requires an access path for removal of the caries lesion, elimination of weak tooth structure that may fracture, refinement of enamel margins to maximize enamel bond strength and minimize a white line around the restoration, and extension into defective areas such as stained grooves and decalcified areas (figs. 11-52 through 11-55; Hudson 2004; McComb 2005;

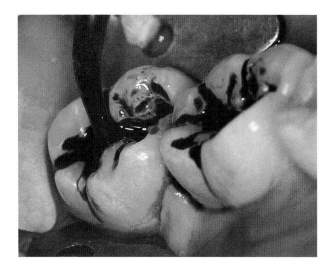

Figure 11-53. Caries indicator is placed on the tooth preparations.

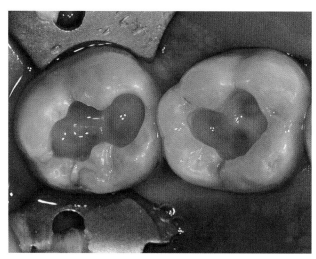

Figure 11-55. Occlusal view of the completed class I preparations for composite on teeth #18 and #19.

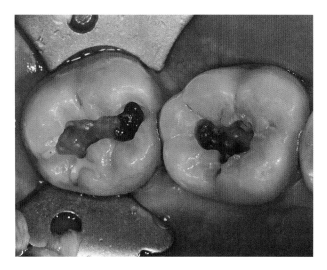

Figure 11-54. Caries indicator dye remains after rinsing with water and air.

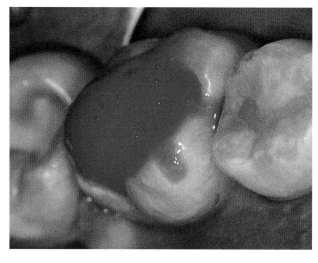

Figure 11-56. The preparations are etched for 15 seconds with 34% phosphoric acid.

Strassler, Porter, and Serio 2005; Lopes and Oliveira 2006; Terry, Leinfelder, and James 2006).

Class I Composite Placement Technique

The goals of direct composite placement are well-adapted margins and walls, minimal polymerization shrinkage, maximum cure of composite, prevention of voids or porosities, minimal postoperative sensitivity, and satisfactory esthetics. These features determine the ultimate success or failure of a restoration. Following the cleaning of the tooth with a prophylaxis cup and pumice, the preparation is etched (15 seconds with 34% phosphoric acid; fig. 11-56). After the completion of the

adhesive process, the composite material is added incrementally. It is essential that the first layer of material be as well adapted and as completely cured as possible. Elimination of voids between the restorative material and the tooth preparation may decrease the likelihood of postoperative sensitivity. Although controversial when used as an intermediate liner between adhesive and composite, a flowable composite with adequate flowability and slump may achieve superior adaptation with fewer voids when applied as the initial, thin (0.5 mm) layer of a class I restoration (fig. 11-57; Chuang et al. 2004; Li et al. 2006; Ruiz and Mitra 2006;). Since most flowable composites have a lower percentage of filler particles compared with regular composite, this

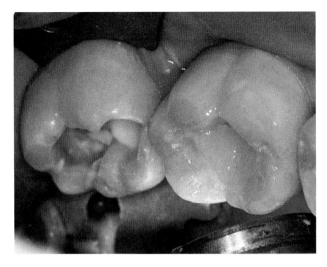

Figure 11-57. An initial, thin (0.5 mm) layer of a flowable composite is placed on the pulpal floor of the class I preparations.

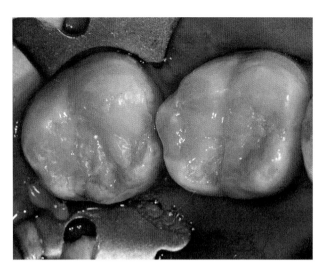

Figure 11-59. A final enamel layer is placed and anatomy is carefully developed prior to light curing.

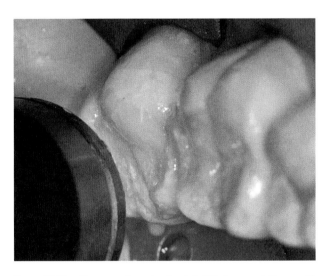

Figure 11-58. The composite restoration is built in incremental layers with dentin being replaced first.

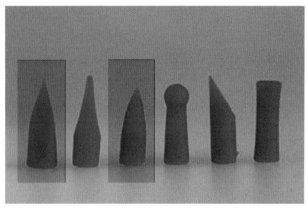

Figure 11-60. The point and pyramid tips of the Optrasculpt composite placement instrument.

layer is light cured twice as long (40 seconds) as subsequent increments. The remainder of the preparation is restored with composite built-in layers that replicate tooth structure by placing dentin (opaque) layers first and then enamel (semitranslucent) layers (fig. 11-58). Tooth stress is created when composite is placed simultaneously on facial and lingual walls then light cured. To minimize stress, an oblique increment should not contact both facial and lingual preparation walls. A final, outer, translucent enamel layer is applied and anatomy is carefully developed prior to light curing, to reduce time and effort in the finishing and polishing phase (fig. 11-59). The Optrasculpt composite placement instrument with a point or pyramid tip is useful for develop-

ing the surface anatomy, pits, and fissures of a class I restoration (fig. 11-60).

If the insertion of composite is done carefully, very little surplus material will need to be removed after placement. If there is excess, it may be removed with appropriate finishing burs. Regular or pointed polishing brushes made of silicon carbide particles may be used to smooth and polish the restoration, followed by rubber points, disks, and cups with polishing paste. It is important not to overheat the composite during finishing and polishing, as overaggressive removal of the composite may cause a white line at the restoration margin. The restoration is completed with a fluoride-releasing composite surface sealant, an unfilled light-cured resin material. The rubber dam is removed and optimal occlusion is verified (fig. 11-61).

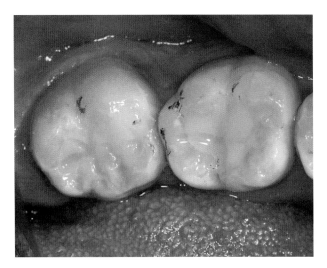

Figure 11-61. The occlusal view of class I-O composite restorations on teeth #18 and #19 after verifying optimal occlusion.

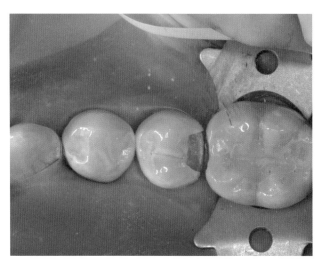

Figure 11-63. A box-only class II composite preparation.

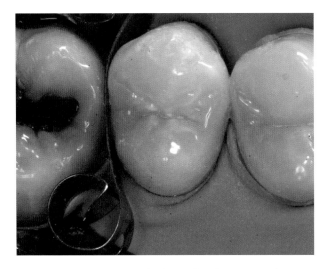

Figure 11-62. Preoperative occlusal view of tooth #4 DO caries lesion.

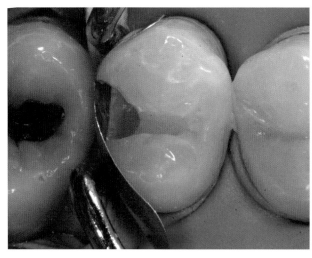

Figure 11-64. A box and occlusal class II preparation connected but narrower than a comparable amalgam preparation.

Class II Composite Preparation

There is no ideal class II composite preparation. The size, depth, and extension of a class II preparation are determined by the characteristics of the caries lesion (fig. 11-62) and/or a defective restoration. Class II treatment may consist exclusively of a proximal box preparation if the occlusal pits and fissures do not need treatment (fig. 11-63), a box and occlusal preparation connected but narrower than a comparable amalgam preparation (fig. 11-64), or a preparation determined by the size of the previous defective restoration. Adjacent tooth structure is protected from iatrogenic damage with a metallic strip. An Interguard is an excellent device (fig. 11-65) because it not only protects adjacent teeth but provides

some tooth separation, which increases the likelihood of obtaining an ideal proximal contact. Another technique is to place a wedge that will separate the teeth, protect the rubber dam and tissues, and increase likelihood of a normal interproximal contact (fig. 11-66). Conservation of tooth structure is the goal. Cavosurface margins should be on enamel. An access path for removal of dentinal caries is created, and unsupported, loose, friable, or demineralized enamel is removed. The preparation is small, shallow, narrow, out of occlusion, with rounded internal line angles (figs. 11-67, 11-68, and 11-69). If the interproximal caries lesion is facially or lingually located it is not necessary to establish both facial and lingual proximal clearance (Giachetti et al. 2006; Hassan and Khier 2006; Boer 2007b). Leaving one

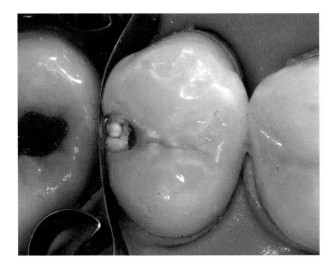

Figure 11-65. An Interguard is used to protect the adjacent tooth and develop the interproximal contact.

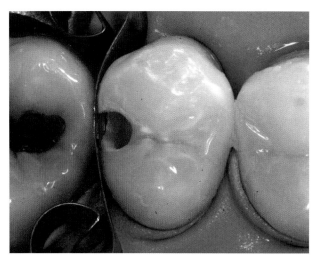

Figure 11-67. Occlusal view of #4 DO (disto-occlusal) composite preparation with proximal decay removed.

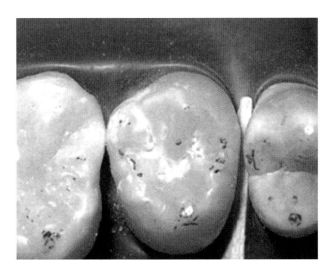

Figure 11-66. A wedge is placed to separate the teeth, protect the rubber dam and tissues, and increase likelihood of a normal interproximal contact.

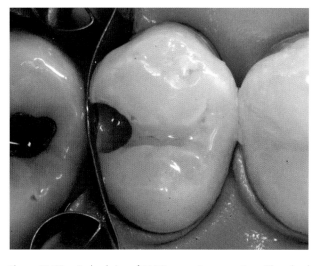

Figure 11-68. Occlusal view of #4 DO composite preparation with occlusal decay removed.

wall in contact (either facial or lingual) will greatly enhance the ability of the clinician to establish a successful proximal contact. Facial and lingual proximal margins receive a 0.5-mm 45-degree bevel (Opdam et al. 1998). A 0.5-mm bevel at 45 degrees is utilized on the gingival margin (fig. 11-70) only if enamel won't be eliminated in the process. The occlusal margin receives a 0.25-mm bevel with a small diamond or hand instrument to eliminate easily chipped, decalcified, or unsupported enamel.

Class II Composite Placement Technique

Restoration with composite of interproximal defects between posterior teeth is troublesome. It is difficult to

create anatomically shaped interproximal contours fitting tightly to adjacent convex surfaces, contain material within a preparation, and compensate for matrix thickness. The best proximal contact areas in class II composite restorations are obtained using a sectional matrix system (Peumans et al. 2001; Loomans et al. 2006). One example of a sectional matrix system is Composi-Tight Gold (Garrison Dental Solutions, Spring Lake, MI). A premolar is commonly restored with an AU 110–sized matrix band, and a molar is frequently treated with an AU 200–sized matrix band (fig. 11-71). A contoured sectional matrix band is applied, a wedge is inserted to prevent a gingival overhang, and a tooth-separating ring is usually positioned between the matrix and wedge. The matrix band is burnished just enough

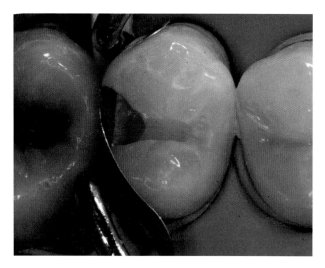

Figure 11-69.   Occlusal view of #4 DO composite preparation completed.

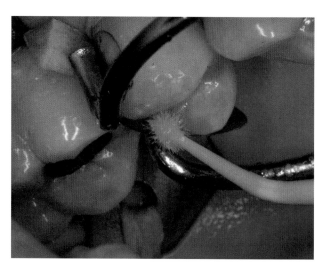

Figure 11-72.   Occlusal view of the application of the dentin bonding agent.

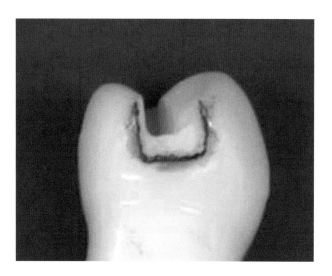

Figure 11-70.   Proximal view of facial and lingual proximal margins with a 0.5-mm 45-degree bevel and a gingival margin bevel of. 5 mm, 45 degrees only if enamel won't be eliminated in the process.

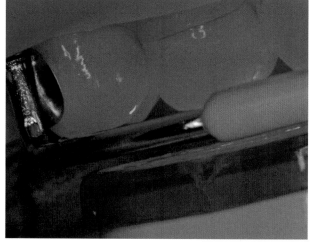

Figure 11-73.   The dentin bonding agent is polymerized with the composite curing light Ultra-Lume LED 5 (Ultradent, South Jordan, UT).

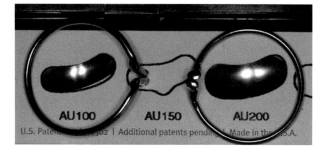

Figure 11-71.   Composi-Tight Gold AU 110–size matrix band, AU 200–size matrix band, and separating rings. Courtesy of Garrison Dental Solutions.

so it touches the adjacent tooth. Following dental prophylaxis of the treatment teeth and the adhesive placement (fig. 11-72), the material is polymerized with a composite curing light such as the Ultra-Lume LED 5 (fig. 11-73; Ultradent Products, South Jordan, UT). A thin (0.5 mm) layer of flowable composite is applied to the gingival, axial, pulpal, and proximal walls (fig. 11-74).

Although controversial when used as an intermediate liner between adhesive and composite, a flowable composite with adequate flowability and slump may achieve superior adaptation with fewer voids, when applied as the initial, thin (0.5 mm) layer (Olmez, Oztas, and Bodur 2004; Koczarski 2005). Flowable composite has greater polymerization shrinkage compared with regular composite, but the shrinkage effect is compensated by a

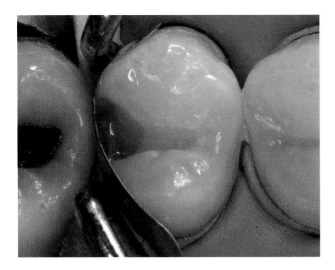

Figure 11-74. A thin (0.5 mm) layer of flowable composite is placed on the gingival, axial, pulpal, and proximal walls.

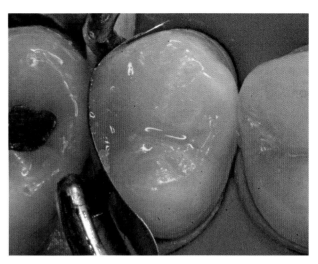

Figure 11-76. A final, outer, translucent enamel layer is placed and anatomy is carefully placed prior to light curing.

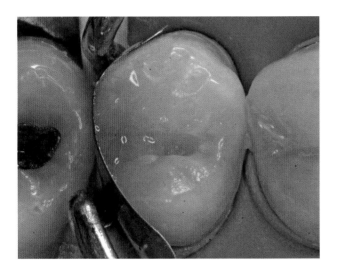

Figure 11-75. The remainder of the preparation is restored with layers of composite starting with the replacement of dentin.

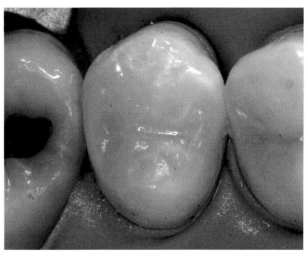

Figure 11-77. Occlusal view of the #4 DO composite restoration following finishing and polishing.

lower modulus of elasticity (more flexibility; Attar, Tam, and McComb 2003). Since most flowable composites have a lower percentage of filler particles compared with regular composite, this layer is light cured twice as long (40 seconds) as subsequent increments. The remainder of the preparation is restored with layers of composite that replicate tooth structure by placing dentin increments first (fig. 11-75) and then enamel additions (fig. 11-76). Tooth stress is created when composite is placed simultaneously on facial and lingual walls then light cured. To minimize stress, an oblique increment should not contact both facial and lingual preparation walls. Composite increments of 2 mm or less are placed

and layered in alternating oblique sections. A final, outer, translucent enamel layer is added and anatomy is carefully developed prior to light curing, to reduce time and effort in the finishing and polishing phase. The Optrasculpt composite placement instrument with a point or pyramid tips may be useful for developing the surface anatomy, pits, and fissures. Following polymerization of the composite, excess composite may be removed with appropriate finishing burs. Regular or pointed polishing brushes made of silicon carbide particles may be used to smooth and polish the restoration, followed by rubber points, disks, and cups with polishing paste (fig. 11-77; Jefferies 2007). It is important not

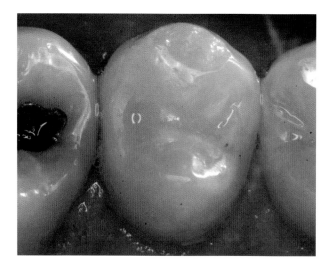

Figure 11-78. Postoperative occlusal view of the definitive restoration exhibits the successful aesthetic result achieved.

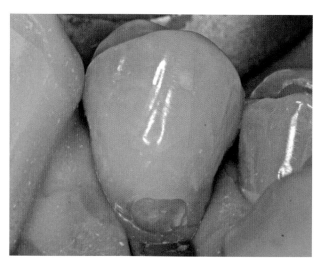

Figure 11-80. Facial view of class V preparation #5-F.

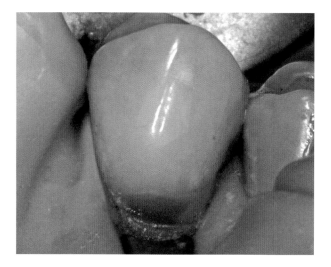

Figure 11-79. Preoperative facial view of class V lesion on tooth #5.

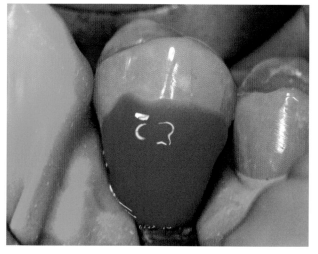

Figure 11-81. Class V preparation is etched with 34% phosphoric acid for 15 seconds.

to overheat the composite during finishing and polishing, as overaggressive removal of the composite may cause a white line at the restoration margin. The restoration is completed with a fluoride-releasing composite surface sealant, an unfilled light-cured resin material. The rubber dam is removed and optimal occlusion is verified (fig. 11-78).

Class V Composite Preparations

There is no ideal class V composite preparation. The size, depth, and extension of the preparation are dictated by the characteristics of the caries lesion (fig. 11-79) and/ or a defective restoration. The axial wall of the preparation is roughened to provide a surface amenable to the

adhesive process. Enamel margins are beveled (fig. 11-80) to achieve a cross-section of enamel rods for improved bond strength. Long bevels create improved strength and show-through of tooth color for composite color matching and a better esthetic result. A root structure margin receives a 90-degree exit angle (Costa et al. 2006). A 0.25-mm retention groove along the gingival wall is considered only if occlusal dysfunction is a contributing factor.

Class V Composite Placement Technique

Following the cleaning of the tooth with a prophylaxis cup and pumice, the preparation is etched (15 seconds with 34% phosphoric acid; fig. 11-81) and the adhesive

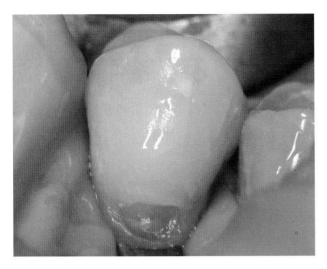

Figure 11-82. A thin (0.5 mm) layer of flowable composite is placed on the gingival wall.

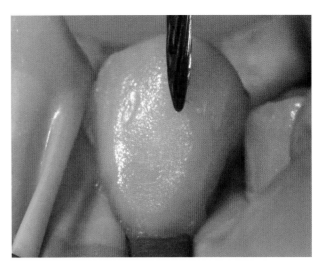

Figure 11-84. Excess composite is removed with a 12-bladed long flame carbide.

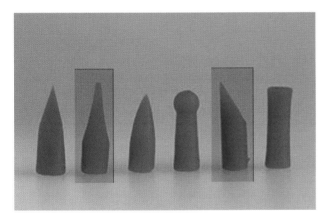

Figure 11-83. The Optrasculpt (Ivoclar Vivadent, Amherst, NY) spatula and chisel are useful for developing the surface of the class V restoration.

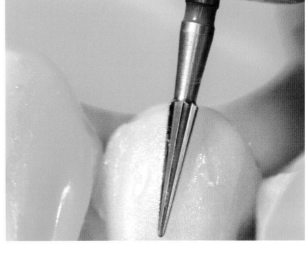

Figure 11-85. Finishing is done with a red-stripe ET4011 multifluted carbide.

process is completed. For a large or root structure preparation, the recommendation is that a thin (0.5 mm) layer of flowable composite be applied to the gingival wall (fig. 11-82) and light cured to increase marginal adaptation and minimize postoperative sensitivity often caused by aggressive finishing of sensitive root structure (Terry 2005a). A mid-gingival-occlusal increment is introduced and light cured, followed by the addition and light curing of an occlusal increment (Owens and Johnson 2005). The Optrasculpt composite placement instrument with a spatula or chisel (fig. 11-83) may be useful for developing the surface of the class V restoration.

Excess composite may be removed by finishing burs such as a 12-bladed long flame carbide (fig. 11-84; Ultra-

dent, South Jordan, UT) and a red-stripe ET4011 multifluted carbide (fig. 11-85; Brasseler, Savannah, GA). Polishing is accomplished with rubber points or a prophylaxis cup with polishing paste (fig. 11-86). Because research indicates that there are no differences in retention rates between hybrid and microfilled composites for class V restorations, either composite type may be used as the restorative material (Browning, Brackett, and Gilpatrick 2000). The restoration is completed with a fluoride-releasing composite surface sealant, an unfilled light-cured resin material (fig. 11-87).

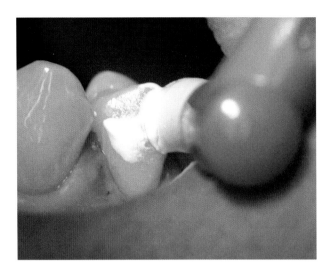

Figure 11-86. The restoration is polished with a prophylaxis cup and polishing paste.

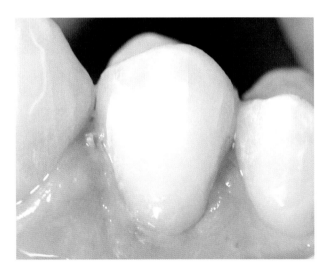

Figure 11-87. Postoperative facial view of the definitive class V composite restoration.

Works Cited

Araujo EM de Jr, Baratieri LN, Monteiro S Jr, Vieira LC, de Andrada MA. 2003. Direct adhesive restoration of anterior teeth: Part 2. Clinical protocol. *Pract Proced Aesthet Dent* Jun; 15(5):351–7.

Attar N, Tam LE, McComb D. 2003. Flow, strength, stiffness and radiopacity of flowable resin composites. *J Can Dent Assoc* 69(8):516–7.

Barghi N, Knight GT, Berry TG. 1991. Comparing two methods of moisture control in bonding to enamel: A clinical study. *Oper Dent* 16(4):130–5.

Boer WM. 2007a. Simple guidelines for aesthetic success with composite resin: Part I. Anterior restorations. *Pract Proced Aesthet Dent* 19(3):145–50.

Boer WM. 2007b. Simple guidelines for aesthetic success with composite resin: Part II. Posterior restorations. *Pract Proced Aesthet Dent* 19(4):243–7.

Browning WD, Brackett WW, Gilpatrick RO. 2000. Two-year clinical comparison of a microfilled and a hybrid resin-based composite in non-carious class V lesions. *Oper Dent* 25(1): 46–50.

Bryant RW. 1992. Direct posterior composite resin restorations: A review. 1. Factors influencing case selection. *Aust Dent J* 37(2):81–7.

Chuang SF, Jin YT, Liu JK, Chang CH, Shieh DB. 2004. Influence of flowable composite lining thickness on class II composite restorations. *Oper Dent* 29(3):301–8.

Costa Pfeifer CS, Braga RR, Cardoso PE. 2006. Influence of cavity dimensions, insertion technique and adhesive system on microleakage of class V restorations. *JADA* 137(2):197–202.

Dietschi D, Scampa U, Campanile G, Holz J. 1995. Marginal adaptation and seal of direct and indirect class II composite resin restorations: An in vitro evaluation. *Quintessence Int* 26(2):127–38.

Fahl N Jr. 2006. A polychromatic composite layering approach for solving a complex class IV/direct veneer-diastema combination: Part I. *Pract Proced Aesthet Dent* 18(10):641–5.

Fahl N Jr. 2007. A polychromatic composite layering approach for solving a complex class IV/direct veneer/diastema combination: Part II. *Pract Proced Aesthet Dent* 19(1):17–22.

Felippe LA, Monteiro S Jr, Baratieri LN, Caldeira de Andrada MA, Ritter AV. 2003. Using opaquers under direct composite resin veneers: An illustrated review of the technique. *J Esthet Restor Dent* 15(6):327–36.

Felippe LA, Monteiro S Jr, De Andrada CA, Di Cerqueira AD, Ritter AV. 2004. Clinical strategies for success in proximoincisal composite restorations: Part I. Understanding color and composite selection. *J Esthet Restor Dent* 16(6):336–47.

Felippe LA, Monteiro S Jr, De Andrada CA, Di Cerqueira AD, Ritter AV. 2005. Clinical strategies for success in proximoincisal composite restorations: Part II. Composite application technique. *J Esthet Restor Dent* 17(1):10–21.

Ferreira Rde S, Lopes GC, Baratieri LN. 2004. Direct posterior resin composite restorations: Considerations on finishing/polishing. Clinical procedures. *Quintessence Int* 35(5):359–66.

Giachetti L, Scaminaci Russo D, Bambi C, Grandini R. 2006. A review of polymerization shrinkage stress: current techniques for posterior direct resin restorations. *J Contemp Dent Pract* 7(4):79–88.

Hassan K, Khier S. 2006. Composite resin restorations of large class II cavities using split-increment horizontal placement technique. *Gen Dent* 54(3):172–7.

Helbig EB, Klimm HW, Schreger IE, Haufe E, Natusch I. 2002. Controlled clinical study of the anterior composite-adhesive system Point 4/OptiBond Solo Plus. *Schweiz Monatsschr Zahnmed* 112(12):1230–35.

Hudson P. 2004. Conservative treatment of the class I lesion: A new paradigm for dentistry. *J Am Dent Assoc* 135(6):760–4.

Jefferies S. 2007. Abrasive finishing and polishing in restorative dentistry: A state-of-the-art review. *Dent Clin N Am* 51: 379–97.

Kawai K. 1993. Effect of surface-penetrating sealant on composite wear. *Dent Mater* 9(2):118.

Koczarski MJ. 2005. Achieving natural aesthetics with direct resin composites: Predictable clinical protocol. *Pract Proced Aesthet Dent* 17(8):523–5.

LeSage BP. 2007. Aesthetic anterior composite restorations: A guide to direct placement. *Dent Clin North Am* 51(2):359–78, viii.

Li Q, Jepsen S, Albers HK, Eberhard J. 2006. Flowable materials as an intermediate layer could improve the marginal and internal adaptation of composite restorations in class-V-cavities. *Dent Mater* 22:250–7.

Loomans BA, Opdam NJ, Roeters FJ, Bronkhorst EM, Burgersdijk RC. 2006. Comparison of proximal contacts of class II resin composite restorations in vitro. *Oper Dent* 31(6): 688–93.

Lopes GC, Oliveira GM. 2006. Direct composite resin restorations in posterior teeth. *Compend Contin Educ Dent* 27(10): 572–9.

McComb D. 2005. Conservative operative management strategies. *Dent Clin North Am* 49(4):847–65.

Milnar FJ. 2004. Selecting nanotechnology-based composites using colorimetric and visual analysis for the restoration of anterior dentition: A case report. *J Esthet Restor Dent* 16(2):89–100.

Munechika T, Suzuki K, Nishiyama M, Ohashi M, Horie K. 1984. A comparison of the tensile bond strengths of composite resins to longitudinal and transverse sections of enamel prisms in human teeth. *J Dent Res* 63(8):1079–82.

Olmez A, Oztas N, Bodur H. 2004. The effect of flowable resin composite on microleakage and internal voids in class II composite restorations. *Oper Dent* 29(6):713–9.

Opdam NJ, Roeters JJ, Kuijs R, Burgersdijk RC. 1998. Necessity of bevels for box only class II composite restorations. *J Prosthet Dent* 80(3):274–9.

Owens BM, Johnson WW. 2005. Effect of insertion technique and adhesive system on microleakage of class V resin composite restorations. *J Adhes Dent* 7(4):303–8.

Peumans M, Van Meerbeek B, Asscherickx K, Simon S, Abe Y, Lambrechts P, Vanherle G. 2001. Do condensable composites help to achieve better proximal contacts? *Dent Mater* 17(6):533–41.

Ruiz JL, Mitra S. 2006. Using cavity liners with direct posterior composite restorations. *Compend Contin Educ Dent* 27(6): 347–51.

Strassler HE, Porter J, Serio CL. 2005. Contemporary treatment of incipient caries and the rationale for conservative operative techniques. *Dent Clin North Am* 49(4):867–87.

Terry DA. 2003. Color matching with composite resin: A synchronized shade comparison. *Pract Proced Aesthet Dent* 15(7):515–21.

Terry DA. 2004. Restoring the interproximal zone using the proximal adaptation technique: Part 1. *Compend Contin Educ Dent* 25(12):965–6, 968, 970–1.

Terry DA. 2005a. Dentin hypersensitivity: Part I. *Pract Proced Aesthet Dent* 17(9):609–10, 612.

Terry DA. 2005b. Restoring the interproximal zone using the proximal adaptation technique: Part 2. *Compend Contin Educ Dent* 26(1):10–2, 15–6.

Terry DA, Geller W. 2004. Selection defines design. *J Esthet Restor Dent* 16(4):213–25.

Terry DA, Leinfelder KF, James A. 2006. A nonmechanical etiology: The adhesive design concept. *Pract Proced Aesthet Dent* 18(6):385–91.

Chapter 12
Selecting Indirect Restorative Materials

Jeffrey P. Miles DDS

Karen A. Schulze DDS, PhD

Daniel Castagna DDS

Having decided which teeth need indirect restorations, the dentist must then choose which materials and techniques to employ. The array of options is at first overwhelming, and the dentist is tempted to leave these decisions to a laboratory technician. While an accomplished technician is an integral part of the restorative team and may have a wealth of knowledge and experience to share, the treating dentist has an ethical, legal, and strategic obligation to make the final decision on materials (Christensen 2003).

This chapter is intended to help the restorative dentist make appropriate decisions in various clinical situations. Our emphasis will be on all-ceramic restorations, expecting that the reader is well trained in gold and metal-ceramic restorations. Gold is still the most durable and long-lasting restorative material available (Donovan et al. 2004), but patient demand for esthetics usually dictates that it be used only where it cannot be seen. Metal-ceramics remain more reliable than all-ceramic restorations but have significant esthetic limitations (Christensen 2005).

The inherent properties of metal copings prevent metal-ceramics from ever looking exactly like tooth structure; a skilled ceramist is needed to make them come close (Shillingberg 1997). Metal-ceramic restorations may be designed with metal occlusal surfaces where interocclusal space is limited and where attrition of opposing natural dentition is expected. Unfortunately, the need to hide these metal surfaces is similar to that of all gold restorations. Options for margin designs include a metal collar, a feather edge porcelain (disappearing metal) margin, or an all-porcelain margin. The first two are unacceptable in the esthetic zone, while the second two are technically difficult to create and often suffer from poor marginal integrity (Limkangwalmongkol et al. 2007; Goldin et al. 2005). The grey color of both noble alloy and base alloy metal-ceramic copings also poses difficulties in recreating lifelike restorations. The heavy layers of opaquing porcelains needed to mask the gray tend to create unnaturally bright restorations, especially when tooth reduction is inadequate (fig. 12-1).

Yellow metals mitigate this problem but with a higher risk of porcelain failure and at a higher cost (O'Brien 1997) (fig. 12-2).

A relatively new restorative system, Captek, replaces the cast metal coping with a platinum and palladium framework infused with pure gold. The warm yellow color and micromechanical retention of the porcelain avoid the need for a thick opaque layer, allowing for a more esthetic restoration. Marginal appearance and integrity are reported to be equal to or superior to traditional metal-ceramic restorations (Shoher 1998).

Resin-based composite indirect restorations have shown promise in patients who have "abusive occlusions." Products such as belleGlass (KerrLab), Sculture/FibreKor (Pentron), Cristobal+ (Dentsply Ceramco), and Sinfony (3M ESPE) limit the wear of opposing dentitions at the sacrifice of their own integrity and should be thought of as having intermediate longevity (Christensen 2003). As such, they are not indicated for cases where long-term esthetic results are required. Our focus will be on all-ceramic restorations.

All-Ceramic Restorations

Ceramics are not intrinsically suited for use as dental restorations, and daunting technical challenges have been overcome to develop the newest generation of materials. The two biggest hurdles to be overcome are the close correlation between translucency and brittleness of ceramic materials and the tendency for ceramics to shrink as they are processed (Guazzato 2004). The results have been sophisticated proprietary systems using a variety of manufacturing strategies. Materials and equipment have typically been developed in tandem; only recently have materials been marketed that can be used in more than one system.

A characteristic of ceramic materials that is often cited in the dental literature and in dental marketing materials is flexural strength. As measured in mega-Pascals (MPa's), flexural strength is a rough but very useful

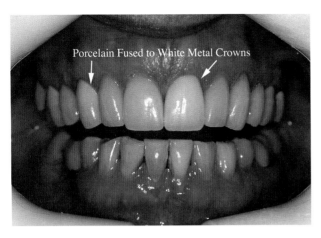

Figure 12-1. Two metal-ceramic restorations adjacent to all-ceramic restorations.

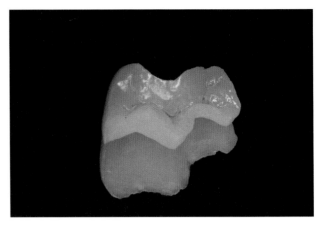

Figure 12-3. Pressed-ceramic inlay.

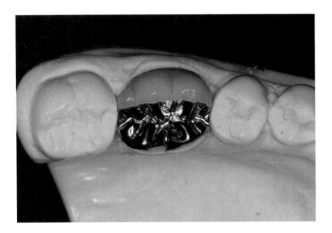

Figure 12-2. Metal-ceramic restoration fabricated with high gold metal.

point of comparison between dental ceramic materials, being well correlated to fracture resistance and hence durability. Dental ceramics in current use have flexural strengths in the range of 140–1300 MPa (Raigrodski 2004). In general, a practitioner should choose a restoration that has the maximum flexural strength obtainable for the given clinical situation.

Single-Component Systems

The least complicated all-ceramic restorative systems deliver a restoration that is a homogenous material throughout. They are limited to feldspathic porcelain or reinforced glass ceramics because of the need for translucency. The structural limitations of these available materials mean these restorations require support from natural tooth structure. Realistically, this restricts them to use as veneers, inlays, or onlays (fig. 12-3).

Traditionally, these restorations have been fabricated by dental technicians on refractory dies or platinum foil

matrices derived from clinical impressions. Of more current interest is using computer-aided design and computer-aided manufacture (CAD/CAM) systems to create restorations in the practitioner's office. This eliminates impressions, temporization, and multiple appointments. CEREC 3D is the most developed and established of in-office CAD/CAM systems and the one we will describe here (Mormann 2006; Reiss 2006).

CEREC 3D consists of two units. The first is the scanning and designing unit, located in the operatory. The second is an automated milling machine typically located elsewhere in the dental office. The preparation guidelines are similar to those of other all-ceramic systems. These include rounded line angles, butt joint margins, and adequate thickness for porcelain. CEREC 3D is designed to fabricate inlays, onlays, veneers, and single-unit crowns, although many question its use for full coverage given the limited strength of its available substrates.

The dentist prepares the affected teeth with conventional instrumentation and then dusts them and the opposing dentition with an opaque powder. Both are then scanned with an infrared scanner linked to the chairside design unit (Luthardt et al. 2005). The computer creates a virtual model of the patient's teeth as well as a proposed restoration. The dentist can modify the restoration design, if necessary, before sending it to the computer-controlled milling machine. CEREC 3D can mill composite resin, feldspathic porcelain, or leucite-reinforced porcelain from solid blocks. Flexural strength is less than 200 MPa for all available blocks (Guazzato et al. 2004). The milling procedure takes less than 20 minutes. Shade selection is good; restorations can be stained and glazed if desired or simply polished (Sadowsky 2006). The intaglio surface is etched with 9% hydrofluoric acid and treated with silane prior to cementing with resin. As with other moderate-strength all-ceramics, CEREC 3D restorations need to be bonded in place before adjusting occlusal contacts.

The CEREC 3D system reliably produces very esthetic restorations with good to excellent marginal fit (Borto-lotto, Onisor, and Krejci 2006). Its chief limitation is the brittleness of its substrates. Adequate available tooth structure and meticulous bonding technique are critical to its success. Its ability to restore teeth in a single appointment appeals to both practitioners and patients (Fasbinder 2006). Unfortunately, the initial investment required of an in-office CAD/CAM system is quite high, while situations appropriate to its use are relatively rare. This introduces a temptation to allow financial pressures to drive treatment planning.

Pressed ceramics, described in more detail below, can also be used for single-component restorations, although they require impressions, temporization, and laboratory procedures. They can be used for veneers, inlays, and onlays, but their translucency and uniform color limit their use to minor cosmetic changes.

Two-Component Ceramic Systems

Traditional feldspathic porcelains remain the material of choice for mimicking natural tooth structure. They have a natural transparency that can be modified with metal oxides to create a wide range of translucencies and shades, but their brittleness means that they cannot be used without some support from tooth structure or a higher-strength coping (O'Brien 1997). The following discussion will focus on high-strength ceramic copings with the understanding that they require veneering by feldspathic porcelains to be cosmetically acceptable. The materials come in three general forms, all of which have a crystalline component lacking in feldspathic porcelain. That component can be suspended within a glass ceramic matrix, part of a crystalline matrix infused with a glass ceramic, or processed to a pure crystalline structure. Like metal-ceramic restorations, most two-component systems are fabricated in dental laboratories from conventional impressions and model work. A more detailed explanation of laboratory procedures can be found in chapter 17.

Pressed Ceramics
Pressed-ceramic copings are the first of the three types. Ivoclar has been a leader in this technology, creating products such as IPS Empress (1 & 2), IPS Eris, and IPS e.Max. Substrates for these products are leucite or lithium disilicate reinforced glass ceramic materials. The reinforcing components are semiliquid at high temperatures but solidify into crystals as they cool inside the molten glass. In function, the crystals act to interrupt

and deflect subcritical crack propagation that would otherwise lead to cohesive failure (Cesar et al. 2005).

Preparations for pressed-ceramic restorations are similar to those of higher-strength ceramics with a few modifications. Reduction needs to be greater than 1 mm on all surfaces, including near the margin. Bevels or chamfers at the margin leave a thin layer of ceramics that could fail during try-in, cementation, or service (Soares et al. 2006). Impression techniques are traditional, as described in chapter 15.

The laboratory process for creating pressed-ceramic copings is very similar to the familiar lost wax technique for casting metals. The dental technician prepares model work in a traditional fashion and waxes a pattern on the die. The pattern is sprued, invested (fig. 12-4), and burned out with dedicated materials and ovens (fig. 12-5). The casting ring is then placed in a "pressing furnace" where a previously selected ceramic ingot is heated to liquid state and pressed into the pattern (fig. 12-6).

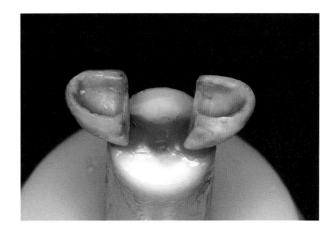

Figure 12-4.   Wax patterns for pressed-ceramic restorations.

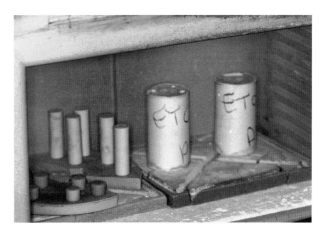

Figure 12-5.   Invested patterns in burn-out oven.

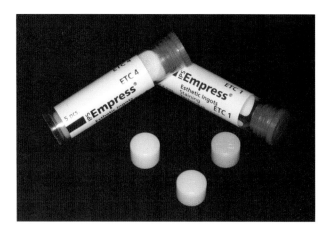

Figure 12-6. Ceramic ingot.

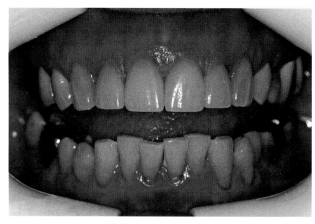

Figure 12-8. Cemented pressed-ceramic restorations.

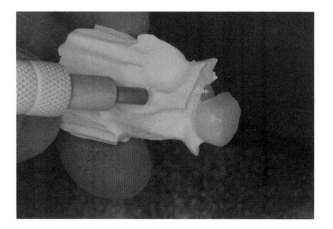

Figure 12-7. Devesting pressed-ceramic restoration.

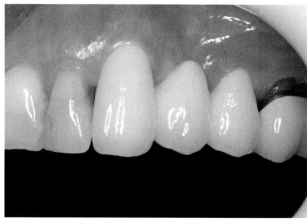

Figure 12-9. Pressed-ceramic three-unit bridge.

Cooling is controlled to ensure marginal integrity and proper crystal formation. Devested with glass bead abrasives (fig. 12-7), the ceramic coping is fit back onto the model and built up with appropriate feldspathic porcelain (Cattel et al. 2002).

Pressed-ceramic restorations can have exceptional esthetics and very good marginal fit (fig. 12-8). They are not, however, extremely strong and need to be placed with appropriate caution. The leucite-reinforced ceramics (e.g., IPS Empress, Finesse) have a flexural strength of 140–180 MPa compared with about 80 MPa for feldspathic porcelain and 1,200 MPa for zirconia materials, to be discussed later (Lawn 2004). Leucite-reinforced pressed ceramics should be restricted to single units in the anterior region and partial-coverage restorations in the posterior. Lithium disilicate reinforced pressed ceramics (e.g., IPS Empress 2, Eris, e.Max Press) have a flexural strength of about 300 MPa (Raigrodski 2004). This allows them to be used for short span bridges ante-

rior to the second premolar, provided space is available for large connectors (>3mm × 3mm; fig. 12-9).

The translucency that allows pressed-ceramic restorations to look so natural can create some problems when the teeth to be crowned have some unnatural coloration after preparation. The practitioner can communicate the underlying shade by choosing a "stump shade" from a specific shade guide (fig. 12-10), allowing the technician to compensate with the choice of ingot.

Adhesively bonded resin cements are required for cementing pressed ceramics in order to maintain their inherent translucency and maximize their fracture resistance (Kramer et al. 2006). The dentist needs to be aware that the shade of the resin cement can affect the final shade of the restoration and choose appropriately. Many resin cements offer multiple shades with try-in pastes, which can help predict and optimize esthetics. The glass component in pressed ceramics is susceptible to etching with hydrofluoric acid. This and silanization can create

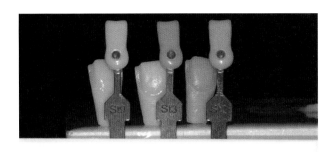

Stumpfmaterial Die Material

Figure 12-10. Stump shade guide.

a tenacious bond between cement, tooth, and restoration. Specific steps for cementing ceramic restorations will be covered in chapter 19.

The leucite and lithium disilicate reinforced glass ceramic materials used in pressed ceramics are also used for CAD/CAM-fabricated two-component systems. The CEREC inLab system—unlike CEREC 3D—uses scans of conventional model work rather than the dentition in vivo. Copings are designed and milled with a variation of the CEREC 3D technology; feldspathic porcelain is added for cosmetics and functional anatomy (Bindl, Luthy, Mormann 2006).

Glass-Infiltrated Ceramics
Zirconia, alumina, and spinel are crystalline ceramic materials that have useful characteristics as dental restorative materials. In their densest and strongest states, though, they are quite opaque and difficult to form. Glass-infiltrated ceramics are materials that make some use of the strength of crystalline ceramics while retaining some of the translucence of glass ceramics. A porous ceramic framework is produced either by computer aided milling (e.g., CEREC InLab, Kavo Everest) or by a slurry application and firing procedure (e.g., InCeram, WolCeram.). The "green state" ceramic framework is then heated in contact with an appropriately tinted glass ceramic, which fills the contiguous porosities by capillary action. Significantly, the firing cycles in this procedure do not produce dimensional change, allowing predictable marginal adaptation. The resulting ceramic copings have an intermediate flexural strength of approximately 350 MPa for spinel, 500 MPa for alumina, and 700 MPa for zirconia, with corresponding increases in opacity.

Similar to pressed-ceramic restorations, preparations for glass-infiltrated ceramics require an even circumferential reduction to allow adequate thickness of restorative material. Deep chamfers are the typically recommended margin design, but they may vary among ceramic systems. Moderate taper and lack of sharp line angles are important for ceramics not only in minimizing stress concentration but also in allowing accurate scanning for those systems using CAD/CAM. This can be a disadvantage of ceramics compared with metal-based restorations when preparing teeth with short or narrow clinical crowns.

Glass-infiltrated ceramics are used mainly as frameworks for full-coverage crowns in the anterior or posterior, and for short span bridges replacing premolars or anterior teeth. Having only moderate strength, they are a questionable choice for bridges replacing molars (Kaiser et al. 2006; Luthy et al. 2005).

Glass-infiltrated ceramics—and the fully sintered ceramics discussed below—are advertised as allowing conventional cementation techniques. This claim implies three properties: high enough strength not to need the intimate support of bonded tooth structure, enough opacity to negate the advantage of resin's translucency and shade selection, and resistance to surface treatment. While the strength is certainly an advantage, the opacity can compromise esthetics. The effectiveness of hydrofluoric acid etching and silane treatment is dependent on the glass present at the surface of the restoration. Glass-infiltrated ceramics have relatively little glass at that surface, and an effective bond between resin cement and restoration can only be achieved by a tribochemical coating process. The Rocatec system by 3M ESPE deposits a thin layer of glass to ceramic substrates, preparing them for silane treatment. This is also effective for the fully sintered ceramics discussed below (Ozcan and Vallittu 2003; Ernst et al. 2005; Amaral et al. 2006).

Fully Sintered Ceramics
Ceramic restorations based on pure crystalline ceramic copings have a significant advantage in strength over pressed or glass-infused ceramics. Their development has required overcoming some daunting technical challenges. Alumina and zirconia have been used in industrial and medical applications for some time, but the ability to economically form precise, individualized structures at a scale appropriate to dentistry has only recently been realized (Reich et al. 2004). Both substances can be formed in bulk at a factory but are difficult to machine in their densest state. At least two systems have been marketed that involved milling zirconium in ·a dense sintered state, but both are largely obsolete due to long milling times, high tool wear, and concerns about imperfections caused by the milling process (Luthart et al. 2002).

Nobel Biocare developed the first commercially successful fully sintered ceramic coping, called Procera All-Ceram. The copings are manufactured at two dedicated sites using information from scans of conventional dies taken at local laboratories. To compensate for the shrinkage that occurs as ceramics are fired from a green state to a fully sintered state, Nobel Biocare fabricates the green state ceramic on a precisely milled oversize refractory die. After final sintering and adjusting, the coping is returned to the local laboratory for application of feldspathic porcelain (Andersson et al. 1998; fig. 12-11). The Procera alumina coping has a flexural strength of 700 MPa, sufficient for a single unit or a short span bridge (Pallis et al. 2004; Fradeani et al. 2005; fig. 12-12).

Fully sintered zirconium is a more appropriate choice for posterior bridges or single units where durability is needed. Nobel Biocare produces a zirconium coping by the same method as described above called Procera All-Zircon. The first commercially available product, though, was Cercon (DCM System Degussa Dental). Unlike Procera, Cercon copings can be fabricated in local dental laboratories with purchased equipment. The Cercon system uses conventional model work and wax patterns (fig. 12-13). The pattern is scanned and an oversized coping is milled from a blank of green-state zirconium that is then sintered to final dimensions (Sturzenegger et al. 2000; fig. 12-14).

The Lava system by 3M dispenses with the waxing step by using a scan of the modelwork to help design the coping. It also mills an oversize green-state coping that is then sintered to fit (figs. 12-15 and 12-16). Eliminating the waxing step has made Lava popular with dental laboratories. Having a coping that can be custom tinted before porcelain stacking has made it popular with dentists and patients. Lava has a flexural strength of 1,100 MPa and can be made as thin as 0.3 mm (Piwowarczyk et al. 2005; Raigrodski 2004). It is limited to six unit spans by the size of the green-state block.

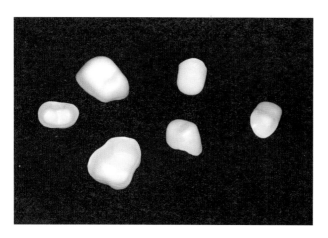

Figure 12-11. Procera copings.

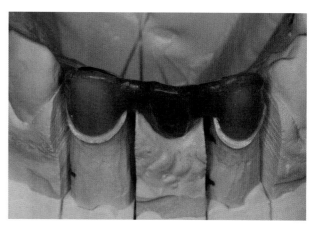

Figure 12-13. Wax-up for Cercon restoration.

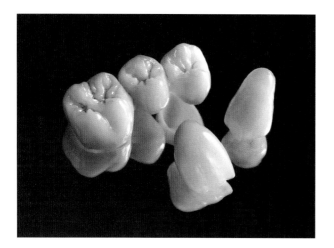

Figure 12-12. Completed Procera restorations.

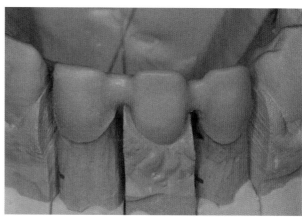

Figure 12-14. Cercon coping.

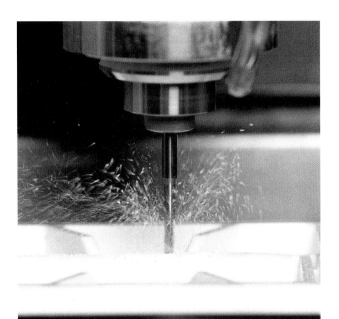

Figure 12-15. Milling Lava coping.

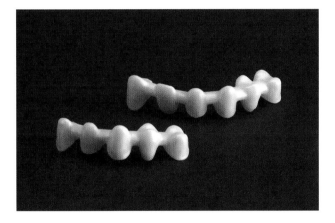

Figure 12-16. Lava copings.

Zeno Tec (Wieland Dental) is a newer system that allows for spans as large as a full arch but at present does not allow for staining. Cercon can now be made with blanks tinted at the factory, which may allow it to regain market share from its newer competitors.

Kavo Everest also offers presintered zirconium blocks with a good range of shades. When fully sintered, these offer a flexural strength similar to Cercon and Lava. These should not be confused with blanks of fully sintered zirconium, which Kavo had marketed as an alternative to milling oversized presintered zirconium blanks. Confusingly, Kavo also offers a zirconium silicate coping structurally similar to InCeram Zirconia (i.e., glass infiltrated), though processed in their CAD/CAM

system. This product, called Everest HPC, has a flexural strength of less than 350 MPa (Heydecke et al. 2007).

Pressed to Zirconium

Feldspathic porcelain as a veneering material over fully sintered zirconium has several drawbacks. It is, of course, brittle. The chipping of porcelain from zirconium-based restorations is similar to that of metal-ceramic restorations, rarely leading to complete delamination or crack propagation into the coping, but sometimes leaving the restoration functionally or esthetically unacceptable. Feldspathic porcelain, when extended to the margin, provides an inferior seal and has a tendency to fracture during try-in. Porcelain margins are also labor intensive, requiring the specialized skills of a ceramist.

For all these reasons, several systems, including Micro Dental's P2Z, Noritake CZR Press, and Ivoclar's Zir-Press have been developed which veneer zirconium copings with pressed ceramics, adding little or no feldspathic porcelain. This allows margins to be placed with a material using a reliable lost-wax technique without a computer needed to estimate the final dimensions of a shrinking ceramic. Considering the impressive accuracy that those estimates have achieved, this may not be a meaningful advantage. Glass ceramics do, though, have a better natural translucence than poly-crystalline ceramics, so pressed-to-zirconium will be superior where esthetics demands a seamless transition from ceramic to tooth structure. Although the pressed ceramic can be made to full contour and stained for realism, a third layer of feldspathic porcelain is needed to make these restorations truly lifelike. Having three components and three methods of fabrication, pressed-to-zirconium restorations are labor intensive and likely to command a higher laboratory fee.

These systems are too new to know for sure if they will suffer fewer fractures and delaminations than porcelain stacked over zirconium. The higher crystalline content in pressed-ceramic substrates, when built to occlusion, may slightly increase wear of opposing dentition compared to feldspathic porcelains.

Making a Selection

Meeting the patient's esthetic needs or desires has to be the first consideration in choosing an indirect restorative material. Every part of a restoration that is readily visible during smiling or talking will need to be made of a natural-looking material.

Consider first the patient's smile line. If the gingival margin of the teeth is exposed during smiling, any metal there will be unacceptable. Similarly, the more opaque copings of alumina or zirconia substrates may look unnatural if extended to a facial margin. A glass ceramic facial margin, whether pressed or stacked, is the only esthetic option for a patient with a high smile line wanting natural-looking anterior teeth. This need can be met with a metal-ceramic restoration (with porcelain margin), a pressed all-ceramic restoration, or a pressed-to-zirconium restoration. The pressed all-ceramic and pressed-to-zirconium provide more reliably accurate margins than the technically demanding hand-stacked porcelain margins of metal-ceramic restorations.

The next consideration should be shade matching. Patients wanting a full smile of bright, white, opaque teeth present little problem in regard to materials selection. All systems have the ability to block out unwanted background color either intrinsically or with opaque modifiers. Matching existing teeth or recreating imperfect natural teeth is a greater challenge. For this, pressed ceramics are the best choice. Their natural translucence and large selection of veneering porcelains allow for a wide range of appearances, limited mainly by communication with the laboratory. This includes choosing a stump shade for prepared teeth with discolored dentin.

When the need for esthetic restorations extends to the posterior teeth, structural considerations increase in importance. Teeth with multiple cusps are subjected to splitting forces to which predominantly glass ceramic restorations are highly vulnerable. Pressed ceramics, therefore, are a questionable choice. Crystalline ceramic substrates, either fully sintered or glass infiltrated, serve better for posterior teeth. Copings of glass-infiltrated alumina or zirconia are durable enough for most single-unit restorations and provide a good translucency and shade selection. Fully sintered zirconia copings offer the highest strength. They can be manufactured to as little as 0.3 mm thick, about the same as a metal coping. This renders them acceptably translucent for most applications. Tinting of copings also helps blend them with natural dentition. The primary drawback to zirconia-based restorations is relatively high cost.

The need for strength is even greater for bridges than for individual uses. Lithium disilicate–based pressed-ceramic frameworks can be used for short spans in the anterior and premolar areas but are not recommended for molar abutments or pontics. Glass-infiltrated ceramic frameworks have similar indications but less natural appearance. Zirconia frameworks should be the first choice for long span or posterior bridges. These have experienced an extremely small incidence of fracture, and current technology allows for thin walls on abutments and excellent marginal adaptation. They can even be used for telescoping bridges and with semiprecision attachments (table 12-1).

Future Trends

All-ceramic restorations currently command a fairly small portion of the indirect dental restorative market. This is due to their relative unfamiliarity and higher cost. As patient demand for all-ceramics inevitably increases, they will increase market share. They may become less costly as the initial investments in research, development, and start-up are amortized.

Zirconia is undoubtedly the material of the present and near future (Blatz et al. 2004). Thin copings now allow for good translucence and very esthetic restorations. Future zirconia substrates are expected to be inherently less opaque. Improvements in CAD/CAM procedures now produce margin fit comparable to metal-based restorations (fig. 12-17). Press-to-zirconia techniques allow for excellent fit and visually seamless margins. Recently, 3M ESPE has introduced new applications for Lava including Maryland bridges and inlay/onlay retained bridges.

Zirconia copings are also increasingly in use as abutments for implant retained restorations with good success. Research is ongoing to develop zirconia implant bodies to eliminate the graying of gingival tissues that can result from placing titanium implant bodies.

Intraoral scanning devices are being developed that propose to eliminate the need for clinical impressions for crown and bridge procedures, improving on the technologies developed for CEREC 3D.

A largely overlooked concern with this relatively new technology is how to deal with all-ceramic restorations when they need to be replaced. All-ceramic restorations are not immune to the problems of fracturing of veneering porcelain or of secondary caries (Aboushelib et al. 2005, 2006; Al Dohan et al. 2004). Removing an inadequate all-ceramic restoration is much more likely to result in a fractured or grossly overreduced tooth than removing a metal-based restoration due to their visual similarity to (Krejci 1995)—and their tenacious, inflexible grip onto—tooth structure. We will need new techniques and equipment to cope with this problem.

Minimum Armamentarium

A dentist practicing esthetic dentistry needs to be able to prescribe a certain minimal selection of available ceramic restorations in addition to any metal-ceramics and full-metal prostheses. A skilled ceramist is required for all restorations with a higher-strength coping veneered with feldspathic porcelain. This includes everything except for the in-office CAD/CAM systems such as CEREC 3D. At a minimum, a laboratory should be able to deliver the following:

Table 12-1. Material selection guide.

Restoration	Material Type	Examples	Advantages	Disadvantages	Cements
Veneer, inlay, onlay	Feldspathic porcelain	Various	Shade and opacity	Brittleness, technique sensitivity	Light-cured resin with shade selection
Anterior single unit	Leucite reinforced	IPS Empress	Esthetics	Low to moderate strength	Dual-cured resin with shade selection
		OPC-3G	Esthetics	Low to moderate strength	
		Finesse	Esthetics	Low to moderate strength	
		CEREC 3D	Single appointment	Low to moderate strength	
		CEREC InLab	Esthetics	Low to moderate strength	
	Aluminous porcelain	HiCeram	Esthetics	Brittleness, technique sensitivity	Dual-cured resin with shade selection
		Vitadur-N		Brittleness, technique sensitivity	
Anterior bridge (<4 units)	Lithium disilicate	IPS Eris	Highly esthetic	Large connectors required	Dual-cured resin with shade selection
Posterior single unit	Glass-infiltrated	InCeram	Low cost	Moderate strength	Resin-modified glass ionomer or self-etching resin cement
		WolCeram	Low cost	Moderate strength	
		CEREC InLab	Low cost	Moderate strength	
		Kavo Everest	Low cost	Moderate strength	
	Alumina	Procera AllCeram	Adequate strength	Opacity, high cost	
Posterior multiple units	Zirconia	LAVA	High strength	Opacity, high cost	
		Cercon	High strength	Opacity, high cost	
		Kavo Everest	High strength	Opacity, high cost	
		Procera AllZircon	High strength	Opacity, high cost	
		ZenoTech	High strength	Opacity, high cost	

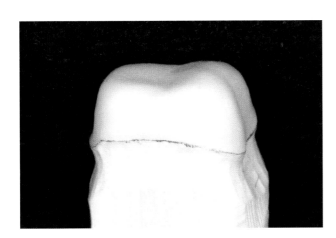

Figure 12-17. Lava coping on die.

- Leucite-reinforced or lithium disilicate–based glass ceramic for veneers, onlays, single units, or short span anterior bridges. Either pressing or milling (CAD/CAM) systems are appropriate.

- Zirconia-based frameworks for posterior fixed bridges and single units in high-load areas.
- Glass-infiltrated ceramics lower-cost option for single posterior units.

Works Cited

Aboushelib MN, de Jager N, Kleverlaan CJ, Feilzer AJ. 2005. Microtensile bond strength of different components of core veneered all-ceramic restorations. *Dent Mater* 21(10):984–91.

Aboushelib MN, de Jager N, Kleverlaan CJ, Feilzer AJ. 2006. Effect of loading method on the fracture mechanics of two layered all-ceramic restorative systems. *Dent Mater* Sep 18.

Al-Dohan HM, Yaman P, Dennison JB, Razzoog ME, Lang BR. 2004. Shear strength of core-veneer interface in bi-layered ceramics. *J Prosthet Dent* 91(4):349–55.

Amaral R, Ozcan M, Bottino MA, Valandro LF. 2006. Microtensile bond strength of a resin cement to glass infiltrated zirconia-reinforced ceramic: The effect of surface conditioning. *Dent Mater* 22(3):283–90.

Andersson M, Razzoog ME, et al. 1998. Procera: A new way to achieve an all-ceramic crown. *Quintessence Int* 29(5):285–96.

Bindl A, Luthy H, Mormann WH. 2006. Strength and fracture pattern of monolithic CAD/CAM-generated posterior crowns. *Dent Mater* 22(1):29–36.

Blatz MB, Sadan A, Martin J, Lang B. 2004. In vitro evaluation of shear bond strengths of resin to densely-sintered high-purity zirconium-oxide ceramic after long-term storage and thermal cycling. *J Prosthet Dent* 91(4):356–62.

Bortolotto T, Onisor I, Krejci I. 2006. Proximal direct composite restorations and chairside CAD/CAM inlays: Marginal adaptation of a two-step self-etch adhesive with and without selective enamel conditioning. *Clin Oral Investig* Oct 10.

Cattell MJ, Palumbo RP, et al. 2002. The effect of veneering and heat treatment on the flexural strength of Empress 2 ceramics. *J Dent* 30(4):161–69.

Cesar PF, Yoshimura HN, et al. 2005. Correlation between fracture toughness and leucite content in dental porcelains. *J Dent* 33(9):721–29.

Christensen GJ. 2003. The confusing array of tooth-colored crowns. *J Am Dent Assoc* 134(9):1253–55.

Christensen GJ. 2005. Longevity of posterior tooth dental restorations. *J Am Dent Assoc* 136(2):201–3.

Donovan T, Simonsen RJ, et al. 2004. Retrospective clinical evaluation of 1,314 cast gold restorations in service from 1 to 52 years. *J Esthet Restor Dent* 16(3):194–204.

Ernst CP, Cohnen U, Stender E, Willershausen B. 2005. In vitro retentive strength of zirconium oxide ceramic crowns using different luting agents. *J Prosthet Dent* 93(6):551–8.

Fasbinder D. 2006. Clinical performance of chairside CAD/CAM restorations. *J Am Dent Assoc* 137(Suppl):22S–31S.

Fradeani M, D'Amelio D, Redemagni M, Corrado M. 2005. Five-year follow-up with Procera all-ceramic crowns. *Quintessence Int* 36(2):105–13.

Goldin EB, Boyd NW III, Goldstein GR, Hittelman EL, Thompson VP. 2005. Marginal fit of leucite-glass pressable ceramic restorations and ceramic-pressed-to-metal restorations. *J Prosthet Dent* 93(2):143–7.

Guazzato M, Albakry M, Ringer SP, Swain MV. 2004. Strength, fracture toughness and microstructure of a selection of all-ceramic materials: Part I. Pressable and alumina glass-infiltrated ceramics. *Dent Mater* 20(5):441–8.

Heydecke G, Butz F, et al. 2007. Material characteristics of a novel shrinkage-free ZrSiO(4) ceramic for the fabrication of posterior crowns. *Dent Mater* 23(7):785–91.

Kaiser M, Wasserman A, et al. 2006. Long-term clinical results of VITA In-Ceram Classic: A systematic review. *Schweiz Monatsschr Zahnmed* 116(2):120–8.

Kramer N, Ebert J, et al. 2006. Ceramic inlays bonded with two adhesives after 4 years. *Dent Mater* 22(1):13–21.

Krejci. 1995. Time required to remove totally bonded tooth-colored posterior restorations and related tooth substance loss. *Dent Mater* 11(1):34–40.

Lawn BR, Pajares A, et al. 2004. Materials design in the performance of all-ceramic crowns. *Biomaterials* 25(14):2885–92.

Limkangwalmongkol P, Chiche GJ, et al. 2007. Precision of fit of two margin designs for metal-ceramic crowns. *J Prosthodont* 16(4):233–7.

Luthardt RG, Holzhuter M, et al. 2002. Reliability and properties of ground Y-TZP-zirconia ceramics. *J Dent Res* 81(7):487–91.

Luthardt RG, Loos R, et al. 2005. Accuracy of intraoral data acquisition in comparison to the conventional impression. *Int J Comput Dent* 8(4):283–94.

Luthy H, Filser F, Loeffel O, Schumacher M, Gauckler LJ, Hammerle CH. 2005. Strength and reliability of four-unit all-ceramic posterior bridges. *Dent Mater* 21(10):930–7.

Mormann W. 2006. The evolution of the CEREC system. *J Am Dent Assoc* 137(Suppl):7S–13S.

O'Brien WJ. 1997. *Dental Materials and Their Selection*, 2nd ed. Chicago: Quintessence.

Ozcan M, Vallittu PK. 2003. Effect of surface conditioning methods on the bond strength of luting cement to ceramics. *Dent Mater* 19(8):725–31.

Pallis K, Griggs JA, et al. 2004. Fracture resistance of three all-ceramic restorative systems for posterior applications. *J Prosthet Dent* 91(6):561–9.

Piwowarczyk A, Ottl P, Lauer HC, Kuretzky T. 2005. A clinical report and overview of scientific studies and clinical procedures conducted on the 3M ESPE Lava All-Ceramic System. *J Prosthodont* 14(1):39–45.

Raigrodski A. 2004. Contemporary materials and technologies for all-ceramic fixed partial dentures: A review of the literature. *J Prosthet Dent* 92(6):557–62.

Reich SM, Wichmann M, et al. 2004. Clinical performance of large, all-ceramic CAD/CAM-generated restorations after three years: A pilot study. *J Am Dent Assoc* 135(5):605–12.

Reiss B. 2006. Clinical results of CEREC inlays in a dental practice over a period of 18 years. *Int J Comput Dent* 9(1):11–22.

Sadowsky SJ. 2006. An overview of treatment considerations for esthetic restorations: A review of the literature. *J Prosthet Dent* 96(6):433–42.

Shillingberg HT, et al. 1997. *Fundamentals of Fixed Prosthodontics*, 3rd ed. Chicago: Quintessence.

Shoher I. 1998. Vital tooth esthetics in Captek restorations. *Dent Clin North Am* 42(4):713–8.

Soares CJ, Marcondes-Martins LR, et al. 2006. Influence on cavity preparation design on fracture resistance of posterior Leucite reinforced ceramic restorations. *J Prosthet Dent* 95(6):9.

Sturzenegger B, Feher A, et al. 2000. Clinical study of zirconium oxide bridges in the posterior segments fabricated with the DCM system. *Schweiz Monatsschr Zahnmed* 110(12):131–9.

Suggested Additional Reading

Raigrodski AJ, Chiche GJ, Potiket N, Hochstedler JL, Mohamed SE, Billiot S, Mercante DE. 2006. The efficacy of posterior three-unit zirconium-oxide-based ceramic fixed partial dental prostheses: A prospective clinical pilot study. *J Prosthet Dent* 96(4):237–44.

Chapter 13
Color and Shade Selection

James Milani DDS, BA

Laura Reid DDS, BS

Richard H. White DDS, BA

Color Perception in Dentistry

To understand basic color theory and how it is used in dental color matching, it is important to know how the human eye works. When an object reflects wavelengths of light back to a viewer, the perception of color occurs. The color of an object is composed of the wavelengths of light being reflected off the surface. The retinal portion of the human eye contains three types of cone cells, each of which perceives one of three wavelengths corresponding to the colors red, green, and blue, respectively (Chu, Devigus, and Mieleszko 2004). With proper lighting intensity, the pupil of the eye opens to a diameter that fully exposes the fovea in the center of the retina that contains a high number of cone cells. This area defines the center of the visual field and provides the best color perception (Chu, Devigus, and Mieleszko 2004).

Color perception is three-dimensional as a result of the three cone types, and a color can be specified by its value, hue, and chroma (Chu, Devigus, and Mieleszko 2004). Value is the brightness or relative lightness or darkness of color. Hue is the color name, such as *red*, *green*, or *blue*. Chroma is the depth or saturation and purity of color. Color order systems are based on the principles of color perception, and the Munsell color wheel is commonly used in dentistry to communicate color qualities (Paravina and Powers 2004).

The color, or hue, perceived by individuals can vary; therefore, it is important to know if your color vision is normal or deficient. A deficiency can result from hereditary disorders, injury, or disease. Poor discrimination between certain colors, usually reds and greens, may be detected by visual testing. The Ishihara test and Farnsworth-Munsell Color 100 (Rosenthal and Phillips 1997) test are commonly used for this purpose (figs. 13-1a and 13-1b).

In addition to color, secondary optical properties found in teeth, such as opalescence, fluorescence, and translucency, influence light reflection and are considered as important in deciding the overall appearance of the tooth (Terry et al. 2002). Opalescence occurs when light is scattered by subsurface areas, causing an incisal halo appearance. Opalescent porcelains can be used in a restoration to recreate this effect (Paravina and Powers 2004).

Opalescence can be found in the incisal edge and proximal incisal areas of anterior teeth (fig. 13-2). Cusp tips and marginal ridges are areas of posterior teeth where this pattern is also found.

Fluorescence is typically assessed in the middle third of an anterior tooth and is generally observed in the yellow/orange color range (Paravina, Powers 2004; see fig. 13-2). Fluorescent ceramic powders in dental porcelain can be used to reproduce this pattern.

Translucency is most evident in the incisal edges of anterior teeth (fig. 13-2). It tends to lower the value of teeth and can also be mimicked with translucent porcelain in a restoration (Priest and Lindke 2000). These three qualities affect the quality and the quantity of light reflected (Winter 1993).

Tooth surface morphology also affects the amount and type of reflection of light (Joiner 2004). Qualities of texture caused by surface imperfections such as perikymata and enamel craze lines have an influence on the way light is reflected and influence the perceived color of teeth. The smoothness or luster of the surface being color matched will also influence appearance (Priest and Lindke 2000; figs. 13-3 and 13-4).

Color Matching Conditions

Illumination quality of the environment can affect the color perception of teeth. To help improve the color match and reduce chances for error, the environmental qualities that most affect shade matching are light intensity (Carsten 2003) and the type of illuminant used. Daylight-corrected lights in the dental operatory can

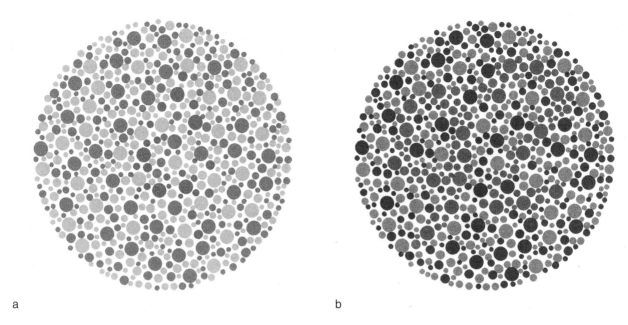

a   b

Figure 13-1.   a. Normal color vision reveals the number 4 in the dot pattern. b. Normal color vision reveals the number 92 in the dot pattern.

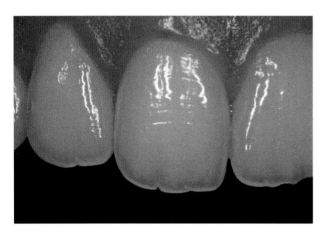

Figure 13-2.   Incisal edges of anterior teeth depicting opalescence and fluorescence.

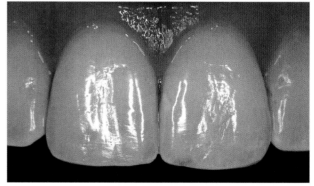

Figure 13-4.   Reflected light is scattered more when surface texture is rough.

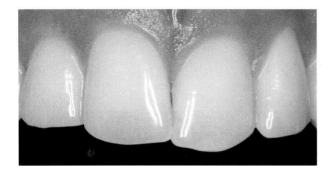

Figure 13-3.   Smooth texture and high luster found on the facial surface of anterior teeth.

help to reduce the differences between artificial light and natural light (Knispel 1991) that contribute to metamerism, or the phenomenon of two objects appearing to match in color under one lighting condition but not under another.

Northern daylight at ten o'clock in the morning is a desirable time of day for color matching in natural light. When natural light is not available, fluorescent bulbs with a color temperature of 5,000–5,500K (D65 illuminants) and a color rendition index greater than 90 out of 100 can be installed (Chu, Devigus, and Mieleszko 2004).

Color Determination in Dentistry

Color Matching

Accurate color matching is important, but the objectives of the patient must also be taken into consideration. Optimally the color analysis will be under color-corrected lights in addition to natural light conditions. Oftentimes, a change of tooth color is what the patient desires, and this must be agreed upon prior to beginning any esthetic restorative treatment. Teeth become dehydrated during preparation as the mouth remains open and compressed air is used to clear the operating field of debris. As a result, the brightness (i.e., value) of the color is increased and the chroma is decreased (Priest and Lindke 2000). Shade matching should be done with the teeth fully hydrated to properly evaluate the natural tooth color.

The type of restorative material to be used will have a direct influence on the shade choices. Matching the relative translucency of the restoration to that of the tooth will give the best chances for an acceptable color match. For example, a zirconium- or alumina-based restoration such as Lava or Procera will have greater opacity than a pressed-ceramic restoration such as Empress I, which will have more translucency. Direct composite materials will have specific techniques or color recipes as given by the manufacturer to achieve the desired esthetic effect.

The color a particular tooth has is the result of varying amounts of dentin and enamel. Dentin influences most of the color while the enamel layer influences translucency, opalescence, and fluorescence. As a result of this mixture, multiple colors of restorative material are often required to restore the tooth back to a natural appearance. The dental lab technician has the ability to use opaquers and color modifiers for internal characterization of the restoration to help achieve this goal.

Dimensions of Color

The three dimensions of color formulated by Munsell in 1898 (Munsell 1961) of value (the lightness or darkness of a color), hue (the basic color), and chroma (the amount or density of a color) form the basis for the majority of current shade matching systems used in dentistry. The Vita shade guide was developed from this system, and many manufacturers of porcelain and composite have adapted it to their materials.

Color Determination Systems

Modern color determination of teeth includes traditional systems that utilize shade tabs and electronic shade systems that utilize digital information capture to map the distribution of facial surface color regions. In addition, photographs can be used to provide supplemental information to the lab in a visual format. Many dentists find it necessary to use a combination of techniques to obtain the best outcome and employ their dental assistant as well in color determination.

Shade Tab Systems

The use of shade tabs for color determination is a very commonly used technique, and many esthetic restorative materials, including denture teeth, are keyed to them. Examples include the VITA Classical Shade Guide (Vident, Brea, CA; fig. 13-5) and the VITA 3D-Master Shade Guide (Vident, Brea, CA; figs. 13-6 and 13-7).

Another common shade tab system is the Chromascop universal shade guide (Ivoclar Vivadent, Amherst, NY; fig. 13-8).

Ivoclar Vivadent products are patterned for use with this guide. Examples include the IPS Empress I and

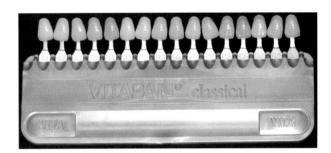

Figure 13-5. Vita Classical shade guide.

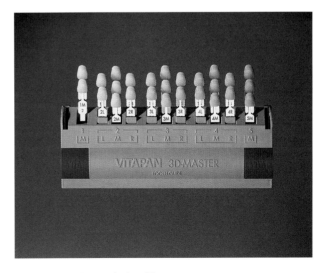

Figure 13-6. Vita 3-D shade guide.

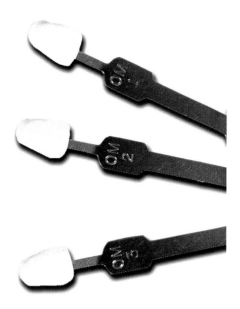

Figure 13-7. Vita 3-D bleach shade tabs.

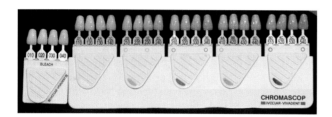

Figure 13-8. Vita 3-D bleach shade tabs.

Empress e.Max system for indirect restorations, and the direct restoratives such as TetricEvoCeram and Artemis composites.

When color matching denture teeth, an additional consideration is the gingival shade of the denture base itself and how the contrast between the two can influence the overall perception of the shade. For example, a relatively dark denture base will result in a lighter appearance of the teeth when compared with the same teeth in a denture base of a lighter shade. Gingival shade guides are available. Examples include the Lucitone 199 shade guide (Dentsply Trubyte) and the Ivocap Plus gingival shade indicator (Ivoclar Vivadent; fig. 13-9).

It is recommended to select the denture tooth shade prior to the ceramic shade when combining a removable prosthesis with a fixed prosthesis. This allows the lab technician to use the denture tooth shade guide as a custom shade guide for matching the ceramic of the fixed units.

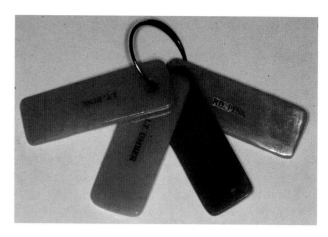

Figure 13-9. Gingival shade guide.

Electronic Shade Systems

As an adjunct to traditional shade tab systems, electronic shade selection systems are especially useful when attempting to blend a restoration into an existing dentition. They can also provide valuable information on the subtleties of value or color proportions as they change over the tooth surface. Results can then be mapped and charted before sending the information to the dental laboratory on a printed prescription form or in an electronic format.

These systems can be divided by type of scanning technology into two main categories: colorimeters and spectrophotometers. Colorimeters store three data points for hue, value, and chroma instead of the sixteen or more data points of reflectance recorded by a spectrophotometer (Paul et al. 2002). The majority of research on natural tooth color has been done with colorimeters (Ishikawa-Nagai et al. 1993; Ishikawa-Nagai et al. 1994; Horn, Bulan-Brady, and Hicks 1998; Freedman 2001; Hunter and Harold 1987; Okubo et al. 1998). An example of this type is the X-Rite ShadeVision system (X-Rite, Grandville, MI) that demonstrates color accuracy similar to that of a spectrophotometer (fig. 13-10). Both of these shade-scanning device categories are keyed to specific ceramic and composite references.

An example of a commonly used spectrophotometer is the Vita Easyshade by Vident (figs. 13-11a and 13-11b).

Software

A third category based on shade analysis software utilizes a digital camera to capture images and then transfer them to a computer where color analysis is managed. An example of this is the ClearMatch system (Smart Technology, Hood River, OR; fig. 13-12).

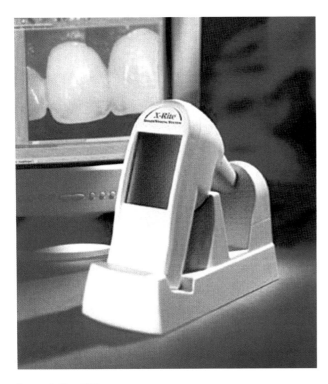

Figure 13-10. X-Rite system.

Color Determination Techniques

Shade Tabs

By dividing the color determination technique into steps, you will ensure a standardized approach to the process and increase your rate of successful shade matching as a result. Each shade guide manufacturer has a recommended approach to this process, and by using a variety of shade guides, your chances of an accurate color determination is improved.

To begin, ensure that all surfaces of the teeth have been thoroughly cleaned. After the teeth are clean, instruct the patient to remove any facial makeup; makeup can influence color matching. Utilize a neutral-colored (light blue or gray) bib to cover any bright clothing (Paravina and Powers 2004). Next, assess the amount of translucency or opacity present to help determine the type of restorative material that will be used. Now determine the value of the teeth you are trying to match. Value is the most important contributor to color matching, and if it is not correct, optimal esthetic results will not be achieved (fig. 13-13). Value is also a major determinant of the type of restorative material to be used with the appropriate underlying preparation.

Acceptable esthetic results can be obtained if the hue is slightly off. If the value is not correct, the restoration will not blend into the existing dentition.

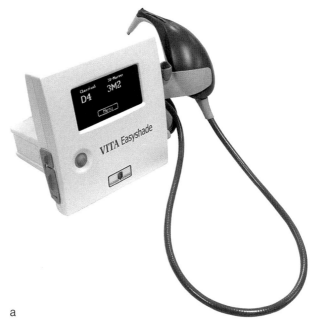

a

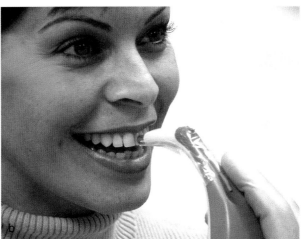

Figure 13-11. a. Vita Easyshade. b. Vita Easyshade close-up.

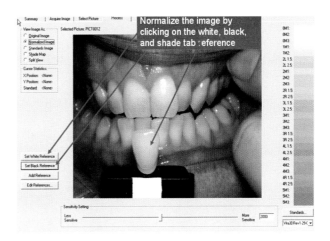

Figure 13-12. ClearMatch screen shot.

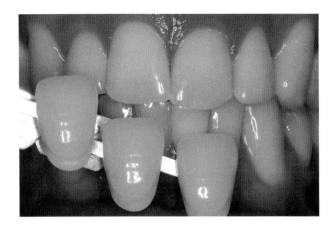

Figure 13-13. Value determination.

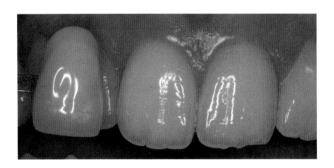

Figure 13-14. Placement of shade tab.

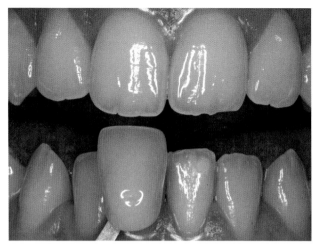

Figure 13-15. Positioning shade tab toward incisal.

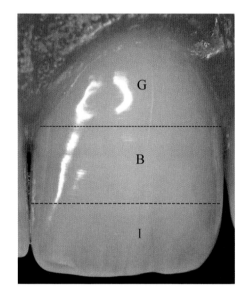

Figure 13-16. Facial surface divided into three sections.

Value Selection

Most companies distribute their shade guides arranged in hue groups. To begin, you may want to rearrange the shade guide tabs by value, starting with the brightest (highest value) and ending with the darkest (lowest value). Here is the arrangement for the standard Vita Shade guide as determined by the manufacturer: B1, A1, B2, D2, A2, C1, C2, D4, A3, D3, B3, A3.5, B4, C3, A4, and C4.

Positioning the shade tab in the following manner will yield the most accurate view:

1. Shade tab at practitioner's eye level
2. At the same incisal edge position as the tooth being matched
3. Parallel to the long axis of the tooth being matched
4. Angled along the same facial plane as the tooth being matched (fig. 13-14).

Place the incisal area of the shade tab closest to the tooth being matched to avoid the hue area in the middle of the tab from influencing your value decision. Incisal shading has the greatest influence on value selection (fig. 13-15).

At this step in the color determination, you are trying to find a value range and not the exact color. Evaluate the chosen tab approximately five to seven seconds and then glance away at a neutral gray card to rest your eyes (Paravina and Powers 2004).

During the value analysis, use various shade tabs in the incisal, body, and gingival areas of the neighboring teeth and the opposing teeth. Learning to see the amount of grayness or value of a tooth takes time, practice, and patience (fig. 13-16).

Hue Selection

Hue is the main or dominant color of the tooth. The most accurate way to use the shade tab is by removing the neck of the tab itself first to eliminate the influence this area has on the color and value selection. The neck area is higher in chroma and lower in value, and eliminating it will ensure that the purest shade is used. You may wish to have an unaltered tab available in the event you want to use the darker, gingival shading to match.

Position the hue area of the shade tab against the area you are trying to match. The dominant hue may be based on the dentin shade and is best found in the middle third of the facial surface. It is possible that the gingival third color selection is close or even the same as the middle third as well. Hue is labeled as A, B, C, or D (fig. 13-17).

The chroma is determined last. This is the amount of color intensity or saturation the tooth has and is indicated by number on the Vita shade guide. For example, A3 has a higher chroma level than A1 within the same hue range (fig. 13-18).

The same steps may be used with the VITAPAN 3D-MASTER (Vident, Brea, CA), although the chroma is selected before the hue with this system. Shade tabs are arranged in an orderly manner by five value groups. Once the value group is chosen, the chroma level, which runs vertically within that group, is decided upon. Hue, which runs horizontally, is then based on whether the comparison tooth is greener or redder than the chosen color. Tabs are marked by number from 1 to 5 to indicate group number and value level; a lower number is given to a higher value or lightness. The number below the group number—1, 1.5, 2, 2.5, or 3—is the chroma level,

a higher number indicating a higher chroma. The letter M represents the middle hue of each group, and the letter L denotes greener, while R is redder, than the M tab (Paravina and Powers 2004). This shade guide system allows value, chroma, and hue to be selected in a systematic manner.

The Chromascop shade determination system is based on Ivoclar dentin shades and is arranged into five subdivided shade or hue groups: group 100 white, group 200 yellow, group 300 light brown, group 400 gray, and group 500 dark brown (Paravina and Powers 2004). The four shade intensities in each group are chromatically arranged. The first step in choosing the color with this guide is to determine the base shade of the patient, remove the corresponding shade group, and then determine the shade intensity within that group.

If you are unsure of the final color selection, it is better to have a restoration returned with a value that is too high and a chroma that is too low. The color may be modified directly through the use of surface staining to bring the differences closer to the intended result.

Teeth change color with time, tending to have a higher value and opacity and a lower chroma at a younger age. The value or translucency decreases and the chroma increases with time, while the hue may stay approximately the same or vary slightly to the redder (Chu, Devigus, and Mieleszko 2004; figs. 13-19a and 13-19b).

For posterior restorations, the Mosaic system (Dental Illusions, Woodland Hills, CA) can be used to communicate information on the characterization of the grooves,

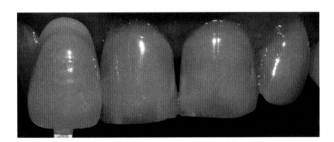

Figure 13-17. Shade tab hue compared to natural tooth hue.

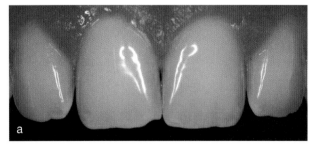

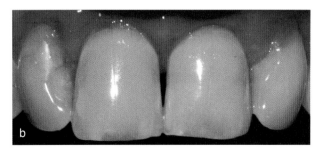

Figure 13-19. a. Example of a younger patient. b. Example of an older patient.

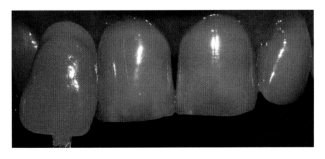

Figure 13-18. Shade tab positioned for chroma determination.

pits, and cuspal coloration to the dental laboratory (Derbabian et al. 2001). The same dimensions of color are used for posterior color matching as those for anterior restorations: value, hue, and chroma.

If there is difficulty in deciding between two values, then choose the lesser or lighter of the two. When choosing chroma, stay within the selected color family: group A (A1–A4) reddish-brown, group B (B1–B4) orange-yellow, group C (C1–C4) greenish-gray, and group D (D2–D4) pinkish-gray (Paravina and Powers 2004). If undecided between two chromas, the one with a higher chroma should be used. The patient should grant approval for pit and fissure staining or areas of hypocalcification that may be incorporated into the restoration (Phelan 2002).

Electronic Scanning

There are two general categories of electronic shade-measuring devices: spectrophotometers and colorimeters. The Vita EasyShade (Vident, Brea, CA) is a commercially available example of a spectrophotometer-type instrument. This device utilizes an image-capture tip the approximate size of a small light-curing tip. As a result, the incisal, middle, and cervical thirds of the tooth must be scanned to complete the color analysis of the entire facial surface (figs. 13-20a and 13-20b).

The X-Rite ShadeVision system (X-Rite, Grandville, MI) is a commercially available example of a colorimeter instrument that captures the entire facial surface of the

tooth being matched. This delivers more information on value, hue, and chroma compared to a spectrophotomer and has the advantage of enabling the lab technician the ability to compare an image of the final restoration with the image captured of the tooth being matched.

Colorimeters are limited in their interpretation of translucency because it is not one of the three attributes of color, namely, value, hue, and chroma (Derbabian et al. 2001)

Software

The ClearMatch system (Smart Technology, Hood River, OR) utilizes computer-based software analysis of an image taken with a digital camera. Detailed shade mapping of the tooth is provided based on dental porcelain shade guide nomenclature (fig. 13-21). Direct composite shading can also be done.

Communication of Color to the Laboratory

With the evolution of dental ceramics and direct composites, numerous tools have been developed to enhance and more accurately communicate the preferred restoration color chosen in the dental office to the dental lab. Communication between the dentist and the laboratory technician becomes critical to meet the expectations of the patient for natural-appearing restorations. It is a good idea to meet with your dental laboratory to discuss

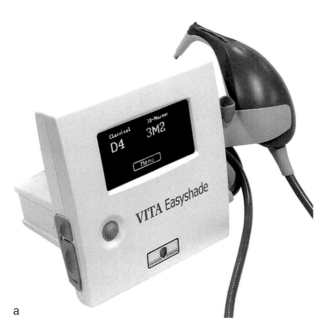

a

Figure 13-20.   a. Vita Easyshade. b. Vita Easyshade placement.

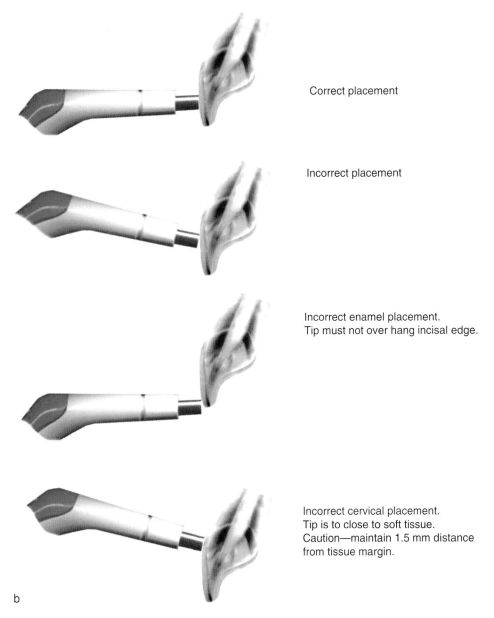

Correct placement

Incorrect placement

Incorrect enamel placement.
Tip must not over hang incisal edge.

Incorrect cervical placement.
Tip is to close to soft tissue.
Caution—maintain 1.5 mm distance
from tissue margin.

b

Figure 13-20. *Continued*

the porcelain systems that they use and the color matching techniques that will need to be used with them.

After choosing the cervical, middle, and incisal shades, photographs can be taken with each tab next to the tooth being matched, followed by a photo of all three tabs close to the teeth (Chu, Devigus, and Mieleszko 2004). Facial photos showing the full smile and face of the patient are also helpful (figs. 13-22a and 13-22b).

If using a laboratory prescription form, diagram the anterior teeth by starting with the cervical region. The color of this area is influenced by the gingival tissue and the root surface. It is the most opaque area of the tooth. The dominant hue or color found in the middle third of

the facial surface is recorded next. The incisal third is recorded last and will have the greatest variation in translucency and color (Priest and Lindke 2000). The amount of translucency and the location of translucent highlights can also be communicated by drawings of the tooth (figs. 13-23a and 13-23b).

Conclusion

Natural tooth color reproduction is the goal of shade matching as part of restoring the dentition. By combining an understanding of basic color science with modern

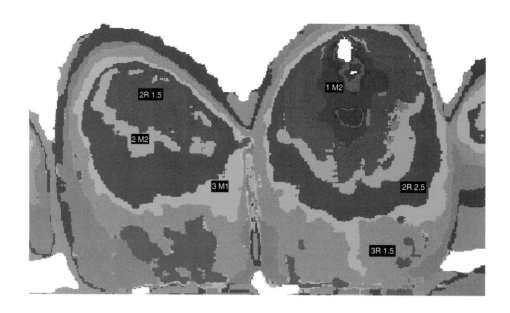

3R 1.5	19.86	2R 2.5	15.93	4M1	12.99	2R 1.5	10.76	3M1	9.73
4R 1.5	6.29	5M1	5.79	2M2	5.53	3L 1.5	4.51	1M2	2.47
2M1	2.25	0M1	0.62	1M1	0.60	4M2	0.56	4L 1.5	0.56
3M2	0.44	0M2	0.33	2L 1.5	0.30	0M3	0.20	5M2	0.14
3R 2.5	0.07	4L 2.5	0.05	3M3	0.01	3L 2.5	0.01		

Figure 13-21. ClearMatch mapping.

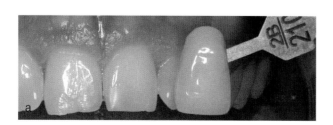
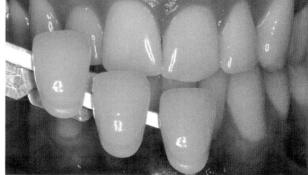

Figure 13-22. a. Digital photo with shade tab. b. Digital photo with three shade tabs.

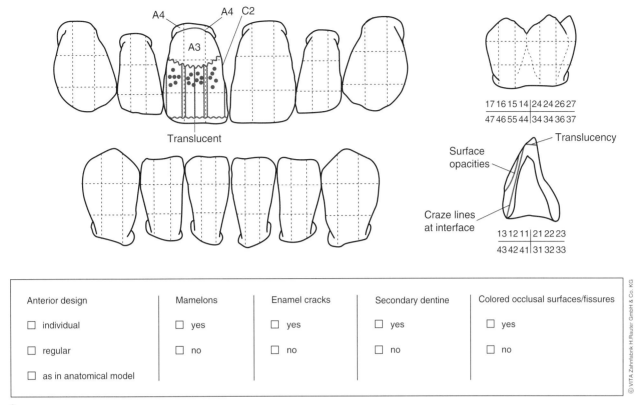

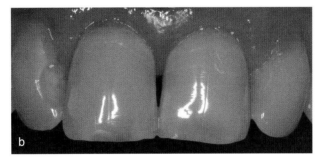

Figure 13-23.   a. Communicating shade and texture to the laboratory technician. Surface characteristics such as craze lines, opacities, and translucency can be included. b. Digital photo.

shade-determining techniques and effectively communicating the requirements to the laboratory technician, the chances of achieving this goal can be improved. Even with these tools available, there will always be the artistic portion that is gained with experience and can only be learned from experience.

Works Cited

Carsten D. 2003. Successful shade matching: What does it take? *Compend Contin Educ Dent* 24:175–8, 180, 182.

Chu SJ, Devigus A, Mieleszko A. 2004. *Fundamentals of Color: Shade Matching and Communication in Esthetic Dentistry.* Chicago: Quintessence.

Derbabian K, Marzola R, Donovan TE, Arcidiacono A. 2001. The science of communicting the art of esthetic dentistry: Part III. Precise shade communication. *J Esthet Restor Dent* 13:154–62.

Freedman G. 2001. Communicating color. *Dent Today* 20:76–80.

Horn DJ, Bulan-Brady J, Hicks ML. 1998. Sphere spectrophotometer versus human evaluation of tooth shade. *J Endod* 24:786–90.

Hunter RS, Harold RW. 1987. *The Measurement of Appearance,* 2nd ed. New York: John Wiley & Sons.

Ishikawa-Nagai S, Sawafuji F, Tsuchitoi H, Sata RR, Ishibashi K. 1993. Using a computer color-matching system in color reproduction or porcelain restorations: Part 2. Color reprocuction of stratiform-layered porcelain samples. *Int J Prosthodont* 6:522–7.

Ishikawa-Nagai S, Sato RR, Shiraishi A, Ishibashi K. 1994. Using a computer color-matching system in color reproduction of porcelain restorations: Part 3. A newly developed spectrophotometer designed for clinical application. *Int J Prosthodont* 7:50–5.

Joiner A. 2004. Tooth colour: A review of the literature. *Journal of Dentistry* 32:3–12.

Knispel G. 1991. Factors affecting the process of color matching restorative materials to natural teeth. *Quint Intl* 22(7): 525–31.

Munsell AH. 1961. *A Color Notation*, 2nd ed. Baltimore: Munsel Color Company.

Okubo SR, Kananwati A, Richards MW, Childress S. 1998. Evaluation of visual and instrument shade matching. *J Prosthet Dent* 80:585–90.

Paravina RD, Powers JM. 2004. *Esthetic color training in dentistry*. St Louis: Elsevier Health Sciences.

Paul S, Peter A, Pietrobon N, Hammerle CH. 2002. Visual and spectrophotometric shade analysis of human teeth. *Dent Res* 81:578–92.

Phelan S. 2002. Use of photographs for communicating with the laboratory in indirect posterior restorations. *J Can Dent Assoc* 68(4):239–42.

Priest G, Lindke L. 2000. Tooth color selection and characterization accomplished with optical mapping. *Pract Periodont Aesthet Dent* 12(5):497–503.

Rosenthal O, Phillips R. 1997. *Coping with Color-Blindness*. New York: Avery.

Terry DA, Geller W, Tric O, Anderson MJ, Tourville M, Kobashigawa A. 2002. Anatomical form defines color: Function, form and aesthetics. *Practical Procedures and Aesthetic Dentistry* 14:59–67.

Winter R. 1993. Visualizing the natural dentition. *Journal of Esthetic Dentistry* 5:102–17.

Suggested Additional Reading

Lee SY, Nathanson D, Giordano R. 2001. Colour stability of a new light-cured ceramic stain system subjected to glazing temperature. *J Oral Rehabil* 28:457.

Leinfelder K. 2000. Porcelain esthetics for the 21st century. *J Am Dent Assoc* 131(Suppl):47S–51S.

Reis RS, et al. 1996. Effect of firing on the color stability of a light-cured ceramic stain. *J Prosthodont* 5:182.

Chapter 14
Preparation Design for Indirect Restorations in Esthetic Dentistry

Foroud Hakim DDS, MBA, BS

Jessie Vallee DDS, BS

This chapter will review the principles of preparation design. Special focus will be placed on preparation design criteria for indirect restoratives that fall under the umbrella of esthetic dentistry. However, successful esthetic preparation design demands more than just knowledge of specific restoration requirements.

"Optimal preparation" encompasses considerations in both design and technique. It not only increases the likelihood of long-term success of restorations but also ensures the relative predictability and efficiency of the steps following preparation. Procedures such as impression making or provisional restoration fabrication may be simplified with appropriate preparation design and technique. On the other hand, poor preparation design, compounded by traumatic technique, can render the same steps difficult and frustrating. The esthetic dentist must therefore pay close attention to the following optimal preparation considerations:

1. Biomechanics
   a. Adjacent tooth preservation
   b. Abutment preservation
   c. Periodontium preservation
   d. Occlusion
2. Restorative mechanics
   a. Retention form
   b. Resistance form
3. Durability of materials
4. Esthetics
   a. Anatomic considerations
   b. Margin location

The challenge of preparation design lies in that optimizing any one consideration for a given preparation often results in the sacrifice of a competing consideration. A classic illustration of this point is the trade-off between the principles of conserving tooth structure versus maximizing tooth reduction to gain esthetic control through porcelain depth.

Ultimately, optimal preparation occurs only when there is a perfect compromise of all considerations, which varies depending on each set of circumstances. Once enamel and dentin are removed, they cannot be replaced or regenerated. There is no substitute for prepreparation planning through case design, which requires consideration of biomechanics, restorative mechanics, and esthetics.

The chapter will begin by covering the optimal preparation guidelines and will follow with specific preparation designs and criteria for indirect restoration that fall under the esthetic category. The categories covered under specific preparation design and criteria for esthetic indirect restorations include the following:

- Ceramo-metal crowns (PFM crowns)
- Full-coverage all-ceramic crowns
- Partial coverage all-ceramic restorations
- Veneers
- Inlays/onlays

Optimal Preparation Guidelines

Biomechanical Considerations

Adjacent Tooth Preservation
Before strategies and precautions are discussed for maintaining the health of a preparation, it is worthwhile to discuss the protection of adjacent teeth during preparation. While preventing damage to proximal teeth is a universal goal, the reality is that postoperative clinical and radiographic evaluations often reveal some alteration or abrasion of the proximal surfaces of teeth adjacent to a crown preparation. Generally, these are inadvertent, minor abrasions that do not materially change the contour of the involved tooth. However, even minimal enamel abrasion may lead to undesirable outcomes such as plaque retention, cavitations, or floss

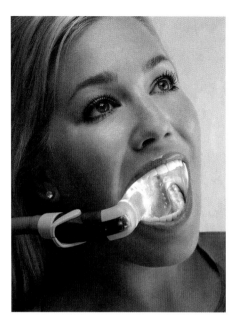

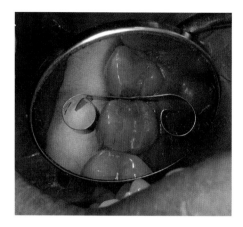

Figure 14-2. Inter-guard placed between bicuspids to protect against inadvertent abrasion of adjacent tooth from Ultradent Corp.

Figure 14-1. Optimized isolation, illumination and retraction achieved in lower left quadrant using the Isolite II Dry Field Illuminator from Isolite Corp. Courtesy of Isolite Corp.

shredding. Adjacent tooth damage can also range to iatrogenic extremes when contour changes are so severe that both tooth health and periodontal status are compromised.

Adjacent tooth to bur contact is unavoidable at times due to difficult access, often experienced while preparing posterior teeth, and patient limitations in opening or obstructive tongues and cheeks. The correct reaction during preparation is to become aware when abrasions occur, employ all strategies possible to minimize reoccurrence, and ultimately, return the abraded surfaces to a high polish. This can be done with any number of proximal polishing flutes, cups, and discs. The significant error lies in leaving an involved surface rough and uncorrected. Of course, a "best practices" goal is to minimize or eliminate bur to adjacent tooth contact. Strategies that an operator may find helpful include the following:

- Maximization of illumination for visualization
- Magnification of the working field (loupes, microscopes)
- Patient environment stabilization (mouth props, Isolite, rubber dams; fig. 14-1)
- Armamentarium selection (smaller-headed handpiece, narrow diamonds for breaking contacts, interguards; fig. 14-2)

Abutment Preservation
Preserving the tooth structure of the abutment tooth involves both preparation integrity maintenance and pulpal health maintenance. While these goals generally go hand in hand, ensuring one does not necessarily ensure the other. For example, an ideal preparation can be attained by standard protocols without the benefit of water mist as a coolant. The preparation geometry may in fact be acceptable, but the pulpal insult, as a result of temperature elevation, jeopardizes the tooth vitality.

Pulpal health may adversely be affected by both heat and overreduction. Excessive heat can be generated as a result of high bur to tooth interface pressure, dull burs that have lost their cutting efficiency, or the lack of adequate water spray as coolant. Pulpal health is also compromised when reduction proximity approaches the pulp. Such a scenario is another good illustration of opposing considerations and compromise in preparation design. In the event that an anterior subject tooth has a narrow profile and width dimension, compounded by a larger pulp dimension, the operator must determine a compromise involving both preparation design and material choice. The goals of pulpal health and idealized ceramic esthetics are balanced, leading to an ideal axial reduction for circumstances at hand. Factors leading to balanced compromise in preparation design are weighted based on radiographic and clinical impression of tooth and pulp dimensions as well as case design and desired esthetic outcomes.

Typically, pulp size decreases with age. Although this varies in patients, radiographs have shown up to 3mm of pulpal body size regression (occurring more occluso-cervically and mesio-distally than facio-lingually) by the age of 60. Optimal preparation is predicated by armamentarium and techniques that reduce the likelihood of pulpal damage (Baldissara, Catapano, and Scotti 1997).

Periodontium Preservation

Gingival inflammation is often associated with the margins of indirect restorations. For example, tissue irritation may be caused by open margins, residual cement, or metal-based allergic reactions. While an ideal preparation does not ensure an ideal restoration, undesirable tissue outcomes are far more likely to occur when preparation principles are violated. The two most likely causes of gingival and periodontal inflammation linked to preparation design are inadequate axial reduction and excessive subgingival margination. Migration of finish lines too far subgingivally can lead to encroachment of the epithelial attachment and violation of biologic width. Inadequate axial reduction may lead to overcontoured restorations. In turn, such restorations can cause gingival inflammation due to compression of crestal gingiva and papillae as well as compromising the patient's ability to perform adequate hygiene and plaque removal (fig. 14-3).

Traditional crown and bridge preparation principles generally advocate supragingival margin placement. Advantages of supragingival margins include the following:

- Easier impression making
- Easier evaluation of both preparations and restorations
- Improved plaque control
- Predictability of marginal seal when terminating on enamel (particularly when bonding)
- Improved access for finishing, recontouring, and cement removal after delivery of a restoration

Despite these advantages, today's esthetically driven restorative arena often dictates that margins be hidden below the gingival crest. In reality, even when a margin is not evident during normal smiling and speaking, patients often scrutinize marginal appearance by lifting their lips and moving their cheeks beyond normal physiological positions. Despite an overall esthetic outcome, a patient may be dissatisfied by even a small band of darker cervical tooth structure, visible only by forced retraction (figs. 14-4a and 14-4b).

Considering the tendency for the gingival migration of margins for esthetic restorations, it is paramount to employ best practices when preparing subgingival margins. These include the following:

- Preoperative sulcular measurements and respect of biologic width
- Appropriate bur diameter selection
- Atraumatic tissue retraction during preparation to minimize laceration (using retraction cord or other adjuncts)

Occlusion

Occlusal considerations are discussed at length in chapter 5.

Restorative-Mechanical Considerations

Retention Form

The ability of a restoration to resist dislodgement in a similar path to placement is defined as retention. Retention form therefore refers to the aspects of a preparation that allow it to be most retentive. The two main factors affecting retention are the convergence angle of opposing walls as well as the total surface area of contact between a restoration and a given preparation.

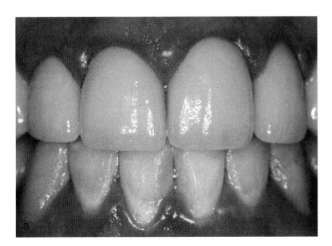
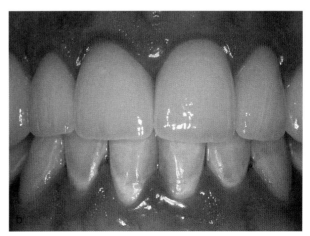

Figure 14-3. a. Marginal tissue inflammation influenced by overcontoured ceramo-metal crowns that violate biologic width in areas with likely influence from patient's metal-based allergy. b. Notice reduction in inflammation in only one week following replacement of ceramo-metal crowns with all ceramic crowns in a lighter shade as directed by patient desires.

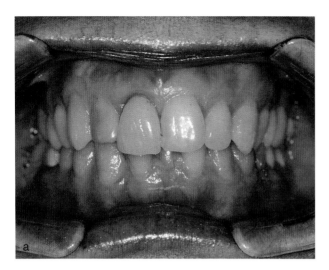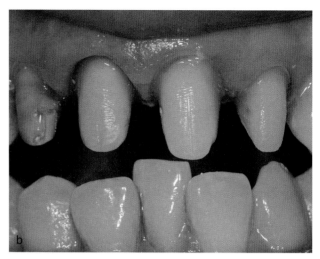

Figure 14-4. a. Preoperative photo highlighting cervical shade discrepancy between numbers 8 and 9 due to cementoenamel junction exposure. b. Notice the subgingival preparation necessitated on tooth number 8 based on the preoperative cervical shade discrepancy.

The convergence angle, also referred to as the taper of a preparation, has an inverse relation to retention quality. As the convergence angle and degree of taper decreases, the retentiveness of the preparation increases (Jorgensen 1955). Universally accepted prosthodontic principles indicate that ideal convergence of opposing walls is 6 degrees. Further, retention form is catastrophically compromised when this angle increases beyond 10 degrees, resulting in an acceptable window of preparation taper between 6 and 10 degrees. Less taper may result in difficulty seating a restoration, while more taper obviously reduces the preparation's retention form. Such recommendations have been made based on studies of traditional indirect restoration held in place by traditional cements like zinc phosphate.

Esthetic dentistry and the emergence of nonmetal-based restorations have led to a host of new indirect restorative options for practitioners and patients alike. This departure from traditional options has led to modifications in preparation criteria. While the principles of retention form and taper still apply, the small and unyielding windows of acceptable taper do not always apply and are counterproductive at times, depending on restoration choice. Pressed ceramic restorations, CAD/CAM-based restorations, and partial coverage ceramic restorations not only have modified preparation design criteria, but the fact that these restorations are typically bonded to tooth structure has led to some departure from traditional notions of retention form. Retention form cannot be ignored, but today's practitioners must have a strategy for optimizing preparation design based on materials, fabrication protocol, and bonding variables.

Resistance Form

Resistance form refers to that quality of a preparation that helps to resist dislodgment of a restoration as a result of horizontal or oblique forces. Normal mastication as well as parafunctional activity can lead to forces that are typically far greater than those that challenge retention. As with retention, traditional resistance form criteria have been dogmatically driven by clinical studies and scientific experimentation based on traditional restorations and cementation protocols. Since ceramo-metal restorations, also referred to as porcelain-fused-to-metal (PFM) restorations, fall into both the traditional and esthetic categories, it is worthwhile to review resistance form criteria. The resistance form necessary for PFM crown preparations dictates particular minimums in preparation geometry. These are universal across prosthodontic education and text. Features that increase preparation resistance form include the following:

- Minimization of taper
- Maximization of axial wall height
- Angular or pyramidal (rather than rounded or conical) preparation line angles
- Addition of adjunctive features such as boxes and grooves

Even when preparing for all-ceramic crowns, these axioms should only be incrementally departed from, based again on material choices and fabrication protocols. A standard rule of thumb for practitioners is to maintain at least a 3-mm wall height assuming a taper of 10 degrees or less to ensure resistance form for a traditional crown and bridge preparation. If these minimums are not achievable or applicable based on clinical circumstance or restorative material choices, dentin and enamel bonding technology becomes paramount for resistance.

Durability of Materials

The durability of indirect esthetic restorations largely refers to those characteristics that resist fracture or premature wear. Precautions should be taken when restoring occlusal and incisal surfaces with porcelain, as the material has the propensity for accelerated wear of opposing natural tooth structure. Traditional ceramics have never presented the liability of rapid wear, which has been a challenge for materials such as resins or extremely soft alloys. In fact, manufacturers consistently strive to develop newer ceramic systems, such as low-fusing porcelains, in hopes of approaching wear rates of natural enamel, about 10 μm per year (Pintado et al. 1997). While rapid or excessive wear of ceramics is not an issue, porcelain fracture is and must be protected against through preparation design.

One cause of porcelain fracture pertaining to PFM restorations is the deformation of the metallic substructure. Individual metal copings as well as connected frameworks have, by nature, the tendency to flex or deflect under load. Thus, precautions are taken during fabrication to minimize flexure, such as adjusting coping thickness and connector size minimums. This relates to minimum reduction requirements during preparation. When the 0.3-mm minimum thickness coping requirement is added to the 1.5-mm ceramic depth required to optimize esthetics for a PFM crown, the ideal reduction criterion approaches 2 mm in the incisal and occlusal zones of preparations. At the same time, overreduction to ensure porcelain thickness and esthetic development is contradicted. Beyond violating the principles of tooth conservation, unsupported porcelain greater than 2 mm in thickness that is suspended too far away from substructure framework is a common cause of ceramic fracture. The same principles apply when the metallic cores of PFM crowns are substituted by bonded tooth structure or ceramic cores like zirconia and alumina. While the cores associated with all-ceramic options have different characteristics than metal, the same limits in porcelain thickness should be adhered to. Strength, durability, and color development criteria result in very similar reduction recommendations for PFM crowns and their all-ceramic counterparts. However, the absence of a metallic core and associated opaquing layer may result in the ability to keep preparations more conservative.

Esthetic Considerations

Anatomic Considerations
Adequate reduction of preparations not only ensures durability, it allows for ceramic layering and optimiza-

tion of esthetics. While practitioners rarely compromise reduction adequacy purposefully, the difficulties of access, intraoral measurement, and evaluation perspective often result in underreduction of crucial esthetic planes. The two most common areas of underreduction are the incisal or occluso-facial plane, often referred to as the esthetic bevel, and the occlusal table. Strategies for ensuring adequate reduction for these areas include the incorporation of depth cuts, reduction templates, and limiting burs (figs. 14-5, 14-6).

In the event that the proposed contours of a final restoration are more prominent than the existing contours,

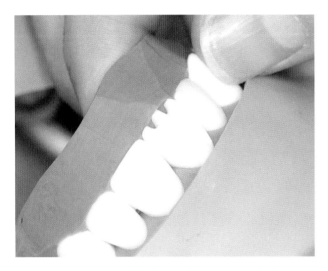

Figure 14-5. Depth cuts and a silicone reduction matrix utilized to ensure adequate reduction for tooth number 8 in a typodont simulation.

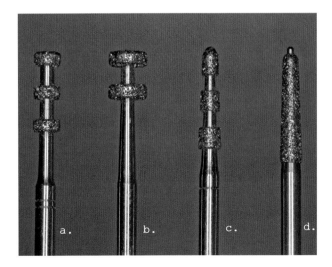

Figure 14-6. Various depth reduction and limiting burs useful in creating adequate reduction while protecting against overreduction: (a) 834A.031 Brasseler, USA; (b) 834.021 LVS1 Brasseler, USA; (c) 868A.018 Brasseler, USA; (d) 856P.018 FG Komet, USA.

for example, lengthening an incisor or increasing the facial profile of lingually positioned bicuspid, a reduction guide or matrix may prove useful. Such guides are made to conform to the idealized contours of a diagnostic wax-up using silicon or thermoplastic sheets and then used intraorally to ensure adequate reduction, prevent the removal of unnecessary tooth structure, and reduce the likelihood of the final restoration having unsupported or overextended porcelain (fig. 14-7).

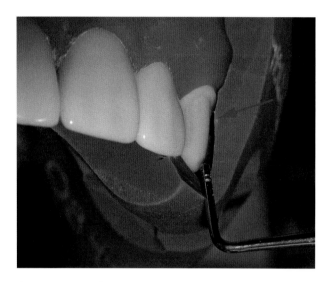

Figure 14-7. Use of a sagitally cut reduction template to check for adequate facial reduction inciso-gingivally of a typodont simulation preparation of tooth #11 for a ceramo-metal restoration. Note: inadequate reduction of less than 1 mm below the height of contour depicted by the arrow.

Margin Location

The preoperative condition of an abutment tooth often dictates margin location during preparation. Examples of this are the necessity to include build-up and core margins, abfraction lesions, or sensitive root surfaces.

As discussed earlier, in cases where preoperative circumstances do not dictate a subgingival margin, patient expectations and desired esthetic outcomes often direct practitioners to place preparation margins at the gingival crest or slightly subgingival.

These patient expectation–driven considerations are particularly crucial in the esthetic zone, which differs from patient to patient. Exceptions to this general strategy may arise in cases where there is significant recession present or where it is clear that the patient does not display the cervical one-third despite extreme lip posturing.

Another important factor to consider is desired restoration shade. Subgingival margins should be considered when the cervical restorative shade of choice differs from that of the natural tooth or root. However, when shade differences between restoration and cervical tooth structure are not drastic, a skillful ceramist, using translucent porcelains and surface staining techniques can render a supragingival margin nearly undetectable.

Subgingival margins should also be considered in the proximal areas of restoration where emergence profile modifications are needed. Examples of cases where profile modifications are indicated include diastema closure or dark triangle correction. Figures 14-8a and 14-8b illustrate correct and incorrect proximal margin locations with resulting restoration contours. It is evident

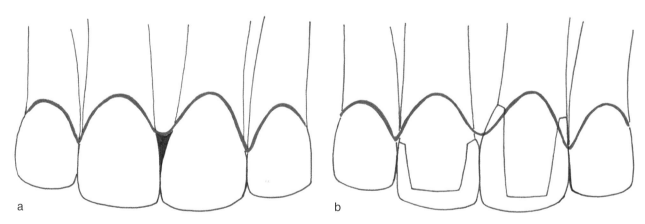

Figure 14-8. Strategy for determining gingival finish line location for proximal aspects of anterior teeth. a. This drawing is a preoperative illustration of a blunted papilla leading to a dark triangle between teeth 8 and 9. b. This drawing compares the appropriate subgingival migration of the finish line for tooth #9 versus the supragingival margin placement for tooth #8. The improved emergence profile and constriction of the dark triangle for tooth #9 is evident as opposed to the abrupt contour of the restoration for tooth #8 leaving the dark triangle unresolved. (Drawings courtesy of Jessie Vallee, DDS)

that underextended margins lead to unnatural and less cleansable proximal contours.

Preparation Design

Ceramo-metal Crown Preparations

Historically, PFM crowns have been the standard of care for teeth under esthetic scrutiny requiring full coverage. Increased demand for cosmetics in dentistry has led to improvements in materials, fabrication systems, and laboratory techniques, which in turn have led to more natural-looking restorations. Even so, the metal core generally renders PFM crowns an inferior choice to their all-ceramic counterparts from a purely cosmetic point of view. Over the last decade, advances in reinforced core–based all-ceramic restorations has led to a decrease in the delivery of PFM crowns. The historic liabilities associated with all-ceramic restorations have largely been overcome. Despite this, ceramo-metal crowns are still a staple of general dentistry. Acceptable fit, excellent durability, and good esthetics can all be achieved with PFM crowns. If for no other indication than to match existing adjacent PFM crowns where similar material is a logical choice, it is worthwhile to review the PFM preparation design criteria.

While basic preparation design principles for PFM crowns are fairly universal, many variations exist. These revolve largely around facial margin design and reduction recommendations for incisal or occlusal areas. Considering the intent of this text, only the most esthetically driven variations of preparation design will be outlined. Criteria for metallic occlusal tables and metallic marginal collars are omitted and can be derived from any prosthodontic text.

The standard PFM crown preparation can generally be divided into two halves when considered from an occlusal or incisal perspective. The facial or buccal half requires greater reduction with a range recommendation between 1 and 1.5 mm, 1.2 mm being the most common recommendation. This reduction should be anatomic so that natural planes are duplicated, resulting in a gingival and esthetic plane. The gingival plane terminates in a shoulder margin design of corresponding depth with two acceptable cavosurface emergence angles. The first is the more esthetic 90-degree shoulder, otherwise called a "porcelain butt joint." The second is the sloping shoulder design where a 120-degree internal line angle is sought, leading to a more acute cavosurface emergence angle. In this variation, a "disappearing metal margin" or "porcelain/metal junction margin" is sought for the final restoration. Unlike the butt joint margin, where only porcelain occupies the terminal

shoulder, as the name implies, the disappearing metal margin has a thin extension of metal that extends to the cavosurface terminus. However, through careful laboratory manipulation, the metal in this area is cut back so thin that it approaches indetectability once veneered with porcelain. Sloping shoulder designs were historically selected despite an esthetic disadvantage to butt joint designs because of easier marginal porcelain manipulation in the laboratory phase as well as decreased fragility. With current ceramic technology, improvements in laboratory techniques, and bonded resin-based cementation, it is currently possible to attain excellent marginal adaptation with pure porcelain butt joints. Because of this, it is not necessary to compromise the esthetics of PFM crown margins, particularly those delivered to the esthetic zone. An added advantage is the increased biocompatibility that is associated with porcelain margins, since inflammatory gingival reactions are often observed where metallic margins approximate gingiva.

The lingual aspects of PFM crown preparations require less discussion. The marginal design of choice is a chamfer. The lingual chamfer and facial shoulder meet and are blended within the proximal area of the preparation. Where this marginal transition occurs is largely a function of the position of the preparation in the dental arches and the esthetic burden of the proposed restoration. Conservation of tooth structure is traded for porcelain depth when color development and translucency are crucial, as in incisor restorations. Shoulder chamfer transitions can occur anywhere from the facial line angles of teeth through the proximal contact areas and are left up to operator discretion considering esthetic demands. As a general rule, the farther posterior a preparation occurs in the dental arch, the less need for lingual extension of the proximal shoulder. Additionally, distal shoulders may often require less lingual extension than mesial shoulders, based on visibility. The lingual chamfer also defines the lingual axial reduction. By definition, a chamfer margin is created by reducing tooth structure to half of the depth of a chamfer diamond bur. This is to assure an acute exit angle to the cavosurface most suitable to metallic margin waxing and casting. Extending axial reduction beyond half of the bur diameter risks creation of undermined enamel. While various chamfer depths are advocated based on circumstances and philosophies, an 878k-016 chamfer bur delivers one of the most universally accepted depths. Whether preparing the lingual, proximal, or facial aspects of a PFM crown preparation, tapered diamonds are recommended. The corresponding tapered shoulder bur, the 847-016, results in a 1.2-mm shoulder when used to its full depth. Tapered diamonds allow the operator to maintain bur and hand piece angulations along the long axis or

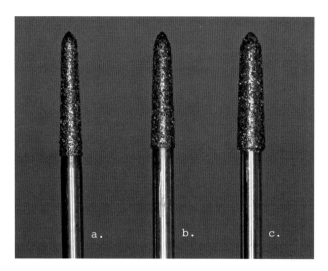

Figure 14-9. Progressively increasing in diameter, these burs are used to one-half of their depth to create a chamfer finish line: (a) 878K.016 Brasseler, USA; (b) 878K.018 Brasseler, USA; (c) 878K.021 Brasseler, USA.

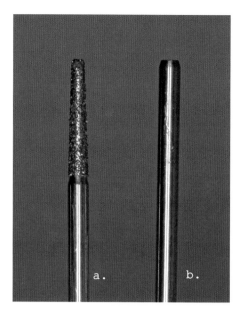

Figure 14-10. These burs are used to prepare and refine a shoulder butt joint: (a) shoulder bur, 847.016, Brassler, USA; (b) "end-cutting" bur, 10839.016, Brasseler, USA.

desired insertion path for a tooth, thus preparing complimentary opposing axial walls with taper ranging from 6 to 10 degrees, while reducing the possibility of creating undercuts. Because PFM crowns that do not display any occlusal metal are the most cosmetic, patients most often demand these. Thus, the traditional junction between porcelain and anatomic metal has migrated from the occlusal table to the lingual aspect. While ceramic depth for translucency is not as crucial on the lingual aspects, space is needed for the thinned metal coping to be veneered with porcelain. A chamfer bur of greater diameter like the 878k-018 is preferred when the porcelain metal junction occurs lingually, as more axial reduction is required. When lingual axial reduction is inadequate, and technicians are asked to deliver occlusal and lingual surfaces in porcelain, the result is often over-bulked, nonanatomic crowns (figs. 14-9 and 14-10).

The occlusal aspect of a posterior PFM crown preparation or the inciso-lingual aspect of an anterior PFM crown preparation should also mimic the natural anatomy of teeth. Reduction planes are created to follow cusp, ridge, and incisal edge anatomy, aiming for 2 mm of reduction on surfaces to be restored with porcelain. The functional and esthetic bevels of PFM preparations merge the axial walls with the occlusal table, paralleling the natural anatomy of teeth. The lingual fossa of anterior teeth should also be prepared anatomically. Where concavity is present as in typical incisors, football-shaped or ovoid diamonds are used to insure anatomic reduction. Minimal reduction of 1.5 mm is required in the lingual fossa, particularly in areas of function or

where porcelain is veneered over the metal coping. This dimension can be reduced to 1 mm as the cingulum approaches the lingual chamfer.

While extremely sharp line or point angles are contra-indicated for any crown preparation due to liabilities associated with waxing and fabrication, defined planes and generally angular geometry is acceptable (figs. 14-11a–c).

Full Coverage All-Ceramic Restorations

Esthetically superior to their PFM counterparts, all-ceramic restorations can be some of the most beautiful and lifelike indirect restorations. Because metal is not present to block light transmission and opaquing is unnecessary, a natural depth of color and translucency can be developed to better mimic natural teeth. Advancements in ceramic technology and the advent of rigid milled cores have essentially eliminated most if not all of the historic limitations associated with early generations of all-ceramic crowns like the porcelain jacket crown or IPS Empress 2 pressed ceramics. Limitations associated with strength, fracture resistance, multiple units, and difficult margin fabrication have been overcome. There are very few clinical circumstances where an all-ceramic restoration is not a suitable choice for providing full coverage.

Despite the already large and ever-growing number of ceramic systems and protocols for fabrication, most

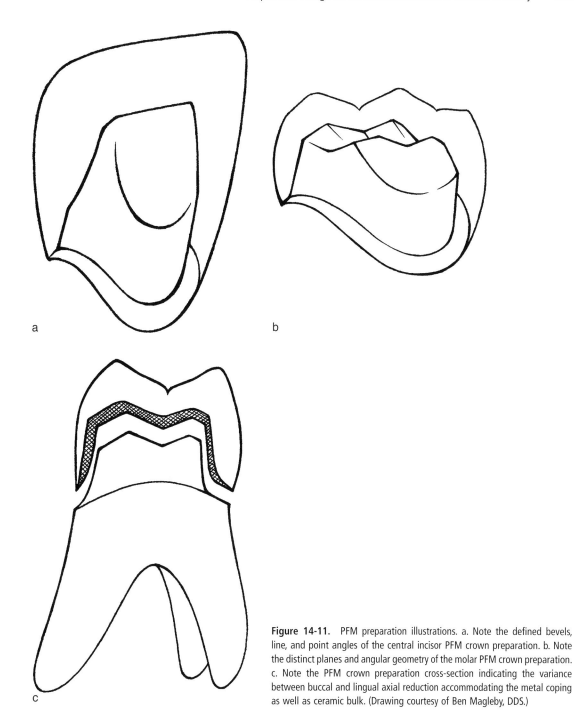

Figure 14-11.   PFM preparation illustrations. a. Note the defined bevels, line, and point angles of the central incisor PFM crown preparation. b. Note the distinct planes and angular geometry of the molar PFM crown preparation. c. Note the PFM crown preparation cross-section indicating the variance between buccal and lingual axial reduction accommodating the metal coping as well as ceramic bulk. (Drawing courtesy of Ben Magleby, DDS.)

preparation design criteria for this class of restoration are fairly similar. A practitioner should always seek manufacturer-recommended preparation design and reduction criteria when preparing for a restoration in this category.

A generic and universal preparation design will be outlined for both anterior and posterior all-ceramic crown preparations. This design is suitable for most

systems available in today's marketplace, including the popular hot-pressed system (e.g., IPS Empress) and milled-core systems (e.g., 3M-LAVA, Procera).

Perhaps the simplest way to define ceramic crown preparation criteria is to compare with PFM crown criteria already mentioned. In general, all-ceramic crowns require more uniform axial reduction along all axial walls. One millimeter of reduction is generally adequate to develop pleasing esthetics and maintain strength in the axial areas of a preparation at or below the height of contour. This axial reduction can be reduced to the range of 0.8 mm in cases where a reinforced zirconia core (3M-LAVA, Porcera) system is utilized or where shade development may not be as crucial such as with less-visible molar restorations. The preparation criterion ranges from 1.0 to 1.5 mm of reduction above the height of contour, as these areas are generally more visible and

esthetically crucial. Finally, the occlusal and incisal reduction ranges are 1.5 to 2.0 mm for all-ceramic crowns and are driven by factors such as bulk requirements for strength, esthetic layering, choosing a core- or noncore-based system, and occlusion (figs. 14-12a–g).

Marginal designs for all-ceramic crowns are also generally uniform circumferentially. Cavosurface exit angles at or approaching 90 degrees are desired, and acute angles are contraindicated. Descriptive terms such as

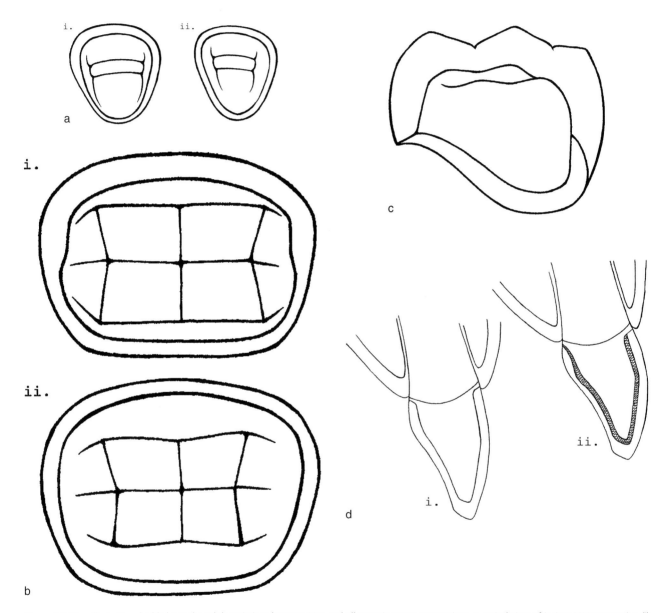

Figure 14-12.   Illustrations highlighting the subtle variations between PFM and all-ceramic crown preparations. a. Incisal view of incisor PFM preparation (i) versus an all-ceramic crown preparation (ii). Note the uniform axial reduction and rounded shoulder depth of (ii) compared to the variable depth of (i) due to a dual-margin design typical of PFM preparations. b. A similar comparison of a molar PFM crown preparation (i), compared with its all-ceramic counterpart (ii). c. The rounded and softer axial and occlusal features of an all-ceramic molar crown preparation are illustrated. (Drawings a–c courtesy of Ben Magleby, D.D.S.) d. Cross-section illutration of an all-ceramic (i) and PFM (i) crown preparation for a maxilary central incisor. Note the checkerboard shading in figure (ii) portrays the relative dimension of the substructure metallic coping (drawings courtesy of Jessie Vallee, DDS). e, f, and g. Facial, incisal, and lingual views of typodont simulation preparation for a PFM (#8) and all-ceramic (#9) crown.

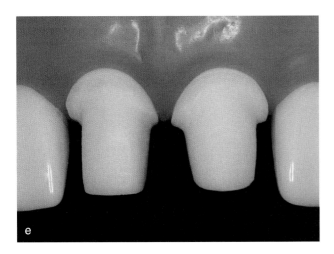

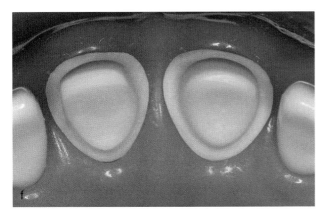

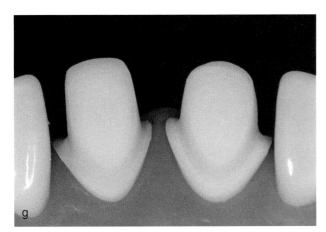

Figure 14-12. *Continued*

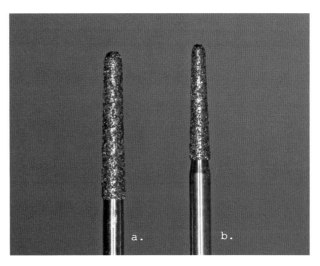

Figure 14-13. Rounded-end tapered diamonds of various diameters are used to create rounded shoulder/modified chamfer margins demanded by most all-ceramic crown criteria: (a) 856.018, Brasseler, USA; (b) 856.016, Brasseler, USA.

ration features. Preparations are described as more flowing and less geometric. The convergence angle or taper range associated with retention form is also extended to 6–15 degrees for all-ceramic preparations. Recommended burs and sample preparations are pictured in figures 14-13, 14-14a–c, and 14-15a–e.

Partial Coverage All-Ceramic Preparation

Several categories of restorations fall under this heading. These include porcelain laminate veneers, porcelain inlays, and porcelain onlays. These restorations not only deliver lifelike esthetics when properly designed and delivered, they may also render excellent function, guidance, and longevity. Multiple units of laminate veneers in the esthetic zone may also lead to esthetic and functional improvements previously achievable only through orthodontic treatment. There is however, a limit to the amount of realignment possible through ceramic manipulation. In many cases, prerestorative orthodontic optimization of abutment positions enables better balance, improved esthetics, and more conservative preparation designs. Case management through prerestorative orthodontics should be considered when tooth positions and angulations are to be altered to a significant degree via ceramic manipulation.

Partial coverage all-ceramic restorations are similar to their full-coverage counterparts in that internal preparation line and point angles require rounding. This is done to eliminate stress-inducing zones within a preparation that are often the cause of fracture and restorative failure.

"rounded shoulder" or "heavy chamfer" are used in manufacturer's literature that indicate 90- or near 90-degree cavosurface angles with rounded internal axiomarginal angles. Unlike PFM preparations, distinct planes and defined angles associated with resistance form are contraindicated with all-ceramic preparations. In fact, great care is taken to soften and round all prepa-

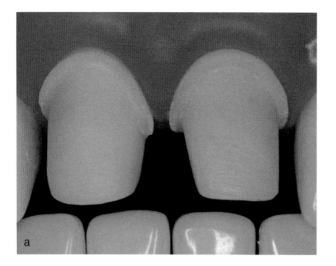

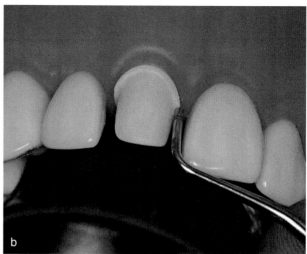

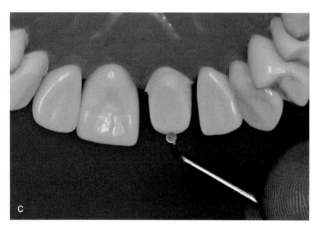

Figure 14-14.   a. Typodont simulation of full-coverage, all-ceramic preparations for teeth 8 and 9. Note the soft, rounded contours and absence of any sharp line or point angles. b. A uniform 0.8- to 1.0-mm marginal reduction is ideal for most typical pressed or milled all-ceramic full-coverage restorations. c. Note the ideal incisal reduction and rounded contours from a lingual view.

Preparation design criteria and variances are outlined for each specific restoration.

Veneer Preparations

Perhaps more than any other class of indirect restoration, ceramic veneer preparations vary based on the involved tooth and the restorative and esthetic objectives. While a group of basic guidelines are followed, operator interpretation and case specifics direct preparation design. Factors such as relative position of abutments, desired final restorative position, length and width modifications, gingival circumstances, smile line, existing restorations, stain or discoloration, and proposed restorative function all play a role in final preparation extensions and reduction. Even the experienced operator benefits from prepreparation case design. This is most commonly accomplished through a wax-up. Once final restorative dimensions and functional require-

ments are developed, preparation extensions become clear. Some of the most common questions practitioners have while prepping for veneers revolve around gingival, inciso-lingual, and proximal extensions. While many variations of porcelain veneer preparations have been proposed, a true understanding of desired esthetic and functional goals usually dictates a unique and ideal preparation for every tooth.

In rare cases, proximal extensions of veneer preparations may terminate before breaking the proximal contact. However, in most cases, particularly in anterior teeth, proximal finish lines are extended beyond the contact and terminate before the lingual line angles. Factors influencing proximal extension include the following:

- Desired width modifications
- Diastema closures and emergence profile modifications

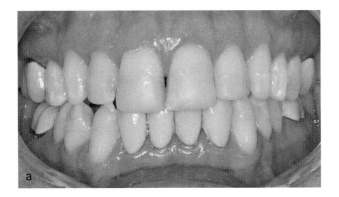

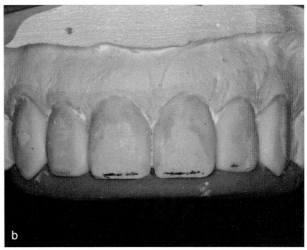

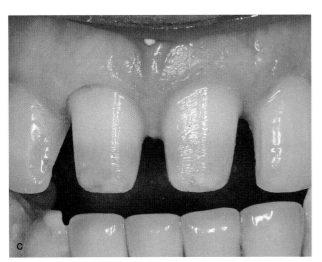

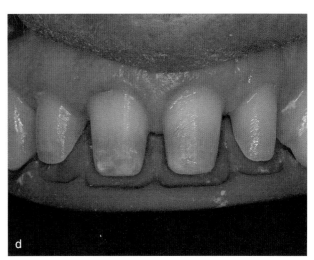

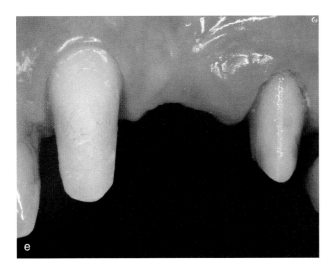

Figure 14-15. a. Preoperative view of maxillary anterior teeth scheduled for all-ceramic full coverage. b. Putty reduction matrix fabricated on idealized wax-up/smile design model. c. 8 and 9 completed preparations. d. Using the reduction matrix to evaluate the four incisor proportions. e. A completed bridge preparation slated for a zirconia-based all-ceramic framework.

- Existing class III restorations
- Proximal tooth discolorations and potential staining
- Esthetic visibility
- Marginal accessibility for laboratory process
- Marginal accessibility for delivery and finish
- Fluidity with inciso-lingual extensions

Inciso-lingual extensions are also determined based on desired restorative outcomes. Some factors influencing inciso-lingual extensions include the following:

- Existing class IV restorations or incisal chips
- Desired length modifications
- Opposing tooth function
- Prescribed guidance changes
- Shade and translucency control

The operator should keep in mind that while the most conservative veneer preparation that satisfies the functional and esthetic objectives is optimal, lingual and proximal extensions are often indicated. Thus, principles of draw and insertion path come into play and cannot be ignored when veneer preparations occupy a greater tooth circumference (figs. 14-16a–e and 14-17a–e).

Gingival extensions are driven by many of the same principles discussed regarding all-ceramic crowns. These include the following:

- Visibility with respect to smile line
- Ideal termination on enamel
- Gingival position and recession
- Shade modifications with respect to cervical tooth and root color
- Existing class V restorations, abfractions, and sensitivity

Reduction depth is another variable in veneer preparation. Without complicating factors, 0.6 mm of facial reduction is generally adequate to attain esthetic shade control. If incisal edges are to be modified or wrapped, the reduction of these areas can range from 1 to 2 mm. When circumstances allow for maintaining veneer preparations entirely on enamel, confidence in bonding protocols and conservation of tooth structure make for best-case scenarios. The most conservative preparations may occur when restoring diastemas, arches with tooth size discrepancies, unstained or discolored teeth, and lingually positioned teeth.

Inevitably, circumstances will often dictate the increase of reduction depth within dentin. Improvements in dentin bonding protocols have made deeper extensions acceptable. However, whenever possible, margins should ideally terminate on enamel. Instances where heavier axial reductions may be indicated include restoring severely discolored teeth (i.e., Tetracycline

stained), teeth with deep existing restorations, and migrating facial profiles lingually.

Ultimately, even when the facial axial reduction can be kept to a minimum, an appropriate finish line depth needs to be developed for the sake of laboratory handling and fabrication, durability through seating and bonding procedures, and to avoid overcontoured cervical profiles. An acceptable marginal depth is 0.5 mm, but this can range in either direction slightly. Perhaps more crucial is the cavosurface emergence profile of the finish line. It is acceptable to have a cavosurface angle approaching 90 degrees, particularly in proximal and lingual or incisal areas. The cervical profile can be somewhat more acute and is sometimes referred to as a "long chamfer" or "rounded shoulder." The margin angle should not drop below 75 degrees; otherwise, thin margins and fragile porcelain will result. As with all other ceramic margin preparations, the internal axial margin angles are rounded (figs. 14-18a–i, 14-19, and 14-20).

Ceramic Inlay and Onlay Preparations

Ceramic inlays and onlays are excellent esthetic options when clinical circumstances call for a restoration more durable than a direct resin or when there is cuspal involvement not justifying full coverage and the unnecessary removal of circumferential enamel or dentin. Since there are various clinical situations where such restorations may be indicated, similar to veneer preparations, it is difficult to provide an ideal preparation diagram. Rather, design criteria are listed that, when followed, should lead to appropriate preparations. Several precautions to choosing ceramic inlays or onlays as the restoration of choice are worth mentioning.

Excessive occlusal forces. While predictability with these restorations has increased, severe occlusal loading commonly associated with bruxism is a contradiction due to fracture risk. This is particularly true as the teeth get closer to the gnasthostomic fulcrum where the forces increase dramatically (i.e., 2nd molars).

Restoring conservative lesions. When a relatively small lesion is to be restored, often a direct restoration can be the most conservative choice. Since seating path and draw are not required for direct resins, a seemingly more durable inlay may come at the expense of unnecessary removal of valuable tooth structure.

Severely broken down teeth. While bonding of onlays is the primary source of reinforcement for both the tooth and restoration, excessive axial and cuspal integrity loss may render a tooth more suitable for core build-up and full coverage.

The basic guidelines for onlay/inlay preparations are as follows (see figs. 14-21, 14-22, and 14-23a and b):

- Outline form should be fluid and is often governed by existing restorations, caries, or fractures. Care

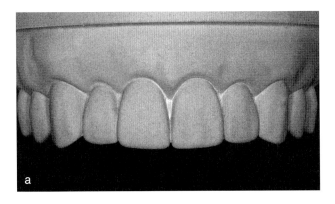
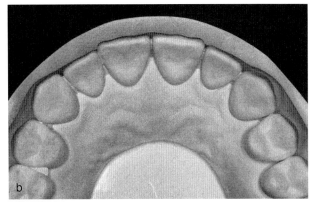
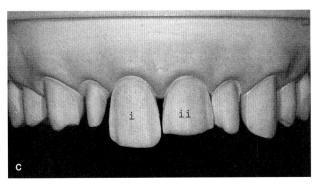
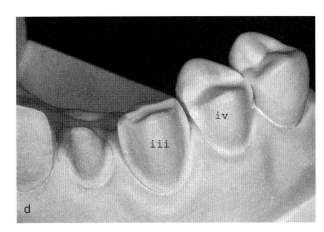
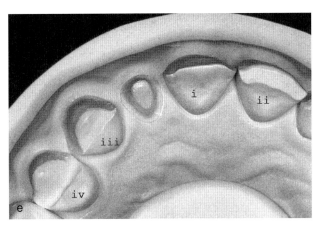

Figure 14-16.   University of the Pacific All-Ceramic Sample Preparation Block. a. Preoperative facial view. b. Preoperative incisal view. c, d, and e. facial (c), angled (d), and incisal (e) views of various veneer preparation designs, including: i. #8 facial-only laminate. ii. #9 incisal shoe veneer prep. iii. #6 incisal wrap veneer prep with broken proximal contacts allowing maximum esthetic and function control. iv. #5 bicuspid veneer preparation extending just beyond central groove with a broken mesial but maintained distal contact.

should be taken to not create ceramic-to-enamel interfaces in areas opposing centric contacts. Preoperative marking with articulating paper may prove useful.

- Pulpal depth along the isthmus should approach 2 mm.
- Load-bearing areas of onlays should have 2 mm of reduction. Occlusal areas not under excessive load may have a minimum of 1.5 mm of reduction through all excursions.

- Proximal box forms should have axial depth of at least 1 mm if not driven deeper by existing restorations.
- All internal angles should be rounded and conducive to buffering stress across a broad area.
- Internal walls should diverge and external walls should converge, consistent with taper and draw principles.
- Proximal box walls should have a minimum of 0.6 mm of clearance from adjacent teeth.

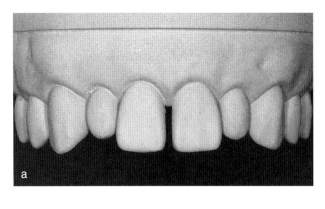
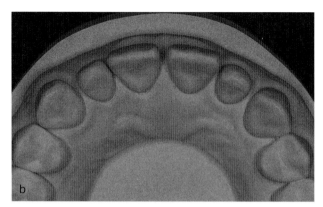
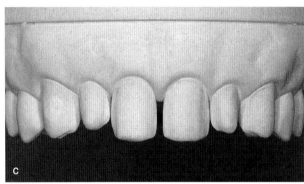
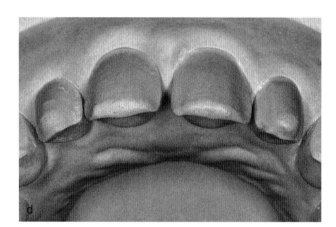
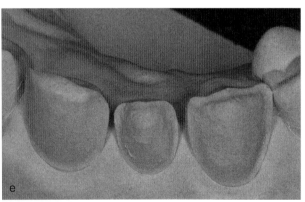

Figure 14-17. University of the Pacific Diastema/Peg Lateral Sample Preparation Block. a. Preoperative facial view. b. Preoperative incisal view. c. Postoperative facial view. d. Postoperative incisal view. Note proximal margin extensions to facilitate appropriate emergence of additional porcelain to be added to close diastema. e. Postoperative angled view.

- All cavosurface exit angles, whether horizontal or vertical, should be at 90 degrees, thus eliminating undermined marginal enamel.
- Excessively tall yet thin retained tooth features should be shortened and restored with porcelain.

Summary

It is important to keep in mind that adjusting occlusion is very difficult considering handling difficulty and fracture vulnerability prior to bonding inlays or onlays. It is prudent to drive laboratory protocol to deliver restorations with optimized occlusion whenever possible. Further, when intraoral adjustments are made postcementation, great diligence should be spent to return the roughened restoration surfaces to a high polish to prevent opposing tooth wear.

Optimal preparation can only consistently be achieved through case design, optimized technique, and appropriate armamentarium. A clear understanding of the restorative burden placed on an abutment by the

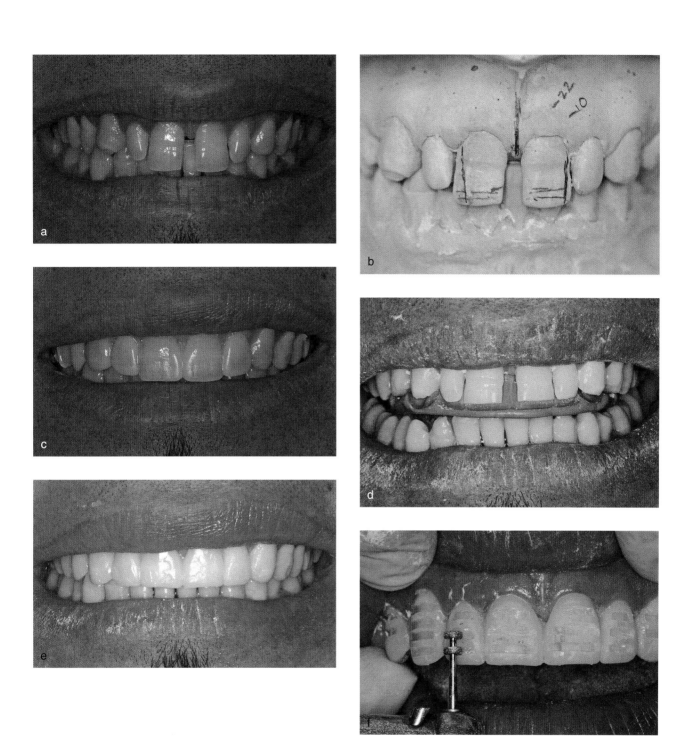

Figure 14-18. a. Preoperative view of 8 unit esthetic and functional rehabilitation. b. Preoperative planning on casts in anticipation of decreasing central incisor length and line angle migration to mesialize and close diastema. c. Overlayed resin smile design. d. Progressive incisal reduction of teeth using reduction template. e. Second overlay of smile design resin with idealized lengths after reduction of numbers 8 and 9. f. Using a veneer depth-reduction wheel directly through the smile design resin to eliminate unnecessary reduction of natural tooth structure. g. Completed preps incisal view. h. Completed preps facial view. i. Final restorations with balanced length-to-width ratios, diastema closure, and optimized guidance facilitated by proper preparation design through smile design.

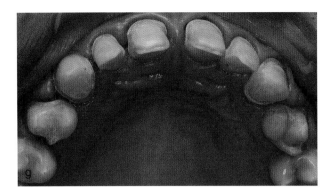

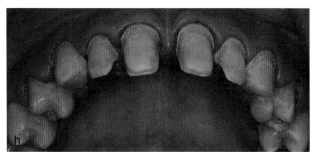

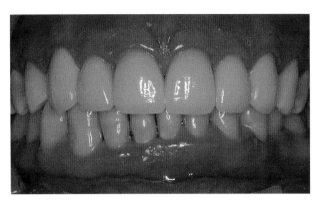

Figure 14-18. *Continued*

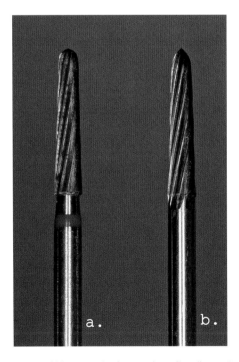

Figure 14-19. Carbide preparation burs used to refine all-ceramic preparation margins: (a) H 375R.016 B Brasseler, USA; (b) H 283K.016 (21) Brasseler, USA.

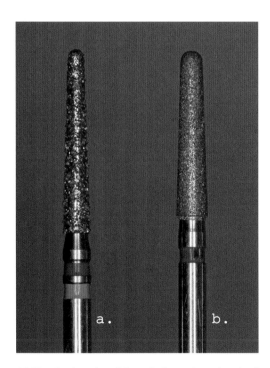

Figure 14-20. Combo grit and fine grit diamonds used to develop final all-ceramic preparation margins: (a) 6844FG.016 Komet, USA; (b) 8856.016 Brasseler, USA.

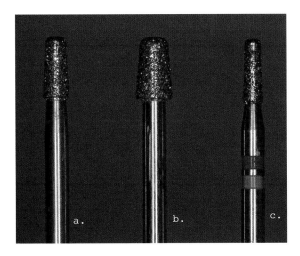

Figure 14-21. Rounded shoulder inlay/onlay diamond burs: (a) 962TG.014 two grit [IP] Brasseler, USA; (b) 845KR.016 Brasseler, USA; (c) b845KR.025 Brasseler, USA.

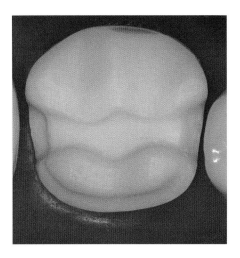

Figure 14-22. Typodont simulation preparation for a ceramic onlay for tooth #19. Note the occlusally diverging internal walls (draw), rounded lingual butt joint, and shoed buccal cusp with rounded cusp anatomy.

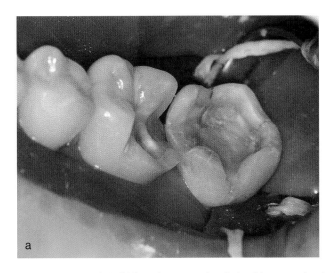

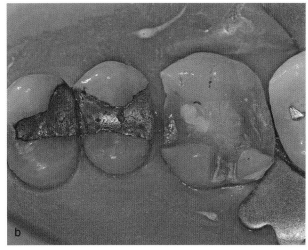

Figure 14-23. a. Clinical inlay/onlay preparations isolated in preparation for bonding of teeth 18 and 19. b. Inlay/onlay preparation for tooth number 14, replacing a large MODBL amalgam with ceramic.

mechanical requirements of the restoration, and in turn, by the functional and esthetic demands placed on the restoration, is necessary for optimal preparation.

The cliché citing dentistry as both an "art and science" particularly applies to the topic of preparation design. This goes beyond the hand skill requirements attained through repetitive practice. The dentist can be equated to a master sculptor, the tooth his block of stone. Just as the accomplished sculptor can envision his masterpiece before any stone is chiseled away, an accomplished practitioner should be able to envision the final preparation before any enamel or dentin is stripped away. The science of dentistry then defines the technical requirements and the steps taken to achieve optimal preparation.

Works Cited

Baldissara P, Catapano S, Scotti R. 1997. Clinical and histological evaluation of thermal injury thresholds in human teeth: A preliminary study. *Journal of Oral Rehabilitation* 24:791–801.

Jorgensen KD. 1955. The relationship between retention and convergence angle in cemented veneer crowns. *Acta Odontol Scand* 13:35–40.

Pintado MR, Anderson GC, DeLong R, Douglas WH. 1997. Variation in tooth wear in young adults over a two-year period. *Journal of Prosthetic Dentistry* 77:313–20.

Chapter 15

Soft Tissue Management, Impression Materials, and Techniques

Gitta Radjaeipour DDS, EdD

Bina Surti DDS, BS

Marc Geissberger DDS, MA, BS, CPT

Esthetic treatment demands accuracy at every stage of the process. Two crucial features for achieving a high-quality indirect restoration are excellent tissue management and impression technique. The restorative dentist has many methods and materials available to achieve an excellent impression. The impression materials available today are extremely accurate, predictable, and durable. Regardless of the material selected, adequate moisture control and soft tissue management are essential. In many situations these factors may be challenging, but with proper techniques, one can achieve optimum, predictable, and consistent results in an efficient, productive manner. This chapter will introduce the reader to techniques for adequate tissue management and impression making.

Periodontal Considerations

A healthy periodontium is essential and contributes significantly to optimal esthetics and function of the dentition. Long-term success of esthetic restorations depends greatly on a healthy periodontium. Before any restorative procedures are considered, a thorough periodontal assessment should be established during the treatment planning phase.

Once the restorative dentist has properly assessed the gingival health of the patient, every effort should be taken to establish and maintain a healthy periodontium throughout the entire restorative treatment. Due to the length of procedure some patients may be in provisional restorations, careful attention to margin design must be employed. Overcountered restorations can cause irreversible changes in the periodontal architecture and ultimately lead to esthetic failure (see fig. 15-1). Additionally, acutely inflamed tissues are difficult to manage during the impression phase of treatment.

Inflamed/Hypertrophic Gingiva

To ensure optimal esthetic results, it is essential to begin the impression process with healthy tissue free of periodontal inflammation and/or bleeding. With healthy gingival tissue, impression taking can be accomplished predictably with relative comfort. Factors that may contribute to gingival inflammation are inadequate periodontal maintenance, poor provisionalization, encroaching on biologic space during preparation, subgingival crown margins, or improper tissue displacement techniques.

Periodontal Maintenance
During extensive treatment plans that span several months to years, it is critical that patients follow a comprehensive periodontal maintenance regimen. Lack of proper periodontal treatment and maintenance can result in inflamed, unhealthy tissue making it extremely challenging for adequate tissue management and successful impressions. Excellent gingival health must be the goal in all phases of esthetic treatment. Meticulous oral hygiene must be stressed during all phases of treatment. This is especially important for patients in provisional restorations awaiting impressions or the delivery of definitive restorations.

Gingival inflammation may also be present from existing crowns with poor contours or marginal discrepancies. Certain cervical marginal configurations have been demonstrated to be inherently rough and thus to increase the potential for plaque accumulation and retention (Donovan and Cho 1998). Sometimes simply removing the source of irritation may rectify any soft tissue inflammation. If this is unsuccessful, the dentist may consider soft tissue excision.

Biologic Width
While subgingival finish lines are not periodontally advantageous, certain clinical situations warrant them:

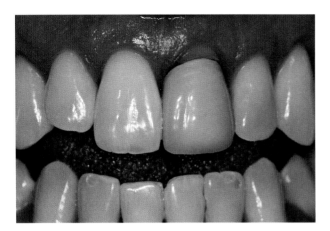

Figure 15-1. Inflamed gingival tissue around an existing porcelain-fused-to-metal restoration.

1. Inadequate retention design without extension subgingivally
2. Preexisting, subgingival margins on an existing restoration
3. Subgingival caries that must be incorporated into preparation design
4. A gummy smile with visible free gingival margins (Goodacre 1990)

Subgingival margins may risk invading the biologic space or width. This not only makes it difficult to take an impression but may lead to chronic gingival inflammation, gingival recession, clinical attachment loss, or bone loss due to the microbial plaque located at the deeply placed restorative margins. Restoration margins that are placed too close to the periodontal attachment will potentially lead to a pronounced chronic inflammatory response. The most common cause of this situation occurs in the interproximal areas of the preparations. Occasionally, clinicians do not follow the anatomic form of the tissue in this area that can lead to bone loss in this region. If the inflammatory process does not lead to bone loss initially, intrabony defects may occur over time (Kois 1996; Newcomb 1974).

Ideal biologic width is the sum of the connective tissue attachment and the junctional epithelium, measured from the crest of the alveolar bone to the base of the sulcus. These dimensions are as follows: sulcus depth of 0.69 mm, epithelial tissue attachment of 0.97 mm and connective tissue attachment of 1.07 mm. The biologic width was determined to be a measurement of 2.04 mm (Gargiulo et al 1961). Ideally, a minimum of 3 mm distance is required from the restorative margin to the alveolar crest (Ingber, Rose, and Doslet 1977). These are average dimensions. Variations exist and should be considered when margins are placed for any restoration.

Provisionalization

A well-fabricated provisional restoration is essential in maintaining a healthy gingival environment prior to making an impression. A quality provisional restoration should have well-adapted and contoured margins, appropriate thickness, esthetics, proximal contacts, occlusion, and possess a smooth and polished surface (Zinner, Trachtenberg, and Miller 1989). While currently available materials for fabricating and luting provisionals are generally non-toxic and hypoallergenic, some may be inherently rough and porous, making them suitable habitats for inflammatory bacteria. Provisional restorations should demonstrate accurate marginal adaptation and physiologic crown contours to provide access for proper oral hygiene (Donovan and Cho 1998). Overextended margins will often cause gingival inflammation and rapid and unpredictable gingival recession. Underextended margins can allow hyperplastic gingiva to grow over the margin, making it very difficult to maintain good tissue health or obtain a suitable final impression. Proper form and contour significantly influence the ability of tissue to resume its proper gingival health (Donovan and Chee 2004). Improper gingival contours, especially in multiple units, can also lead to gingival inflammation and potentially to gingival recession (Donaldson 1974). In addition to possessing mediocre esthetics, poorly finished and polished provisionals will promote plaque and bacterial accumulation. For extensive esthetic cases, a laboratory-proceeded provisional restoration may prove advantageous. Regardless of which type of provisional restoration is utilized, meticulous attention to the removal of excess provisional cement must be employed to prevent tissue inflammation.

Having the patient rinse with chlorhexidine gluconate for two weeks before treatment and during the period of provisionalization can be helpful in minimizing gingival inflammation (Sorensen et al. 1991; Christensen 2005).

Improper tissue displacement can also cause tissue irritation and inflammation to the periodontium (Feng et al. 2006). Improper and aggressive retraction technique can cause irreversible gingival trauma that may compromise the esthetic outcome. During the placement of retraction cord, care must be taken to treat the gingiva as gently as possible. If the tissue is excessively traumatized, it may be necessary to postpone the procedure and allow the tissue to properly heal.

Soft Tissue Removal

Intentional removal of tissue using a rotary instrument may provide the most convenient method of minor soft tissue removal. However, if used improperly or aggressively, gingival tissue can be irreversibly traumatized. The interdental papilla is particularly susceptible and very easily traumatized (Goodacre 1990). The unpredictable healing or heavy bleeding that may result can make impression taking at the same appointment difficult. The dentist may consider other modes of tissue excision such as electrosurgery (to be discussed later in this chapter), soft tissue laser (to be discussed later in this chapter), or periodontal surgery. Before removing or recontouring any soft tissue, the dentist must determine if the proposed tissue modification will leave adequate attached gingiva, maintain biologic width, and prevent compromised esthetics.

Tissue Management Prior to Impression Fabrication

One of the most significant but often overlooked steps in impression fabrication is tissue management and temporary displacement. Because most esthetic restoration margins are placed near the crest of the gingiva or slightly apical to that position (subgingival), tissue retraction and temporary displacement is usually required. There are several techniques that may be employed. There is no universal technique that can be used for every clinical procedure. Rather, clinicians must be able to make the appropriate selection from various techniques. Often a combination of tissue management techniques can be utilized to enhance the impression fabrication process. The following is a list of techniques for consideration. Particular care must be employed with esthetic restorations, as improper tissue retraction can have deleterious results to the surrounding tissues.

1. Single cord retraction
2. Dual cord retraction
3. Electrosurgery
4. Laser

Retraction cord may be placed in the periodontal sulcus to provide temporary retraction (both apically and laterally) of the soft tissues surrounding prepared teeth, creating adequate space and access for impression material. For precise fitting restorations, exact reproduction of prepared teeth is essential. Failure to obtain an accurate impression can result in poorly fitting restorations, recurrent decay, or early catastrophic failure.

Gingival retraction cords are fabricated from two or more strands that are interlocked to form a knitted, braided, woven, or twisted pattern. Knitted cords are preferred, since they resist unraveling during insertion (fig. 15-2). Retraction cords usually possess one strand

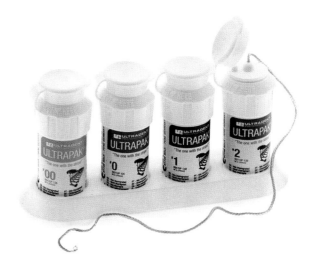

Figure 15-2. Ultradent's knitted retraction cord in four different sizes.

made from an absorbent material. Additionally, there are strands made from degradation-resistant materials, such as nylon, polyester, fiberglass, or metal. Some cords may possess epinephrine (adrenaline), a vasoconstrictor, or aluminum trichloride, a hemostatic agent.

Tissue Retraction Utilizing Cord

To obtain a good impression, soft tissue should be adequately retracted. In some cases, the process of retraction or gingival displacement is rushed and, as a result, the margins may be poorly captured, producing an inferior impression. Once retraction cord has been placed, adequate time must be provided to allow complete retraction. It is recommended to leave the retraction cord in place for a minimum of five minutes in order to temporarily remove tissue memory.

Single Cord Technique
Generally speaking, the use of a single cord retraction technique is reserved for clinical situations where the margin of the preparation is incisal to or at the free crest of the gingival (fig. 15-3). Additionally, a single cord technique should be considered for thin gingival types and tissue with limited sulcus depth (figs. 15-4 and 15-5). If minimal amounts of bleeding are present, hemostatic material should be considered. Evaluate the tissue prior to cord placement. Areas that appear inflamed or edematous may begin to bleed once cord placement is initiated. It is advantageous to scrub these areas with a hemostatic agent prior to initiating cord placement. A product such a ViscoStat (Ultradent; fig. 15-6) is recommended because of its strong hemostatic properties and well-designed delivery system.

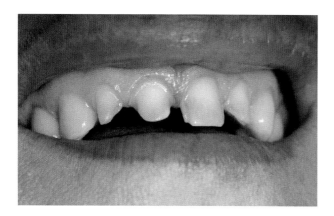

Figure 15-3. Four anterior veneer preparations prior to tissue retraction.

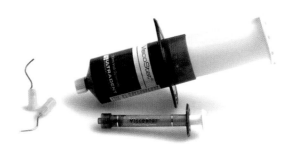

Figure 15-6. Hemostatic agent, ViscoStat (Ultradent).

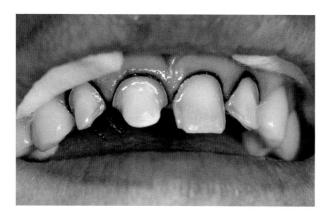

Figure 15-4. Single #00 cord in place.

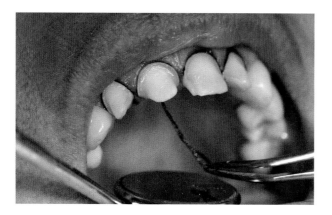

Figure 15-5. Removal of the cord #00 prior to impression.

It is essential that good instrumentation is utilized. Improper instrumentation can damage surrounding tissues and often leads to frustration. When selecting the size of the cord, it should be predetermined if the cord is to be removed prior to the introduction of impression material. If the cord will remain in the sulcus during

impression fabrication, the cord must be small enough to be placed apically to the margin without obscuring any portion of the margin. If the cord will be removed just prior to the introduction of impression material, it is advantageous to select a cord that is slightly larger and occupies the space both apically and adjacent to the prepared margin.

Proper instrumentation is crucial when placing cord. Begin with the cord-packing instrument at 45 degrees to the axial surface of the tooth. Roll the cord into the sulcus by rotating the instrument parallel to the axial surface. This technique will "tuck" the cord into place.

Dual Cord Technique

There are various clinical situations where a dual cord technique will prove advantageous. Thick gingival types often require additional retraction to provide adequate space for impression material. Margins that are placed subgingivally often require the use of a double cord technique. Additionally, teeth with periodontal pockets of 3–4 mm depth often require two cords to provide adequate retraction. The selection of the size of both cords is of critical importance. The first cord should be placed apical to the margins circumferentially after the preparations are near completion. It is critical that this cord sit below the margin as it will allow the practitioner easy access to final margin refinement. The largest cord that fits apically to the margins should be selected. A common error practitioners make is to select a cord that is too small. If this is done, the cord is difficult to place and will tend to "float" in the sulcus. Using a larger cord will help lock the cord in place by engaging the walls of the sulcus. Figures 15-7 through 15-12 depict the use of the dual cord technique on a single tooth preparation.

Once the margin position has been finalized and refined, the second cord may be placed. It is important to recognize that this cord will be removed prior to impression material placement; therefore, it is advantageous to utilize a cord that is 5–10 mm longer than the

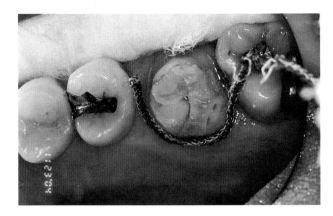

Figure 15-7. Dual cord technique, cord #00 placement.

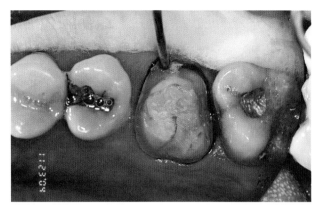

Figure 15-10. Application of hemostatic agent around the sulcus.

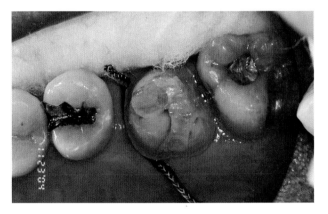

Figure 15-8. Dual cord technique, initial placement of first cord.

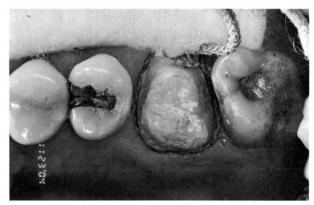

Figure 15-11. Dual cord technique, second cord placement.

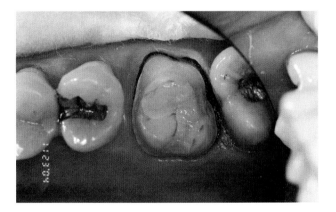

Figure 15-9. Dual cord technique, first cord complete placement.

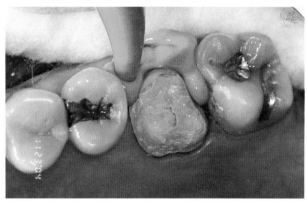

Figure 15-12. Syringing impression material.

circumference of the margin and slightly larger than the space directly adjacent and apical to the margin. An ideally placed second cord will sit immediately adjacent to the margin, providing both apical and lateral retraction. The excess length of cord should be positioned buccally for simple and efficient removal. Once all cords

have been placed, a waiting period of 5 minutes should be observed. This will allow for adequate tissue displacement and decrease the likelihood that the tissue will collapse on the margins upon removal of the second cord. Figures 15-13 through 15-20 depict the use of the dual cord technique on multiple tooth preparations.

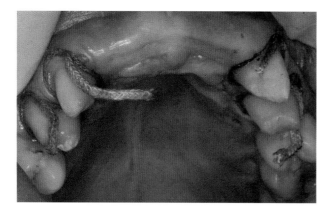

Figure 15-13. Dual cord technique, multiple teeth.

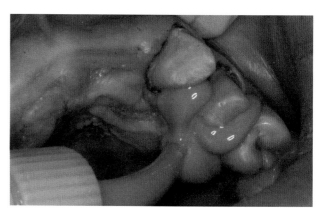

Figure 15-16. Syringing of impression material, lingual view.

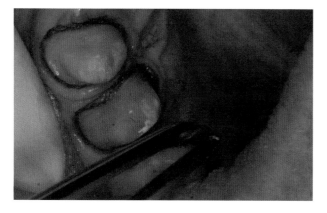

Figure 15-14. Dual cord technique, multiple teeth, removal of cord #2.

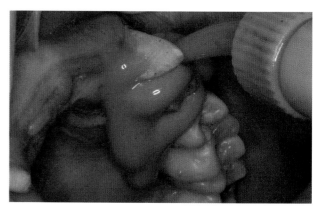

Figure 15-17. Syringing of impression material, facial.

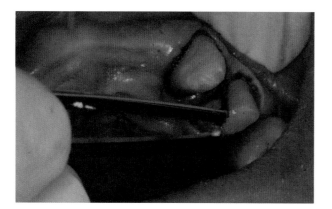

Figure 15-15. Dual cord technique, multiple teeth, removal of cord #1.

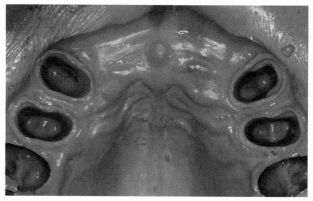

Figure 15-18. Impression of multiple teeth, dual cord technique.

Electrosurgery

Electrosurgical techniques offer predictable results, and when used skillfully can create a blood-free operative site ready for impressing. There are many different units available on the market, but all work in the same fashion (fig. 15-21).

Electrosurgery excises and coagulates tissue using high-frequency current through a circuit completed by contact between the patient and a ground electrode. The electrode produces a high-current density and rapid temperature rise at its point of contact within the precise affected tissue. Some indications for electrosurgery are to remove hypertrophic tissue to gain access for tooth

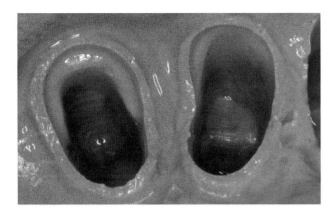

Figure 15-19. Left side, impression of multiple teeth, flash on margin area and absence of voids.

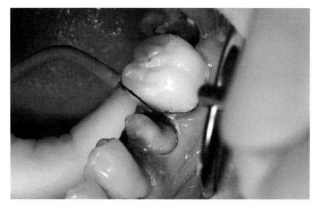

Figure 15-22. Using electrosurgical technique for reshaping of soft tissue.

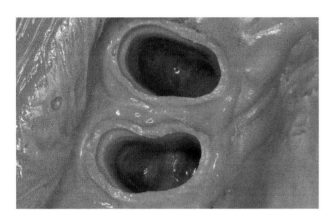

Figure 15-20. Right side, impression of multiple teeth absences of voids.

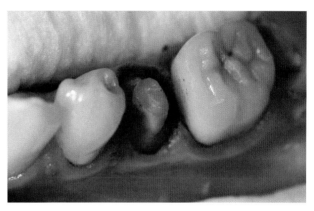

Figure 15-23. Image of soft tissue immediately after electrosurgical reshaping.

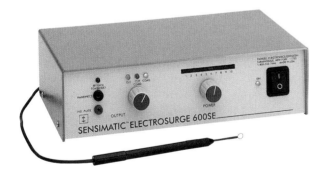

Figure 15-21. Electrosurge unit.

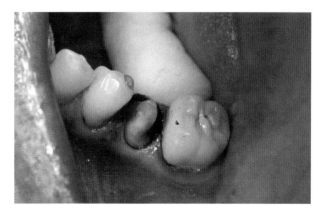

Figure 15-24. Soft tissue image prior to impression.

preparation, develop a gingival trough around the margins of a prepared tooth, control hemorrhage, or reshape tissue of pontic area (Patel 1986) with minimum postoperative healing or discomfort (figs. 15-22, 15-23, and 15-24).

Electrosurgery is contraindicated in patients with any electronic medical devices or patients who are immuno-compromised. The electrode should stay clear of any metal in the vicinity of the procedure. This may result in sparking or an electric shock. Sparking may also appear if the setting is too high. The electrode should not contact bone for long periods of time or it may initiate bone loss or sequestration of bone. Always follow the manufacturer's instructions.

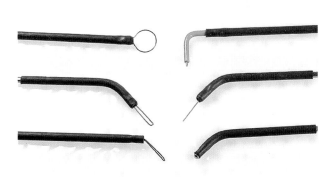

Figure 15-25.   Different tip sizes and shapes for electrosurge unit.

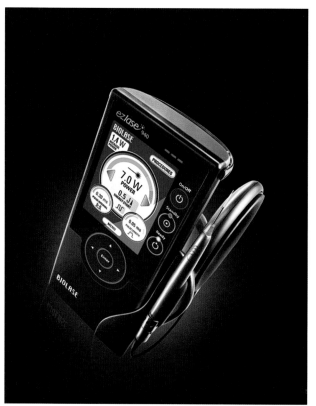

Figure 15-26.   ezlase laser unit (Biolase Technology, Inc).

Electrosurgery Technique

The electrosurgery equipment includes the unit, various types of electrodes, and the conductive plate. Before the procedure begins, anesthesia must be given and verified. The grounding plate is placed under the back of the patient. Proper tip should be selected based on the needs of excision (fig. 15-25). A straight or very narrow loop electrode is most appropriate for sulcular enlargement. Larger loop electrodes are useful for preparing ovate pontic sites where adequate tissue is present and for gingival contouring. Once the proper electrode is selected and proper setting is established, the procedure is initiated. The foot switch should be depressed before placing the tip on the tissue. The tip is then lightly placed on the tissue. The electrode should move at a speed of no less than 7mm per second. It is necessary to retrace the initial cut within 8- to 10-second intervals (Shillingburg 1997, Kalkwarf et al. 1983). The tip should move smoothly without pulling, dragging, or charring of the tissue. The electrode should be constantly moving with light, uniform strokes.

It is best to cut on moist tissue; however, avoid excess pooling of water around the surgical site. A high-volume suction tip should be kept adjacent to the tissue being cauterized. Intermittent stops should be made to wipe off any excess tissue fragments from the electrode. A cotton pellet dipped in hydrogen peroxide may be used to wipe off loose cauterized tissue (Shillingburg 1997; Rosenstiel, Land, and Fujimoto 2006).

Soft Tissue Laser

Soft tissue lasers are routinely used in esthetic cases for procedures such as gingival troughing, gingival recontouring, removal of granulation tissue, hemorrhage control, and crown lengthening. They may be used with minimum anesthesia and produce little to no postoperative discomfort (fig. 15-26).

Unlike electrosurgery, where the tissue may become discolored, the laser allows one to excise tissue with no visible tissue charring or discoloration. This is especially important when fabricating restorations in the esthetic zone. The cut is more precise than a scalpel or electrosurgery, with less bleeding. The laser coagulates and seals tissue to provide better visualization, cleaner impressions, and more predictable healing. Lasers are faster, more effective esthetically, more comfortable postoperatively, and can reduce overall treatment time (Sulewski 2000; Sarver and Yanosky 2005; figs. 15-27 and 15-28).

Some general types of soft tissue lasers marketed for dental uses are carbon dioxide laser, Nd:YAG laser, and diode laser. The carbon dioxide laser is effective for removing shallow but wide areas of soft tissue such as frenula, aphthae, or leukoplakia (Sulewski 2000). These lasers cannot be delivered through the optic fiber, so precise tactile sensation is very difficult to achieve (Dederich and Bushnick 2004). While Nd:YAG lasers are able to cut hard tissue as well as soft tissue, they have a mode of operation that may make it difficult to achieve

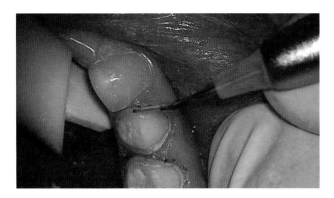

Figure 15-27. Soft tissue contouring using laser unit.

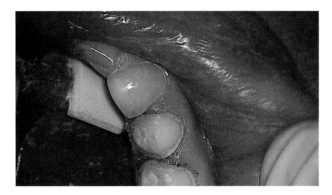

Figure 15-28. Soft tissue immediately after reshaping with laser unit.

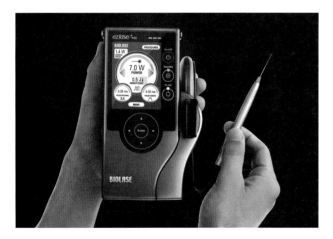

Figure 15-29. ezlase 940 (Biolase Technology, Inc).

certain precise esthetic procedures such as gingival contouring. Diode lasers cut soft tissues equally well, are cost effective, and are compact in design, making them an ideal choice for esthetic soft tissue procedures (fig. 15-29).

Diode lasers have a wavelength of 600–980 nanometers. The laser energy is absorbed by pigmentation in the soft tissues, making this laser an excellent hemostatic agent (Sarver and Yanosky 2005). The diode laser may be used with the fiber tip either in contact to cut or in close proximity to treat the target area. Placing the tip in direct contact with the tissue will enhance tactile feedback (Lee 2006).

"A laser creates a light beam that is monochromatic (narrow wavelength) and highly collimated through a filamentous tube. The tube or fiber has a cladding layer that collimates the light energy, and has a protective jacket outside. The laser delivers concentrated energy through the fine tip of the fiber to tissue, where energy is absorbed. The degree of absorption is based on the wavelength (measured in nanometers), the power output, and the characteristics of the tissue, including water content" (Rossman and Cobb 1995). This energy transmitted through the tip cuts soft tissue through ablation of tissue (Research Committee 2002). Ablation means the separation of the tissue, which results in an incision that is sealed, coagulated, and sanitized. Lasers can deliver energy in either continuous mode or pulse mode. In the continuous mode, the tissues may absorb more energy, which results in greater heat and potentially more postoperative discomfort (Sarver and Yanosky 2005). For this reason, pulse mode is recommended. The cut is sterile due to the destruction of all bacteria by the laser energy, and bacteremia is greatly reduced due to the sealing of blood vessels and lymphatics (Sarver and Yanosky 2005).

Laser Technique

Depending on the type of laser unit used, fiber optics can be either disposable or may come in a long coil. While disposable tips require no preparation, the coiled fiber optics only require minimal preparation.

The laser beam in the fiber optic is encased in a jacket or sheath. The sheath needs to be cleaved with a glass cutter to create a 90-degree edge. This creates a precise beam of light that will result in precise cutting of the tissue. First, place the energy settings according to the manufacturer's recommendations and the operator's experience. The setting should be in pulse mode to better control the ablation. The laser hand piece should be held firmly with a modified pen grasp (Lee 2006). The fiber should be placed parallel to the long axis of the tooth (figs. 15-30 and 15-31). Once proper positioning is established, quick featherlike strokes should be used. The laser hand piece should be kept moving to prevent thermal damage to underlying tissue. The operator should not attempt to remove tissue by dragging the glass fiber; instead, the laser light energy should do all the ablation. As the tissue is ablated, hemostatis occurs due to the photochemical interaction with the biologic tissue (Sulewski 2000).

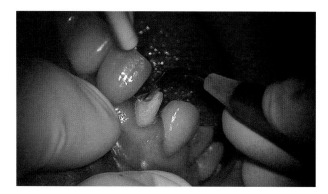

Figure 15-30. Proper positioning of the fiber tip with pen grasp.

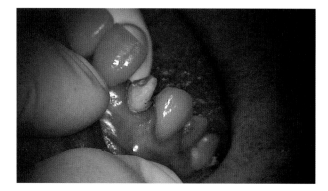

Figure 15-31. Reshaped soft tissue, prior to impression.

Though using a soft tissue laser may be straightforward, nevertheless, formal training is recommended to become familiar with the appropriate protocols.

Impression Materials

To fabricate an accurate fitting indirect restoration, such as a crown, practitioners need an exact reproduction of the form and relation of the teeth and surrounding oral tissue. It is neither possible nor desirable to make patterns for fixed prostheses directly in the mouth (Rosenstiel, Land, and Fujimoto 2006). Impression materials are used to record the shape of the teeth and alveolar ridges. There is a wide variety of impression materials available, each with their own physical properties, advantages, and disadvantages.

The fit of any indirect restoration depends on a precise working model and a skilled technician. A precise replication of a tooth preparation is achieved through a quality impression. New impression materials with different properties are continuously introduced to the dental market. Impression materials that are in common use can be classified as elastic or nonelastic. Elastic impression materials dominate the marketplace and are the most common choice for indirect restorations. The primary reason for their popularity is that they can be stretched and bent to a large degree without suffering any permanent deformation. They are particularly useful in clinical situations where undercuts may be present.

There are several types of elastic impression materials. The challenge that clinicians often face is what type of impression material to use in varying clinical situations. Impression materials should possess certain properties to ensure clinical success. Ideal properties of an impression material include the following:

1. Safety
2. Accuracy
3. Easy handling
4. Dimensionally stable
5. Capacity to be poured multiple times
6. Tolerable taste
7. Nonirritating to human tissues
8. High degree of detail reproduction

Additionally, impression material should be compatible with materials used for model work. Although all final impression materials are relatively expensive, cost of material is also a factor.

Not all impression materials have ideal physical properties, and no one impression material is perfectly suited for all clinical situations. One must keep in mind that the precision of impression will ultimately dictate the precision of the die and subsequent restoration. An ideal impression material possesses hydrophilic properties, allowing the material to tolerate moisture. In contrast, impression materials that are hydrophobic possess lower affinity for moisture, high contact angles, and may possess lower degrees of surface detail. Materials of this type are less desirable than the aforementioned.

Contact Angle

Contact angle is the angle at which a liquid interface meets a solid surface. On a hydrophilic surface, a water droplet will completely spread, whereas on hydrophobic surfaces, a water droplet will simply rest on the surface without actually wetting the surface to any significant extent. The lower the contact angle for an impression material, the more desired it becomes, since low contact angles minimize voids and bubbles.

Elasticity

Elasticity is a variable that describes the relationship of stress to strain within the elastic region. The modulus of elasticity describes a material's stiffness. The elasticity of an impression material is a factor that works to prevent permanent distortion. As impression materials become more elastic, they become more tear resistant.

Flowability

An imperative factor in choosing an impression material is the flowability of the impression. Viscosity is a measure of the resistance of a fluid to deform. It is the thickness or resistance to flow. The lower the viscosity of the impression material, the better the flowability.

Handling

The handling characteristics of an impression material are one of the most significant factors practitioners must assess when choosing a given impression material for any procedure. In general, impression materials should be easy to mix and have reasonable working and setting time.

Ability to Be Disinfected

Impression materials should have the capacity to be disinfected without loss of surface detail or accuracy. The surface must be resistant to chemical degradation from any commercially available surface disinfectants.

Types of Impression Material

There are several types of impression material available commercially for use in clinical practice. A good working knowledge of the handling characteristics of each type of material is essential for today's practitioner. Each type of material will have benefits and drawbacks that must be weighed during the selection process. There are six common types of impression materials:

1. Irreversible hydrocolloid
2. Reversible hydrocolloid
3. Polysulfide
4. Polyether
5. Condensation reaction silicones
6. Addition reaction silicones

Although there are several categories of impression materials to choose from, this chapter will limit its discussion to the two most commonly used categories: addition reaction silicones and polyethers. Polysulfides and reversible hydrocolloids are hydrophilic by nature but require careful timing and pouring protocols. This fact makes them less desirable when shipping or transportation to a laboratory will be utilized. Furthermore, they are less dimensionally stable when stored for any

prolonged period of time compared to addition reaction silicones (polyvinyl siloxanes) and polyethers.

Addition Reaction Silicone (Polyvinyl Siloxane)

Polyvinyl siloxane was introduced in the mid-1970s, and it is an addition reaction silicon elastomer (figs. 15-32, 15-33, 15-34, and 15-35). Addition silicones are the most

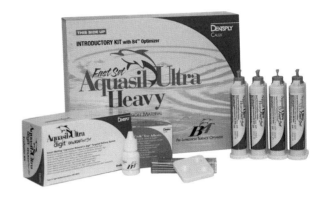

Figure 15-32.   Aquasil Ultra Heavy, fast set (Dentsply).

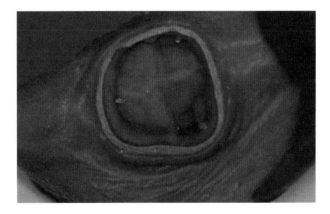

Figure 15-33.   Impression of single tooth using polyvinyl siloxane.

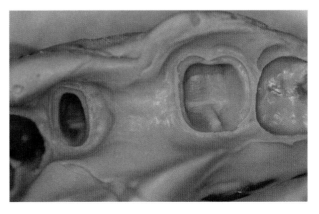

Figure 15-34.   Impression of multiple teeth using polyvinyl siloxane.

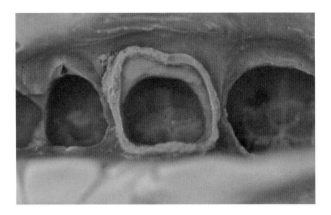

Figure 15-35.   Impression of single tooth using polyvinyl siloxane.

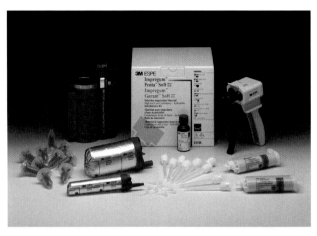

Figure 15-37.   Polyether impression material, Impregum (3M ESPE).

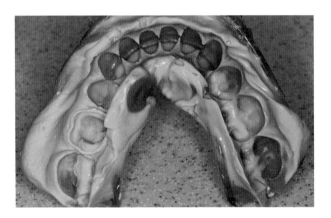

Figure 15-36.   Full arch impression using polyvinyl siloxane.

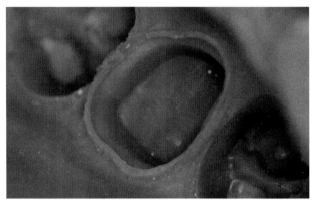

Figure 15-38.   Polyether impression of a single tooth, Impregum (3M ESPE).

versatile and widely used due to their dimensional stability and accuracy. This stability allows for delayed pouring without the risk of distortion (fig. 15-36). They are well tolerated by patients due to their relatively innocuous taste and smell. They are quite elastic, which makes them relatively easy to remove once set. They have a high tear strength and ability to be disinfected with minimal dimension change. Addition silicones provide excellent surface detail and resist deformation.

There are some drawbacks to these materials. Their set is inhibited by the presence of sulphur-containing products. They are hydrophobic by nature, and surfactants are commonly added to improve wetability.

Polyether

Polyether impression materials are popular among practitioners due to several favorable characteristics. Polyether material consistently yields superior results with or without a custom tray when compared with the other impression materials (Ciesco et al. 1981). Impregum (3M ESPE; fig. 15-37) was the first elastomer to be introduced specifically for restorative dentistry in the late 1970s. Polyethers are hydrophilic by nature, are dimensionally stable for short periods of time, have a low contact angle, can be poured several times, and are relatively tear resistant (fig. 15-38). They may be the material of choice over addition reaction silicones when moisture control issues or copious salivation are anticipated clinically. They are not a perfect impression material. Polyether impression material should be poured within forty-eight hours and stored dry, since they can absorb water. After several weeks of storage they begin to degrade.

Additionally, polyether's high elastic module makes it a rigid material when set. Caution must be utilized when significant undercuts are present as the material can become "locked" in the patient's mouth. Laboratory technicians must employ caution when separating casts from polyether impressions. There is an increased risk of breaking stone teeth when using polyether impression material.

Armamentarium for Final Impressions

Impression Tray

There are several choices and decisions that must be made when selecting the appropriate impression tray for a final impression. There are universal characteristics that must be present regardless of the type of impression tray selected. The impression tray must

1. be rigid enough to resist bending or distortion during insertion and removal,
2. possess mechanical retentive features that help resist separation of impression material,
3. extend far enough into the vestibules to capture all necessary anatomy,
4. have adequate room for impression material on all sides of the prepared teeth, and
5. be comfortable for the patient.

Initially, the clinician needs to determine whether a custom tray or stock tray is desired. If it is determined that a stock tray is to be utilized, the clinician must select a full arch, quadrant, or dual-arch impression tray. Generally speaking, the type of tray selected is based on the number of prepared teeth to be impressed and the complexity of the occlusal scheme present. If limited opening is present, or the patient has difficulty during impression making, a custom tray may be indicated. Although custom trays require fabrication, they utilize far less impression material, and the overall cost of impressions captured is less compared with full-arch stock tray impressions.

Full-Arch Impression Trays

For fixed or removable prosthetic restorations that include more than three units, large esthetic cases, and long-span fixed partial dentures, a full-arch impression is suggested. This will provide the laboratory technician with the maximum amount of detail and information. For this type of impression a metal tray, rigid plastic tray, or custom tray may be utilized. The tray selected must closely conform to the arch curvature of the patient's mouth. This will ensure a complete, accurate detail reproduction and aid the practitioner with seating the tray.

Quadrant or Dual-Arch Impression Trays

For simple cases involving a limited number of restorations, a quadrant or dual-arch tray can be utilized. Double-arch impression trays should be sufficiently sized to include the canine tooth. Dual-arch impression trays are preferred because they offer the advantage of capturing the opposing dentition, occlusion, and bite registration simultaneously. Double impression trays should be evaluated in the mouth to ensure the patient can completely close when the tray is in position. The double-arch impression method has proved to produce crowns with equivalent margin accuracy and superior occlusal accuracy, compared to crowns fabricated from the conventional complete-arch impression technique (Cox, Brandt, and Hughes 2002).

Tray Dimensions

It is essential to have approximately 5 mm of space between internal walls of the tray and the prepared teeth to eliminate the possibility of deformation or distortion of the impression. In the event that there is inadequate space between the tooth and the internal aspect of the tray, the likelihood of tearing the impression upon removal is increased. Furthermore, there is a greater chance that permanent distortion may occur if there is not adequate room for impression material to flow freely between the tray borders and the prepared tooth.

Distortion Resistance

It is important that impression trays be strong enough to resist bending and flexing while the setting process of impression material occurs. Additionally, trays must resist permanent deformation upon removal from the oral cavity and upon separation of master casts after they have been poured. Some trays are constructed of inferior materials and may distort during use. Dentists and dental assistants must avoid altering pressure on impression trays during setting. It is essential to note that even heavy body impression material is not strong enough to resist changes in pressure during their set. Potential for distortion greatly increases if pressure on the setting material is altered as it sets.

General Impression Techniques

The use of a two-stage putty/wash technique was advocated for years. In a randomized controlled trial, Luthardt et al. (2005) concluded that the two-stage putty and wash impression showed significantly reduced accuracy compared with a one-stage technique. With the introduction of various viscosity impression materials and dramatic improvements in delivery techniques, the need for a two-stage impression has vanished and will not be discussed. In their in-vitro study of surface defects in mono phase and two-phase addition reaction silicone (polyvinyl siloxane) impressions, Millar, Dunne, and Robinson (1998) concluded that mono phase materials in stock trays carry an increased risk of void formation on the surface of the impression when compared with two-phase addition silicone in custom trays. Today, the most favorable and accurate techniques employ either a monophase material in a stock tray, a monophase material in a stock tray with a low-viscosity wash, or a low-viscosity wash in a custom tray. The latter two will be discussed in detail.

Regardless of the tissue management technique employed, the impression material delivery technique will not vary. There are several rules that should be observed during impression material placement. They can greatly enhance the likelihood of capturing a flawless impression.

1. For mandibular teeth, always start the impression on the distal lingual portion of the prep and work mesially. This will decrease the likelihood that fluid is introduced from submandibular salivary glands at a critical time.
2. For multiple unit impressions of anterior teeth, capture the lingual surfaces of each preparation first. Too often the authors have observed clinicians starting with the buccal surfaces of anterior teeth. This technique predisposes the impression to possess bubbles, as the wash material will tend to slump to the lingual and trap air. Additionally, having material covering the buccal will obscure the view of the lingual surface and complicate the process unnecessarily.
3. Concentrate on delivering the impression material to the sulcus, not to the margin. This will greatly increase the likelihood that the final impression will possess adequate amounts of flash.
4. For multiple-unit posterior impressions, capture all the lingual or palatal surfaces first, beginning with the distalmost preparation. Once completed, move to the distalmost buccal surface and express material into the proximal surface until visible movement of the lingual material is observed. Continue expressing material around the buccal sulcus into the mesial proximal surface and watch for movement of the lingual impression material. Continue this sequence with all remaining preparations.
5. Difficult tongues may be managed with retraction devices such as the Isolite or Hygroformic.
6. Salivary control is critical and must be well controlled for successful impressions. For posterior impressions, a dryaide is extremely helpful. For multiple-unit anterior and posterior preparations, horseshoe cotton rolls are beneficial.

Low-Viscosity Wash in a Custom Tray

A low-viscosity polyether or polyvinyl siloxane wash material may be used with a custom tray. The use of a custom tray with low-viscosity wash may be used for any of the following clinical situations:

1. Single-unit crown, inlay, or onlay preparations
2. Multiple-unit crown preparations
3. Closed-tray implant impressions
4. Fixed partial denture impressions

Prior to commencing the impression, it is essential that the custom tray be checked for appropriate fit. Once the preparations have been finalized, the following steps should be followed to obtain an acceptable impression:

1. Obtain necessary tissue retracted using one of the aforementioned techniques.
2. Apply adhesive to the tray.
3. Rinse the preparations to ensure a clean surface. Keep the preparations dry and well isolated.
4. Load the impression tray and impression syringe with low-viscosity impression material. It is best to load the tray and then the syringe to maximize working time.
5. Syringe low-viscosity impression material around each preparation.
6. Seat the tray from posterior to anterior to prevent excess material from passing to the back of the throat. It is crucial that the tray be kept immobile during the setting process to prevent distortion.
7. Once thoroughly set, remove the impression and evaluate it for accuracy. If acceptable, apply a surface disinfectant and ship to the laboratory.

One-Step Low-Viscosity Wash and Tray Material in a Stock Tray

This technique will use a low-viscosity wash material in conjunction with a medium-body (monophase) tray material. The advantages of using a prefabricated stock tray are that they allow for easy removal and are less likely to lock in than are custom trays. They can be used in a wide variety of clinical situations, including the following:

1. Single-unit crown, inlay, or onlay preparations
2. Multiple-unit crown preparations
3. Closed tray implant impressions
4. Open tray implant impressions
5. Fixed partial denture impressions

A medium body (tray) and low viscosity (wash) or either a polyvinyl siloxane or a polyether may be utilized for this technique. Figure 15-39 shows an impression of multiple preparations using polyether for this technique. Figure 15-40 shows the corresponding model.

1. Try-in and select the appropriate stock tray. Ensure that adequate space is present on both the buccal and lingual aspects of all preparations.

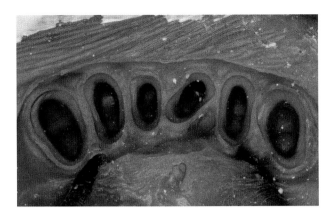

Figure 15-39. Polyether impression of multiple teeth, Impregum (3M ESPE).

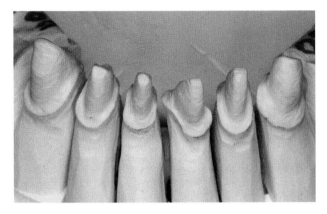

Figure 15-40. Master cast fabricated from a high-quality impression. Note the clarity and detail of each preparation.

2. Obtain necessary tissue retracted using one of the aforementioned techniques.
3. Apply adhesive to the tray.
4. Rinse the preparations to ensure a clean surface. Keep the preparations dry and well isolated. This is critically important if a polyvinyl siloxane impression material is selected.
5. Load the impression syringe with low-viscosity impression material. This is handed to the clinician to begin the application of impression material while the tray is being loaded.
6. Load the impression tray with monophase (tray) impression material and a thin wash of low-viscosity impression material.
7. Syringe low-viscosity impression material around each preparation.
8. Seat the tray from posterior to anterior to prevent excess material from passing to the back of the throat. Increasing the velocity at which the tray is seated will assist in advancing the impression material gingivally. It is critical that the tray be kept immobile during the setting process to prevent distortion.
9. Once thoroughly set, remove the impression and evaluate it for accuracy. If acceptable, apply a surface disinfectant and ship to the laboratory.

Disinfection of Impressions

Studies have revealed that placing elastomeric impression material such as polyether, polysulfide, addition reaction silicone, and condensation silicone in 5.25% NaOCl for ten minutes or 2% glutaraldehyde for thirty minutes has no negative effect on dimensional accuracy. The accuracy of impression materials is adversely affected with eighteen hours of immersion disinfection (Lepe and Johnson 1997). Another study by Jagger et al. in 2004 concluded that "various disinfection treatments had different effects on the impression material; with few individual exceptions, the impressions which were immersed in different solutions expanded and therefore produced casts with smaller dimensions than standard."

Long-term (18 hours) immersion disinfection affected the fit of fixed partial prostheses and is not recommended. To minimize the potential for distortion of impressions, place surface disinfectants for the amount of time prescribed by the manufacturer.

Salivary Control for Copious Salivators

Sal-Tropine, the anticholinergic drug atropine sulfate, has been shown to reduce secretions by more than 50% of the baseline levels at rest (Dworkin and Nadal, 1991). Atropine-induced inhibition of salivation occurs within thirty minutes to one hour after the drug has been introduced. Anticholinergics should not be prescribed to any patient with heart disease or glaucoma. In cases of glaucoma, permanent blindness can occur. These medications should be reserved for extremely difficult clinical situations and rarely utilized.

Works Cited

Christensen GJ. 2005. The state of fixed prosthodontic impressions: Room for improvement. *J Am Dent Assoc* 136(3):343–6.

Ciesco JN, Malone WF, Sandrik JL, Mazur B. 1981. Comparison of elastomeric impression materials used in fixed prosthodontics. *J Prosthet Dent* 45(1):89–94.

Cox JR, Brandt RL, Hughes HJ. 2002. A clinical pilot study of the dimensional accuracy of double-arch and complete-arch impressions. *J Prosthet Dent* 87(5):510–5.

Dederich DN, Bushnick RD. 2004. Lasers in dentistry separating science from hype. *JADA* no. 135, 204–9.

Donaldson D. 1974. The etiology of gingival recession associated with temporary crowns. *J Periodontol* 45:468–71.

Donovan TE, Chee W. 2004. current concepts in gingival displacement. *Dent Clin N Am* 48:433–44.

Donovan TE, Cho GC. 1998. Soft tissue management with metal-ceramic and all-ceramic restorations. *CDA Journal* 26(2):107–12.

Dworkin J, Nadal J. 1991. Nonsurgical treatment of drooling in a patient with closed head injury and severe dysarthria. *Dysphagia* 6:40–9.

Feng J, Aboyoussef H, et al. 2006. The effect of gingival retraction procedures on periodontal indices and crevicular fluid cytokine levels: A pilot study. *J Prosthodont* 15(2):108–12.

Gargiulo AW, et al. 1961. Dimensions and relationships of the dentogingival junction in humans. *J Periodontol* 32:261–7.

Goodacre CJ. 1990. Gingival esthetics. *J Prosthet Dent* 64(1): 1–12.

Ingber JS, Rose LF, Doslet JG. 1977. The "biologic width": A concept in periodontics and restorative dentistry. *Alpha Omegan* 70(3):62–5.

Jagger DC, Al Jabra O, Harrison A, Vowles RW, McNally L. 2004. The effect of a range of disinfectants on the dimensional accuracy of some impression materials. *Eur J Prosthodont Restor Dent* 12(4):154–60.

Kalkwarf KL, Krejci RF, Edison AR, Reinhardt RA. 1983. Lateral heat production secondary to electrosurgical incision. *Oral Surg Med Oral Pathol* 55:344–8.

Kois JC. 1996. The restorative-periodontal interface: Biological parameters. *Periodontology 2000* 11:29–38.

Lee EA. 2006. Laser-assisted gingival tissue procedure in esthetic dentistry. *Pract Proced Aesthetic Dent* 18(9):2–6.

Lepe X, Johnson GH. 1997. Accuracy of polyether and addition silicone after long-term immersion disinfection. *J Prosthet Dent* 78(3):245–9.

Luthardt RG, Koch R, Rudolph H, Walter MH. 2005. Qualitative computer aided evaluation of dental impressions in vivo. *Dent Mater* 22(1):69–76.

Millar BJ, Dunne SM, Robinson PB. 1998. In vitro study of the number of surface defects in mono phase and two-phase addition silicone impressions. *J Prosthet Dent* 80(1):32–5.

Newcomb GM. 1974. The relationship between the location of subgingival crown margins and gingival inflammation. *J Periodontol* 45(3):151–6.

Patel, Marzbung. 1986. Electrosurgical management of hyperplastic tissue. *J Prosthet Dent* 56(2):145–7.

Research, Science and Therapy Committee of the American Academy of Periodontology. 2002. Lasers in periodontics. *J Periodontol* 73:1231–9.

Rosenstiel SF, Land MF, Fujimoto J. 2006. *Contemporary Fixed Prosthodontics*, 4th ed. Maryland Heights, MO: Mosby Elsevier.

Rossman JA, Cobb CM. 1995. Lasers in periodontal therapy. *Periodontology 2000* 9:150–64.

Sarver DM, Yanosky M. 2005. Principles of cosmetic dentistry in orthodontics: Part 2. Soft tissue laser technology and cosmetic gingival contouring. *Am J Orthod Dentofacial Orthop* 127(1):85–90.

Shillingburg HT. 1997. *Fundamentals of Fixed Prosthodontics*, 3rd ed., edited by LA Bateman. Chicago: Quintessence.

Sorensen JA, Doherty FA, Newman MG, Flemming TF. 1991. Gingival enhancement in fixed prosthodontics. Part I: Clinical finding. *J Prosthet Dent* 65:100–7.

Sulewski JG. 2000. Historical survey of laser dentistry. *Dent Clin North Am* 44(4):771–2.

Zinner I, Trachtenberg D, Miller R. 1989. Provisional restorations in fixed partial prosthodontics. *Dent Clin North Am* 33(3):355–77.

Suggested Reading

Block PL. 1987. Restorative margins and periodontal health: A new look at an old perspective. *J Prosthet Dent* 6(57): 683–9.

Breeding LC, Dixon DL. 2000. Accuracy of casts generated from dual-arch impressions. *J Prosthet Dent* 84(4):403–7.

Ceyhan JA, Johnson GH, Lepe X, Phillips KM. 2003. A clinical study comparing the three-dimensional accuracy of a working die generated from two dual-arch trays and a complete-arch custom tray. *J Prosthet Dent* 90(3):228–34.

Ceyhan JA, Johnson GH, Lepe X. 2003. The effect of tray selection, viscosity of impression material, and sequence of pour on the accuracy of dies made from dual-arch impressions. *J Prosthet Dent* 90(2):143–9.

Cho GC, Chee WW. 2004. Distortion of disposable plastic stock trays when used with putty vinyl polysiloxane impression materials. *J Prosthet Dent* 92(4):354–8.

Christensen GJ. 2000. Improving the quality of fixed prosthodontic services. *J Am Dent Assoc* 131(11):1631–2.

Cox JR. 2005. A clinical study comparing marginal and occlusal accuracy of crowns fabricated from double-arch and complete-arch impressions. *Austrian Dentistry Journal* 50(2):904.

Department of Plastic and Maxillofacial Surgery. *Saliva Control in Children*. Melbourne, Australia: The Royal Children's Hospital.

Herfort TW, Gerberich WW, Macosko CW, Goodkind RJ. 1978. Tear strength of elastomeric impression materials. *J Prosthet Dent* 39(1):59–62.

Hope Pharmaceuticals. 1994. *Sal-Tropine prescribing information*. Scottsdale, AZ: Author.

Ifran Ahmad. 2006. *Protocols for Predictable Aesthetic Dental Restorations*. Lackwell.

Johnson GH, Chellis KD, Gordon GE, Lapel X. 1998. Dimensional stability and detail reproduction of irreversible hydrocolloid and elastomeric impressions disinfected by immersion. *J Prosthet Dent* 79(4):446–53.

Johnson GH, Lepe X, Aw TC. 2003. The effect of surface moisture on detail reproduction of elastomeric impressions. *J Prosthet Dent* 90(4):354–64.

Lai JY, Silvestri L, Girard B. 2001. Anterior esthetic crown-lengthening surgery: A case report. *J Can Dent Assoc* 67(10):600–3.

Larson TD, Nielsen MA, Brackett WW. 2002. The accuracy of dual-arch impressions: A Pilot Study. *J Prosthet Dent* 87(6):625–7.

Lowe RA. 2006. Clinical use of the Er, Cr:YSGG laser for osseous crown lengthening: Redefining the standard of care. *Pract Proced Aesthet Dent* 18(4):S2–9; quiz S13.

Magid KS, Strauss RA. 2007. Laser use for esthetic soft tissue modification. *Dent Clin North Am* 51(2):525–45.

Millstein P, Maya A, Segura C. 1998. Determining the accuracy of stock and custom tray impression/casts. *J Oral Rehabil* 25(8):645–8.

Nissan J, Gross M, Shifman A, Assif D. 2002. Effect of wash bulk on the accuracy of polyvinyl siloxane putty-wash impressions. *J Oral Rehabil* 29(4):357–61.

Padbury A Jr, Eber R, Wang HL. 2003. Interactions between the gingiva and the margin of restorations. *J Clin Periodontal* 30(5):379–85.

Petrie CS, Walker MP, O'Mahony AM, Spencer P. 2003. Dimensional accuracy and surface detail reproduction of two hydrophilic vinyl polysiloxane impression materials tested under dry, moist, and wet conditions. *J Prosthet Dent* 90(4):365–72.

Reddy MS. 2003. Achieving gingival esthetics. *J Am Dent Assoc* 134(3):295–304; quiz 337–38.

Teraoka F, Takahashi J. 2000. Dimensional changes and pressure of dental stones set in silicone rubber impressions. *Dent Mater* 16(2):145–9.

Wadhwani CP, Johnson GH, Lepe X, Raigrodski AJ. 2005. Accuracy of newly formulated fast-setting elastomeric impression materials. *J Prosthet Dent* 93(6):530–9.

Walker MP, Petrie CS, Haj-Ali R, Spencer P, Dumas C, Williams K. 2005. Moisture effect on polyether and polyvinylsiloxane dimensional accuracy and detail reproduction. *J Prosthodont* 14(3):158–63.

Wostmann B, Blosser T, Gouentenoudis M, Balkenhol M, Ferger P. 2005. Influence of margin design on the fit of high-precious alloy restorations in patients. *J Dent* 33(7):611–8.

Chapter 16
Provisional Restorations

Jeffrey P. Miles DDS

Dudley Cheu DDS, MBA

Daniel Castagna DDS

In the practice of general dentistry, provisional restorations are usually referred to as "temporaries" and are often made to a quality appropriate to that term. The minimal functions of protecting open dentinal tubules, preventing tooth movement, and providing a chewing surface can be met by a wide range of materials and techniques. Each has its advantages and disadvantages, and all do some minor and hopefully reversible harm to surrounding structures (Wassell and St. George 2002).

Provisional restorations in esthetic dentistry, though, need to be much more sophisticated, approximating the final restorations much more closely in function, durability, and appearance. They need to be able to function for extended periods of time, they need to be gentle to periodontal tissues, and they need to provide a preview of the final restorations (Nejatidanesh et al. 2006; Small 2005).

Treatment Planning

It is tempting to send a patient home with provisional restorations that replicate the forms of the preoperative dentition. This certainly minimizes the chances of functional problems, phonetic changes, esthetic concerns, decementation, and breakage, but it dispenses with all the information these problems would illustrate (Fondriest 2006). Instead, provisionals must be an important part of esthetic dentistry, included in the initial treatment planning (Derbabian et al. 2000). Chapter 6 describes the steps in creating a smile design from diagnostic models. Planning for provisional restorations is a natural extension of this process. With input from the patient, wax is added to mounted models to simulate the desired tooth shapes. These models, duplicated if necessary, will guide the laboratory fabrication of the final restorations and serve as a template for provisional restorations. The dentist should decide early in the treatment planning whether provisional restorations are to

be fabricated directly (intraorally) or indirectly. Although most provisionals placed in routine dentistry are fabricated directly, as the number of teeth prepared and the patient's demand for maximum esthetics increase, the need for indirect techniques also increase.

Direct Provisional Restorations

The starting point for fabricating direct provisionals is a well-thought-out, high-quality wax-up on a modified preliminary model (Psichogios and Monaco 2003; figs. 16-1 and 16-2). A template is made from this model to carry the self-curing acrylic to the mouth and form the provisionals. Many materials have been used to create templates; we will discuss the two that produce the best, most predictable results.

A silicone or vinyl polysiloxane putty can be pressed directly onto a stone and wax model for this purpose (fig. 16-3). This is a fairly quick procedure and can be performed several times if the practitioner wishes to section one or more of the matrices to create reduction guides (Fondriest 2006). A slight relief of the putty material at the gingival constriction or on the gingival margin of the cast can help to create a bulk of acrylic that is more easily finished (Bohnenkamp and Garcia 2004; fig. 16-4). A major disadvantage of using most kinds of putty as a matrix is that their opacity makes it impossible to see if the matrix is seated properly. An error in placement usually requires the provisional be made again, since there will be some thin areas, some thick areas, and some distortion of the crown forms. Of course, the more prepared teeth and fewer unprepared teeth remain in the area, the more difficult it becomes to ensure proper seating. Discus Dental has recently introduced a clear bite registration material that can be used as a see-through matrix that may overcome this problem. Nevertheless, a putty matrix has no provision for venting the acrylic as it is dispensed, which can lead to voids in

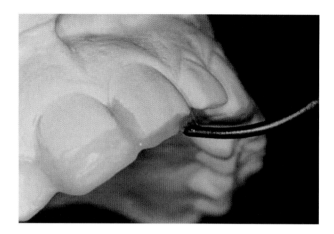

Figure 16-1. Adding wax to preoperative models.

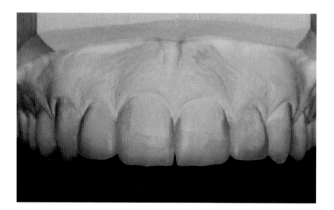

Figure 16-2. Completed wax-up for direct provisional restorations.

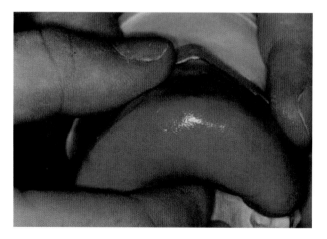

Figure 16-3. Vinyl polysiloxane putty matrix fabrication.

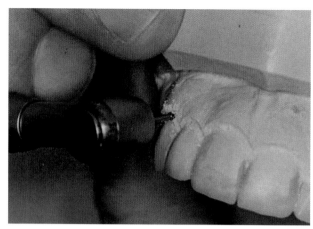

Figure 16-4. No. 4 round bur creating a trough cervical to completed wax-up.

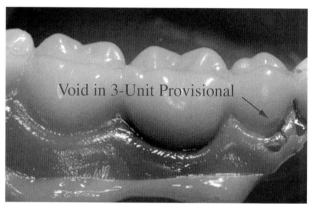

Figure 16-5. Void in bis-acrylic provisional restoration.

the occlusal or incisal areas, requiring repair with a fresh mix or flowable composite (fig. 16-5).

Using a clear thermoplastic matrix may help with these problems. This technique requires that the stone and wax model be reproduced as a well-trimmed stone model (Small 2005).

A clear plastic sheet is heated in a vacuum-forming machine and pulled down onto the model. After cooling, the plastic is removed from the model and excess is trimmed away. The clear matrix should include several unprepared teeth and some of the soft tissue areas of the model to help locate the matrix. Being clear, the matrix can be tried in the mouth to check for accuracy and tooth reduction (Fondriest 2006). Vent holes can be placed in the occlusal or incisal areas of the matrix to allow trapped air to escape, minimizing voids (Schwedhelm 2006). Unfortunately, the plastic sheet needs to be fairly thin to give adequate detail and is therefore flexible and prone to distortion (Wassell et al. 2002).

Regardless of the matrix used, direct provisionals should be made from a bis-acrylic material (Temphase, Luxatemp, Integrity, etc.; see figs. 16-6 and 16-7). These are filled composite resin materials with acceptable

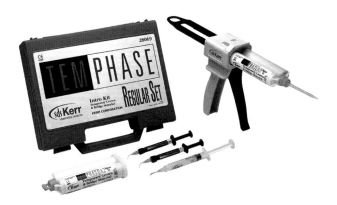

Figure 16-6.   Bis-acrylic provisional material.

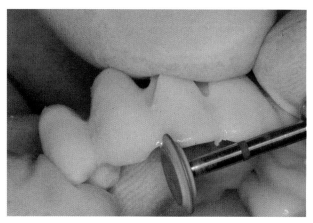

Figure 16-8.   Initial trimming of bis-acrylic provisional.

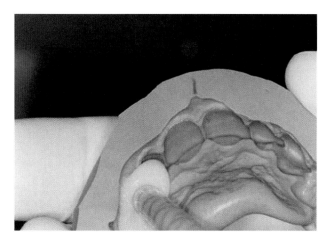

Figure 16-7.   Bis-acrylic material dispensed into Vinyl polysiloxane putty.

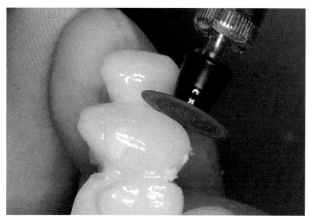

Figure 16-9.   Trimming line angles of provisional.

polymerization shrinkage and heat production (Nejati-danesh et al. 2006). Methacrylate resins, when placed in bulk, create enough heat to be dangerous to the pulp and undergo enough shrinkage to require a second mix (Burke et al. 2005). These materials should be limited to extraoral use except for the relining of laboratory-fabricated provisionals and for customizing bis-acrylic, as in the following example (Castelnuovo and Tjan 1997).

Figures 16-8 through 16-14 show the making of a bis-acrylic provisional. After the initial bulk reduction had been accomplished, the incisal embrasures were formed using a bur designed to establish anatomically correct incisal embrasures (fig. 16-8). Composite finishing disks were used to create the facial line angles of this eight-unit provisional restoration (fig. 16-9). Composite finishing burs were used to further refine the anatomical features (fig. 16-10). Due to the large soft tissue defect present in the anterior segment of this case, the prosthetic design of this restoration included the incorpora-

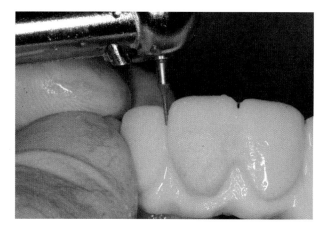

Figure 16-10.   Perfecting incisal embrasures.

tion of gingival tissue on the definitive prosthesis. The provisional restoration was contoured to receive gingival methacrylate acrylic to reproduce gingival esthetics (fig. 16-11). Cold-cured pink methacrylate acrylic was

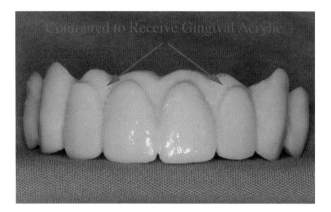

Figure 16-11. Extensions to correct gingival defect.

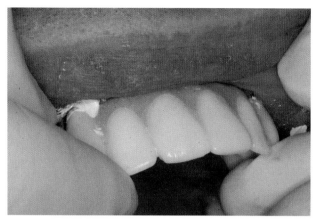

Figure 16-14. Cementing anterior provisional.

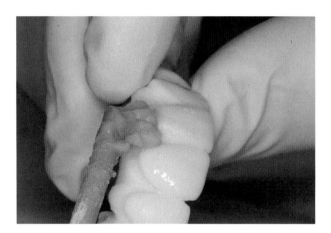

Figure 16-12. Pink acrylic added to gingival extension.

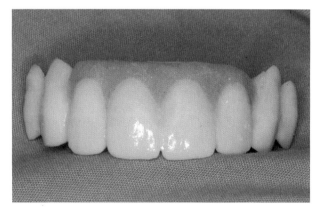

Figure 16-13. Finished provisional restoration.

placed in the gingival area and introduced to the oral cavity to capture the ridge anatomy (fig. 16-12). The provisional was given a final contouring and polishing, then cemented with provisional cement (figs. 16-13 and 16-14).

Bis-acrylics are made in a modest range of shades that should not be considered representative of the final restorations. They dispense as a fairly runny gel and spend very little time in a malleable phase before becoming very rigid. If allowed to set completely before removing, they can lock into adjacent embrasures or other undercuts, needing to be broken out (Wassell et al. 2002). Timing the placement, removal, modification, and reseating of bis-acrylic provisionals takes some practice.

Direct provisionals will usually need a fair amount of adjustment and finishing before cementation. The margins are typically bulky and will need to be carefully trimmed (Schwedhelm 2006). Some skill is required to "read" the margin of the preparation in the provisional and to trim precisely to that margin. Overtrimming will expose prepared tooth structure and temporary cement. Undertrimming will leave bulk or flash at the margin, causing gingival inflammation between appointments. Particularly in the anteriors, flash on provisional restorations can quickly cause irreversible gingival recession and compromise final esthetics.

Light-cured flowable composite can be used to fill gaps and voids and to add contour to provisionals. This works well immediately after polymerization, less well when provisionals have been in the mouth for some time (Bohnenkamp and Garcia 2004).

Multiple units deserve careful consideration. Ideally, provisionals should anticipate the final restorations in both number and contours. Teeth that are abutments for a bridge should receive a provisional bridge. Teeth that will not be splinted in the final restorations should not be splinted in the provisionals. The latter presents some difficulties since acrylic in a matrix will create a single solid unit wherever it can (Wassell et al. 2002).

There are several solutions for this problem. A solid piece of acrylic as recovered from the template can be sectioned with a thin diamond disc, taking a lingual approach and gently breaking through to the facial embrasure. This may leave an unnatural lingual embrasure that can be troublesome for the patient.

Another strategy is to place short pieces of celluloid strip between the teeth before preparation and capture them in a preoperative alginate or silicone wash impression. The impression is used as a matrix while the celluloid strips keep the resulting provisionals from adhering to each other. As with the first method, it may be necessary to add a small amount of extra material to completely close all contacts (Wassell et al. 2002).

Both of these methods are time consuming and technique sensitive, but the alternative of cementing splinted provisionals risks leaving gingival embrasures filled with acrylic and temporary cement, likely to cause unpredictable and unpleasant gingival changes. When multiple-unit temporaries, whether direct or indirect, need to be cemented as a single unit, extra effort must be taken to open gingival embrasures to an extent that might be unacceptable in permanent restorations.

Indirect Provisional Restorations

The alternative to fabricating provisionals intraorally is to create them from models. This can be done either at the dentist's office or at a dental laboratory. The in-office procedures present many of the same difficulties as direct provisionals (Shillingberg et al. 1997). Considering the demanding nature of patients interested in esthetic dentistry, the predictability and convenience of laboratory-fabricated provisionals justify their increased cost. Generally, if the case is too large to comfortably fabricate direct provisionals—four or more units—the dentist should delegate fabricating provisionals to an experienced dental laboratory.

Even with laboratory support, the dentist needs to be involved in the design of the provisionals. Once again, diagnostically mounted casts and a simulated smile design are the staring point. With the patient committed to the treatment, the casts are sent to the laboratory to prepare indirect provisionals. While the laboratory will perform many of the same steps described above for direct provisionals, all phases will be accomplished more precisely and with more durable materials (Derbabian et al. 2000).

Laboratories have several strategies available to them, most of which begin with a rigid condensation silicone putty matrix registering the contours of the waxed models. Typically, the diagnostic cast is duplicated and the teeth that will be prepared in the mouth are prepared on the cast (fig. 16-15). Since the provisionals will need to fit over the preparations in the mouth without modi-

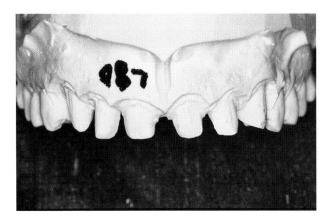

Figure 16-15. Trimmed preoperative model.

fication, it is important that the preparations on the model be carefully underreduced. This takes some skill and knowledge of preparation design. Laboratories can offer the option of structural reinforcements that would be difficult or impossible to create in direct provisionals. Frameworks cast from nonprecious metal can be used to reinforce provisionals for bridges or multiple splinted units. The cost of this option is easily justified considering the lost chair time and patient confidence that result from fractured multiunit provisionals (Galindo et al. 1998; Amet and Phinney 1995). Fiber reinforcement is a helpful and less expensive alternative (Hamza et al. 2006). Single units generally do not need any sort of reinforcement.

All indirect provisionals use some form of polymethyl methacrylate resin (PMMA) as the main structural component. PMMA, also used for denture bases, is the most durable of the resins available for dental use. It is less brittle and more color stable than either bisacrylic or poly-ethyl methacrylate and is available as either a heat-cured or cold-cured material (Haselton et al. 2005). Heat-cured PMMA is preferred for the bulk of the provisionals, with cold-cured PMMA being used for filling voids and gaps. Neither is appropriate for intraoral fabrication due to their high exotherm and unpleasant odor.

Laboratory-fabricated provisionals allow for a greater degree of shade matching than is available with direct provisionals. PMMA is available in a large selection of shades that a skilled technician can layer and blend to preview the gradations that will be present in the final restorations (Magne 2006; fig. 16-16). Subtler shades can be achieved by incorporating the shells of plastic denture teeth into the facial surface of the provisionals. When polished and glazed, laboratory-fabricated provisionals should look similar to the final restorations.

After preparation of the patient's teeth, the provisionals will be tried on to make sure they seat completely,

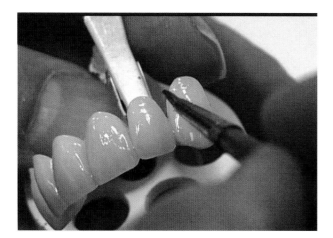

Figure 16-16. Stained and glazed laboratory-fabricated provisionals.

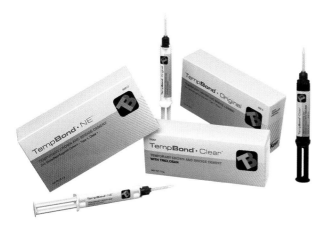

Figure 16-17. Noneugenol provisional cement.

relieved if necessary, and relined with a cold-cured resin (Christensen 2003). Laboratories may provide a clear splint fabricated from their prepared models to try over the tooth preparations to check for clearance. The resin should be of the polyethyl methacrylate or polyvinyl methacrylate type (Galindo et al. 1998). In thin layers used for relining, they do not produce enough heat to endanger pulp health, although it is still a good idea to remove and replace the provisionals during the setting period to make sure they do not lock into undercuts. The chairside resins can also be used to add to the outer surfaces of the provisionals if needed for esthetics or function. Trimming margins, opening embrasures, and polishing the fresh acrylic require the same techniques as for direct provisionals.

As with direct provisionals, laboratory-fabricated provisionals should be cemented with eugenol-free temporary cement (Wassell et al. 2002; fig. 16-17). If extra retention is needed, zinc phosphate or zinc polycarbox-

ylate cements may be used. If resin or glass ionomer cements are used, they may be impossible to remove without altering the preparations (Burke et al. 2005).

When the dentist and patient are satisfied with the function and esthetics of the provisional restorations, an alginate impression should be taken. A model is poured and sent to the laboratory as a guide for the fabrication of the permanent restorations (Derbabian et al. 2000; figs. 16-18, 16-19, 16-20).

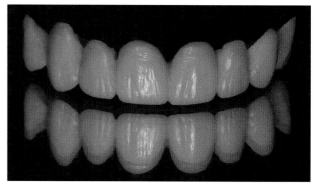

Figure 16-18. Laboratory-fabricated provisional bridge.

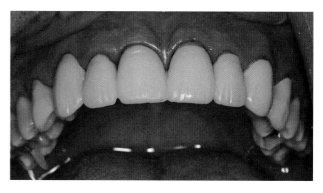

Figure 16-19. Cemented provisional bridge.

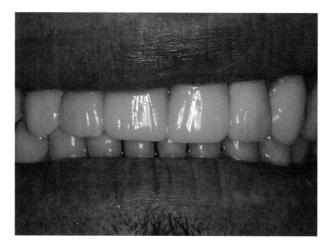

Figure 16-20. Cemented provisional bridge.

Provisionals for Porcelain Veneers

Making provisional restorations for porcelain veneers presents some unique difficulties due to their intrinsically unretentive design. While occasionally provisionals may be unnecessary when tooth reduction is minimal, most extensive veneer cases will involve some teeth that need to be more aggressively reduced. These teeth, without provisionals, will be sensitive and unsightly (Raigrodski et al. 1999).

Because of the difficulty of anticipating the depth of tooth preparation, laboratory-fabricated provisionals for veneers are impractical (Burke et al. 2005). Needing to fabricate provisionals directly, the dentist must decide if they should be made from the unaltered cast or from the diagnostic wax-up. As noted earlier, provisionals should provide a useful preview of the permanent restorations, but with the minimal retention available on veneers, that information may need to be sacrificed for the reliability of provisionally restoring to the preoperative contours.

A matrix may be made from either vinyl polysiloxane putty or clear thermoplastic. Advantages and disadvantages of each are the same as described above for full-coverage restorations. Fortunately, because of the greater amount of remaining tooth structure, the matrices seat more predictably, yielding provisionals that should require less adjustment. While bis-acrylic is typically used, flowable or hybrid composites have been advocated for their superior shade selection and polishability (Christensen 2003; Raigrodski et al. 1999).

When the provisionals have been finished, tried in, and approved, they need to be bonded to the teeth. A small spot of phosphoric acid gel is placed in the center of the facial aspect of each tooth (Burke et al. 2005). This is rinsed and a total-etch bonding agent is placed, thinned, and light cured. A conventional resin cement or flowable composite is used as a luting agent. Care must be taken to remove all excess material before it has a chance to fully cure. Self-etching bonding agents and cements need to be avoided. When the provisional restorations are removed, only the small spots of tooth structure that were etched should retain any resin; these may need to be carefully removed with a smooth diamond bur.

Summary

Provisional restorations tend not to get the attention they deserve. All practicing dentists are aware of the inconvenience and loss of patient confidence that failing provisionals can cause, but most are unwilling to adequately plan ahead or spend the chairside time necessary to fabricate high-quality provisionals. The methods described above take some time, skill, and expense but are necessary to stabilize extensive, complex, and lengthy esthetic restorative cases.

Dentists also tend to underestimate the amount of information that can be gained by placing provisionals that preview the proposed permanent restorations. Rarely is it possible to anticipate all of the functional, phonetic, and esthetic needs and desires of a patient. High-quality provisionals allow us to gather much of that input and ultimately to communicate that to the laboratory. As frustrating as it may be to throw away a provisional restoration that has taken so much effort to produce after a relatively short period of service, destroying and remaking permanent restorations is much more traumatic.

Works Cited

Amet EM, Phinney TL. 1995. Fixed provisional restorations for extended prosthodontic treatment. *J Oral Implantol* 21(3): 201–6.

Bohnenkamp DM, Garcia LT. 2004. Repair of bis-acryl provisional restorations using flowable composite resin. *J Prosthet Dent* 92(5):500–2.

Burke FJ, Murray MC, et al. 2005. Trends in indirect dentistry: 6. Provisional restorations, more than just a temporary. *Dent Update* 32(8):443–4, 447–8, 450–2.

Castelnuovo J, Tjan AH. 1997. Temperature rise in pulpal chamber during fabrication of provisional resinous crowns. *J Prosthet Dent* 78(5):441–6.

Christensen GJ. 2003. The fastest and best provisional restorations. *J Am Dent Assoc* 134(5):637–9.

Derbabian K, Marzola R, et al. 2000. The science of communicating the art of esthetic dentistry: Part II. Diagnostic provisional restorations. *J Esthet Dent* 12(5):238–47.

Fondriest JF. 2006. Using provisional restorations to improve results in complex aesthetic restorative cases. *Pract Proced Aesthet Dent* 18(4):217–23.

Galindo D, Soltys JL, et al. 1998. Long-term reinforced fixed provisional restorations. *J Prosthet Dent* 79(6):698–701.

Hamza TA, Rosenstiel SF, et al. 2006. Fracture resistance of fiber-reinforced PMMA interim fixed partial dentures. *J Prosthodont* 15(4):223–8.

Haselton DR, Diaz-Arnold AM, et al. 2005. Color stability of provisional crown and fixed partial denture resins. *J Prosthet Dent* 93(1):70–5.

Magne P, Magne M. 2006. Use of additive waxup and direct intraoral mock-up for enamel preservation with porcelain veneers. *Eur J Esthet Dent* 1(1):10–19.

Nejatidanesh F, Lotfi HR, et al. 2006. Marginal accuracy of interim restorations fabricated from four interim autopolymerizing resins. *J Prosthet Dent* 95(5):364–7.

Psichogios PC, Monaco EJ. 2003. Expedient direct approach for esthetic and functional provisional restorations. *J Prosthet Dent* 89(3):319–22.

Raigrodski AJ, Sadan A, et al. 1999. Use of a customized rigid clear matrix for fabricating provisional veneers. *J Esthet Dent* 11(1):16–22.

Schwedhelm ER. 2006. Direct technique for the fabrication of acrylic provisional restorations. *J Contemp Dent Pract* 7(1):157–73.

Shillingberg HT, et al. 1997. *Fundamentals of Fixed Prosthodontics*, 3rd ed. Chicago: Quintessence.

Small BW. 2005. Pretreatment wax-ups and provisionals for restorative dentistry. *Gen Dent* 53(2):98–100.

Wassell RW, St George G, et al. 2002. Crowns and other extracoronal restorations: Provisional restorations. *Br Dent J* 192(11):619–22, 625–30.

Chapter 17
Laboratory Fabrication of Esthetic Restorations

Jeffrey P. Miles DDS

Karen A. Schulze DDS, PhD

Daniel Castagna DDS

Dentists are confronted with a rapidly evolving array of choices for fabricating esthetic restorations. Fortunately each successive generation of materials has provided a genuine improvement over previous materials as manufacturers overcome the considerable difficulties presented in adapting ceramics to function as teeth. Marketing materials, however, whether distributed by manufacturers or by laboratories, are designed to entice rather than edify, and should be treated with a healthy dose of skepticism. An important tool in evaluating new materials is a meaningful knowledge of existing materials, including a familiarity with the laboratory procedures that go into making esthetic restorations (Christensen 2003).

Every development in esthetic restorations since the maturation of metal-ceramic technology has been in the form of vertically integrated proprietary restorative systems. This phenomenon has several ramifications that need to be considered by prescribing dentists. First, it requires a discreet choice. Dentists rarely request that specific metal alloys or specific brands of porcelain be used in their restorations, but a dentist who does not specify a ceramic system to be used is delegating an important responsibility. Second, the dentist should be generally aware of the investments made by dental laboratories in the equipment, materials, and training required to fabricate each type of restoration. Dentists need to be aware of potential biases in recommendations from laboratories and suppliers, appropriately balancing the interests of patient, practitioner, and technician in choosing restorative systems. Significantly, some systems allow for the high-strength ceramic coping to be produced at a facility other than the local laboratory, allowing a technician with a reduced financial stake to continue to provide the personalized service valued by many practitioners. The practitioner who understands all aspects of esthetic restorations is much more likely to make appropriate choices than one who relies solely on the advice of others.

Historical Perspective

While the goal of this chapter is not to teach the history of dental materials, the authors feel that a general understanding of the evolution of esthetic restorations provides a basis for evaluating current systems as well as an understanding of the improvements pursued by emerging systems.

Glass-based ceramics have provided a visual substitution for tooth structure for decades. Fracture resistance has been the elusive goal. Adding metal oxide crystals to glass ceramics has been a way to modify optical characteristics as well as inhibit the propagation of cracks within the ceramic mass. Aluminous porcelain combined feldspathic porcelain and alumina crystals to form the substructure of "porcelain jacket crowns" (Shillingberg et al. 1997; O'Brien 1997). Now largely obsolete, these restorations combined superior esthetics with poor marginal fit and fracture resistance. The dentin bonding techniques that may have improved their clinical performance were developed too late to rescue these restorations.

Leucite-reinforced glass ceramics represented an improvement over aluminous porcelain, not only in their intrinsic physical properties but also in their potential fabrication techniques. Aluminous porcelains, being hand stacked, contained unavoidable imperfections that tended to initiate and propagate fractures, leading to structural failure. Leucite materials can be heated to a semiliquid state and forced into molds of the required shape. Imperfections are drastically reduced, resulting in much improved durability. The first system widely marketed using this technique, Dicor, used a centrifugal casting system nearly identical to that used for casting metals. These restorations were homogenous ceramic units with color and opacity variations provided solely by surface staining (Malament and Socransky 1999). While enjoying modest success for some years after introduction, Dicor failed to displace the cosmetically inferior but much stronger metal-ceramic crowns.

Pressable Ceramics

The next generation of leucite-reinforced glass ceramics incorporated two significant improvements over the castable ceramics. The most obvious to the patient and practitioner was the use of separate coping and veneering ceramics to make a more visually complex and realistic restoration. Copings can be fabricated in a modest selection of shades, while the veneering porcelains can replicate all shades and characteristics available for metal-ceramic restorations.

Ivoclar Vivadent has marketed the most successful of the pressed ceramic systems, IPS Empress. Empress cases arrive at the laboratory with conventional impressions and mounting information. Preparation designs, discussed in chapter 14, are similar to those of other all-ceramic restorations in their need for adequate reduction on all surfaces, including margins, and rounded angles. Copings are waxed onto stone dies with a minimum thickness of 0.8 mm (fig. 17-1). Large-gauge sprues are needed to allow movement of the semiliquid glass into the burned-out wax pattern. Multiple units can be invested together, provided they are all of the same shade. Burn-out is similar to the lost wax technique for metal casting, but as with most all-ceramic systems, all equipment is unique to the proprietary system being used. Rather than using a centrifugal casting technique, high heat and pressure are used to force molten glass into the pattern in a "press furnace" (fig. 17-2). Fortunately, these furnaces are affordable to local laboratories; many are designed to function also as conventional porcelain ovens. Once cooled, the patterns are devested with a glass bead abrasive and fit back onto stone dies (fig. 17-3). A ceramist must then stack feldspathic porcelain to complete esthetic and functional requirements (fig. 17-4).

IPS Empress, with a flexural strength of about 100 MPa (Tinschert et al. 2000; Guazzato et al. 2004b), is recommended strictly for single units, typically in the anterior. Short-span all-ceramic bridges near the anterior can be fabricated in the same manner, with a stronger substrate,

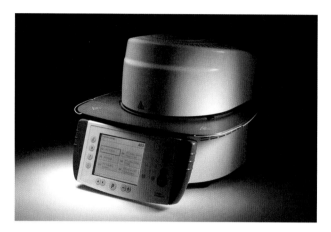

Figure 17-2.   Press furnace.

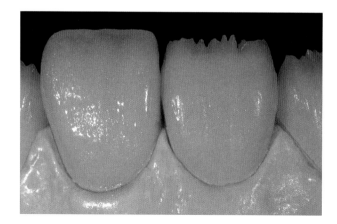

Figure 17-3.   Pressed ceramic coping.

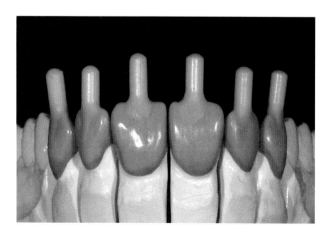

Figure 17-1.   Wax-ups for pressed ceramic restorations.

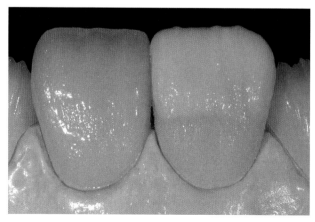

Figure 17-4.   Feldspathic porcelain added to pressed ceramic coping.

lithium disilicate. Ivoclar's system was initially designated IPS Empress II; an improved system is named IPS Eris. The substrate is visually similar to leucite-reinforced glass but forms a more crystalline structure on cooling. Requiring a significant bulk for strength, connectors between abutments and pontics must be large occluso-gingivally and facio-lingually. This limits the cases that can be fabricated with this system (Della Bona, Mecholsky, and Anusavice 2004).

Other pressable ceramic systems include Finesse by Ceramco and OPC G-3 by Pentron. These two claim that a reduced leucite component in their veneering porcelains leads to reduced wear of opposing tooth structure (Elmaria 2006).

Pressed ceramics can be used for veneers, either as single-component restorations or characterized with feldspathic porcelain (Garber and Adar 1997). They can also be used as single-component ceramic inlays or onlays, although these applications have been largely supplanted by CAD/CAM systems. Reinforced-glass ceramics can also be pressed onto zirconia copings, as described below.

The substrates used for pressed ceramic copings—leucite-reinforced glass and lithium disilicate—are also available for use in CAD/CAM applications. They are mounted on metal spindles for processing in a computer-controlled milling machine such as Cerec 3D and Cerec InLab.

Glass-Infiltrated Ceramics

Glass-infiltrated crystalline ceramics represent a step up in fracture resistance from the reinforced-glass substrates described above. Several pathways have been developed to create these materials, but all arrive at a structurally similar product. Like pressed ceramic, these materials form the coping of restorations, being veneered with feldspathic porcelain for esthetics and function.

The first commercially successful glass-infiltrated ceramic material was Vita's In-Ceram. The crystalline phase, which could be spinell ($MgAl_2O_4$), alumina (Al_2O_3), or zirconia (ZnO_2), arrives as a fine powder. This is mixed in a proprietary liquid to create a suspension, or slip (fig. 17-5). The slip is applied to a refractory die, shaped, and fired at a controlled temperature. Critically, the ceramic particles bond to each other without coalescing, creating a porous structure with contiguous voids (fig. 17-6). This is referred to as a "green-state" ceramic. At this stage the ceramic is opaque, somewhat soft, and can be easily adjusted with rotary instruments. The coping is brought to its final state by heating in contact with a tinted glass. This glass saturates the porous structure, filling the voids and imparting an appropriate color (fig. 17-7).

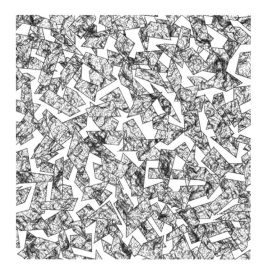

Figure 17-5. Diagram of ceramic slip.

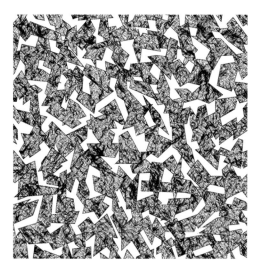

Figure 17-6. Diagram of green-state ceramic.

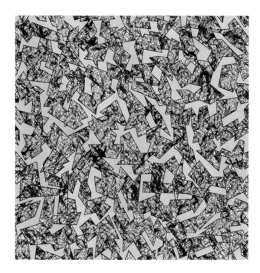

Figure 17-7. Diagram of glass-infiltrated ceramic.

Glass-infiltrated ceramics are attractive options for several reasons. First, neither firing of the materials results in dimensional change, allowing predictable fit without computer manipulations. Second, they achieve a fracture resistance superior to reinforced glass (e.g., pressed ceramics) due to the contiguous crystalline scaffolding. In-Ceram Spinell achieves a flexural strength of 350 MPa, In-Ceram Alumina 250–600 MPa, and In-Ceram Zirconia 420–800 MPa (Raigrodski 2004). Finally, the copings have an appealing translucency and range of shades greater than the dense sintered ceramics discussed below.

Applying the slip by hand has largely been replaced by more automated techniques for producing glass-infiltrated ceramics. Vita developed a process, called Wol-Ceram, for electrostatically applying slip to a stone die, which produces a rigid presintered coping. This is sintered to a green state without a refractory die, and then infiltrated with glass by the same method as In-Ceram, and achieves corresponding fracture strengths.

CAD/CAM systems such as Cerec InLab can mill copings from blocks manufactured in the green state preparatory to glass infiltration, or from blocks of previously infiltrated substrates. Kavo markets a "shrink-free zirconia" coping that is milled in a silica-infiltrated green state. Oxidizing the silica during firing provides the glass component. Flexural strength is about 350 MPa (Heydecke et al. 2007).

Fully Sintered Ceramics

The quest for dental ceramics with strength to rival metal ceramics has led to the development of fully sintered alumina and zirconia copings. The crystalline components of these materials are the same as those used in glass infiltrated ceramics, but rather than having interstices filled with glass, these products are fired at a temperature high enough to condense the crystals into a solid mass. When this happens, they shrink. Being able to fashion an oversized coping that will predictably shrink to the needed dimensions has been a significant technological achievement.

Nobel-Biocare came first to market with Procera, a dense sintered alumina coping produced exclusively at their facilities. A local laboratory creates conventional models with removable dies. These dies are mounted in a specially designed scanning device that records the shape by turning it and physically probing the surface. This "touch-probe scanning" is analogous to the optical and laser scanners used in other CAD/CAM systems. The information is digitally relayed to the Nobel-Biocare facilities where the coping is manufactured. An over-

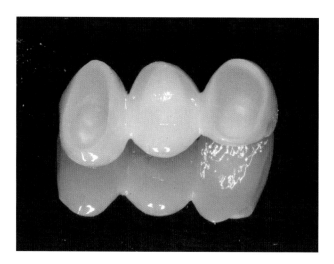

Figure 17-8. Intaglio surface of Procera restorations.

sized refractory die is milled, onto which an alumina slip is applied. The slip is sintered to a green-state ceramic while on the die, and milled to an appropriate thickness. It is then removed from the die and further sintered to its final size and shape and shipped to the local laboratory. A ceramist then adds dedicated feldspathic porcelain to final form and appearance (Andersson et al. 1998). Procera crowns provide good strength and acceptable marginal fit but suffer from an opacity that could be difficult to disguise, especially at the margin (Heffernan et al. 2002; fig. 17-8). Nobel Biocare has further improved the Procera system by introducing zirconia as a substrate, allowing for greater strength, a range of shades, and the ability to fabricate bridges.

The first commercially available system to use fully sintered zirconia was Densply's Cercon. Cercon fabrication begins with conventional modelwork and the preparation of a wax pattern of the desired framework. Rather than being invested, the wax pattern is sprued into an aluminum frame and dusted with a reflective metallic powder. The Cercon "brain" optically scans the pattern (fig. 17-9), calculates the shape an oversized coping will need to take, and mills that shape out of a green-state zirconia blank. The coping is then removed from its framework and fully sintered in a high-temperature oven. Feldspathic porcelain is added to complete the restoration. Cercon copings, like all fully sintered zirconia copings, are virtually indestructible (Guazzato et al. 2004a). Unfortunately, as originally developed they were also quite bright and fairly opaque. While always appearing more natural than metal-ceramic restorations, early Cercon crowns and bridges displayed brightness, especially at the margin, which was sometimes cosmetically unacceptable (Raigrodski 2004). Cercon has since

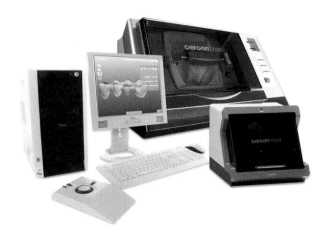

Figure 17-9.   Cercon Brain.

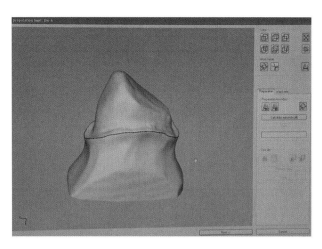

Figure 17-11.   Digital image of scanned die.

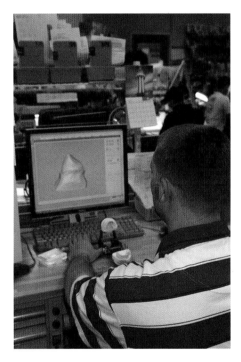

Figure 17-10.   Designing Lava coping.

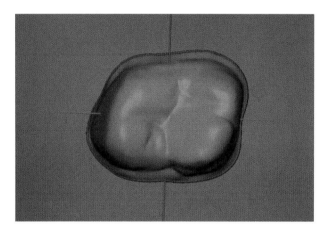

Figure 17-12.   Digital image of scanned die.

addressed this problem with green-state zirconia blanks in a range of dentin shades, but not before losing market share to 3M's zirconia product, Lava.

3M overcame two objections to the pioneering Cercon system. First, they answered the desire for a selection of dentin shades in the zirconia framework. Second, they delegated all of the design work to computer control (figs. 17-10, 17-11, 17-12). Conventional model work is thoroughly scanned (fig. 17-13) and displayed on a monitor. A technician designs the desired coping, having control over material thickness, connector size and shape,

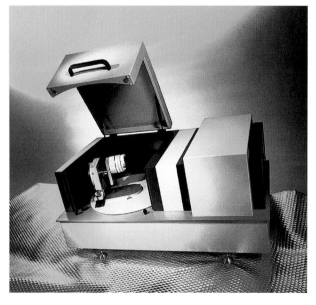

Figure 17-13.   Lava scanning machine.

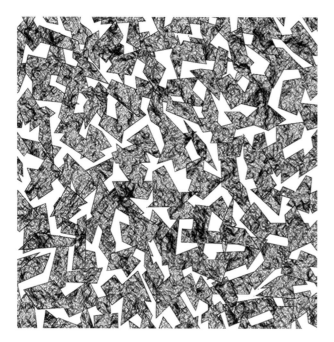

Figure 17-14.   Diagram of green-state ceramic.

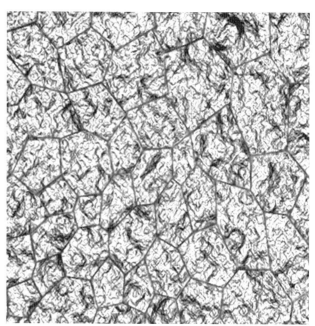

Figure 17-15.   Diagram of fully sintered ceramic.

and margin design. An appropriately sized green-state blank (fig. 17-14) is milled to the needed shape. Released from its framework, the still-porous coping is briefly soaked in a tinted liquid, imparting the desired shade to the final product. Full sintering is similar to the Cercon process (fig. 17-15). Feldspathic porcelain is added to full contour (Piwowarczyk et al. 2005; fig. 17-16).

This sequence eliminates the need for the technically demanding, and costly, waxing and mounting steps used by Cercon. The result is a more predictable coping fit, but not, at present, a reduced cost. The Lava copings, while being virtually indestructible (fig. 17-17), achieve marginal accuracy comparable to metal-ceramic restorations (fig. 17-18), allow for a good range of dentin colors, and exhibit good translucency when fabricated to their minimum thickness of 0.3 mm (fig. 17-19).

The Kavo Everest system and others use a very similar CAD/CAM procedure to fabricate fully sintered zirconia copings of comparable quality. All, though, display some opacity at the margin, which may be unacceptable to a patient with anterior gingival display. Overcoming this problem without sacrificing the impressive strength of zirconia required a clever hybrid of CAD/CAM and pressable techniques.

Press to Zirconia

MicroDental's P2Z (press to zirconia) and Ivoclar's e. ZirPress are very similar systems. Each begins with a fully sintered zirconia coping that has been produced by

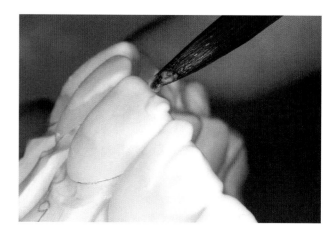

Figure 17-16.   Feldspathic porcelain added to Lava coping.

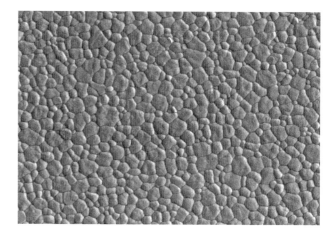

Figure 17-17.   Scanning electron micrograph of Lava surface.

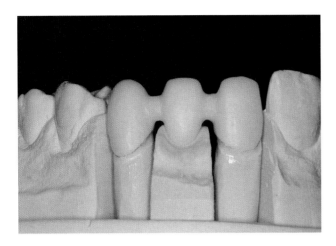

Figure 17-18. Lava copings on dies.

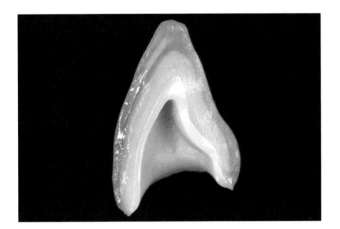

Figure 17-19. Cross-section of Lava crown.

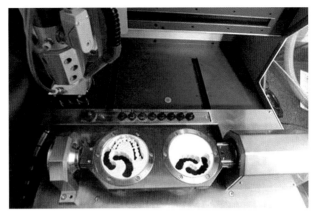

Figure 17-20. ZenoTech zirconia blanks.

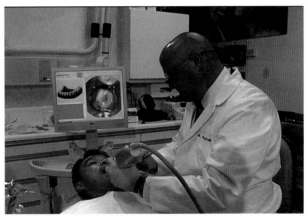

Figure 17-21. Chairside scanning. Photo courtesy of Glidewell Laboratories. Reprinted with permission.

any of the preceding methods and designed to extend short of the facial margin. The zirconia surface is treated with a proprietary liquid to prepare it for bonding to the pressed ceramic. Wax is added to the treated coping to the desired contour including the facial margin. For optimal esthetics, the wax-up may be cut back to leave room for a final increment of feldspathic porcelain. The coping, with wax, is invested and burned out as described above for pressable ceramics. The desired shade of ceramic is loaded into the press furnace and pressed onto the zirconia coping. The pressed substrate is translucent but monochromatic. It can be stained to increase realism or receive a final layer of feldspathic porcelain.

Pressing to zirconia is a labor-intensive procedure and is sure to demand higher laboratory fees. It does, though, allow for the strength of zirconia with the natural marginal appearance of pressed ceramics, a combination not possible with other products. These restorations have not been in service long enough to determine their durability in the mouth.

Future Trends

While neither dentists nor laboratory technicians should make an unexamined assumption of the superiority of CAD/CAM over handmade ceramic copings, the latter are unlikely to show great leaps in quality and productivity. Computer-driven processes, though, certainly will. Already, systems such as Weiland Dental's ZenoTech use larger zirconia blanks, allowing for milling full-arch restorations or several multiple-unit restorations in one step (fig. 17-20). Computer designed and milled plastic veneers can be substituted for the waxed component in pressed-to-zirconia restorations, cutting labor costs.

Scanning technology will continue to improve, allowing for quality restorations to be placed on less-than-ideal preparations. Intraoral scanning will progress beyond the technologies developed for CEREC 3D, ultimately leading to the elimination of clinical impressions for routine restorative procedures (fig. 17-21). This could also reduce the need for plaster and stone model work. Ceramists trained to artfully apply feldspathic porcelain to the multitude of reinforced ceramic copings seem to have a secure place in the evolving world of dental technology. Less-skilled technicians may find their tasks usurped by computers needing progressively less human input and producing more accurate and durable restorations.

Works Cited

Andersson M, Razzoog ME, et al. 1998. Procera: A new way to achieve an all-ceramic crown. *Quintessence Int* 29(5):285–96.

Christensen GJ. 2003. The confusing array of tooth-colored crowns. *J Am Dent Assoc.* 134(9):1253–35.

Della Bona A, Mecholsky JJ, Anusavice KJ. 2004. Fracture behavior of lithia disilicate- and leucite-based ceramics. *Dent Mater* 20(10):956–62.

Elmaria 2006. An evaluation of wear when enamel is opposed by various ceramic materials and gold. *J Prosthet Dent* 96(5):345–53.

Garber DA, Adar P. 1997. Securing the position of ceramic veneers in dentistry. *Signature* 4(2):2–4.

Guazzato M, Albakry M, Ringer SP, Swain MV. 2004a. Strength, fracture toughness and microstructure of a selection of all-ceramic materials: Part I. Pressable and alumina glass-infiltrated ceramics. *Dent Mater* 20(5):441–8.

Guazzato M, Albakry M, et al. 2004b. Strength, fracture toughness and microstructure of a selection of all-ceramic materials: Part II. Zirconia-based dental ceramics. *Dent Mater* 20(5):449–56.

Heffernan MJ, Aquilino SA, et al. 2002. Relative translucency of six all-ceramic systems: Part II. Core and veneer materials. *J Prosthet Dent* 88(1):10–15.

Heydecke G, Butz F, et al. 2007. Material characteristics of a novel shrinkage-free ZrSiO(4) ceramic for the fabrication of posterior crowns. *Dent Mater* 23(7):785–91.

Malament KA, Socransky SS. 1999. Survival of Dicor glass-ceramic dental restorations over 14 years: Part I. Survival of Dicor complete coverage restorations and effect of internal surface acid etching, tooth position, gender, and age. *J Prosthet Dent* 81(1):23–32.

O'Brien WJ. 1997. *Dental Materials and Their Selection*, 2nd ed. Chicago: Quintessence.

Piwowarczyk A, Ott P, Lauer HC, Kuretzky T. 2005. A clinical report and overview of scientific studies and clinical procedures conducted on the 3M ESPE Lava All-Ceramic System. *J Prosthodont* 14(1):39–45.

Raigrodski A. 2004. Contemporary materials and technologies for all-ceramic fixed partial dentures: A review of the literature. *J Prosthet Dent* 92(6):557–62.

Shillingberg HT, et al. 1997. *Fundamentals of Fixed Prosthodontics*, 3rd ed. Chicago: Quintessence.

Tinschert J, Zwez D, et al. 2000. Structural reliability of alumina-, feldspar-, leucite-, mica- and zirconia-based ceramics. *J Dent* 28(7):529–35.

Chapter 18
Luting Agents for Dental Restorations

Karen A. Schulze DDS, PhD

Richard G. Lubman DDS

The main goal for cementation or luting is the joining of an externally fabricated restoration to tooth structure. Adhesion is defined as the bonding together of particles of different substances. The term *cementation* has been used over centuries for the process of fixing a metallic or ceramic restoration to tooth structure. However, during the last thirty years, things began to change with the introduction of more adhesive materials. In this context, the word *cementation* hardly does justice to the range of materials on the market. Another term for fixing a restoration in place is *luting*. The word *lute* means a material used as a protective layer to fill the gap and prevent the entrance of fluids. Because the term *cementation* is not specific to a cement and includes contemporary products such as adhesive resins, it is perhaps more appropriate to use the term *luting agent* (Noort 2002).

Ideally, the restoration precisely matches the prepared tooth margin and establishes a perfect seal with the tooth. In reality, a variety of factors influence this outcome, such as the type of luting agent, the preparation design, and the type of restorative material used. The use of full-ceramic restorations demands a very technically challenging handling of the luting cement as well as the dental hard tissue or an implant abutment (Kerby, McGlumphy, and Holloway 1992; Lüthy, Loeffel, and Hammerle 2006).

The history of cemented dental restorations goes back to the mid-nineteenth century. At the beginning of the twentieth century, materials such as zinc oxide eugenol, zinc phosphate, and silicate cements were introduced and are still used today in some dental practices. Increased research in the last two decades has led to the development of new materials with improved adhesive properties. In addition to the traditional use for cementation, some of the new materials have the capability to chemically bond and/or micromechanically bond to tooth structure. This chapter will explain the properties and the uses of luting cements for a variety of restorations.

General Requirements for Luting Agents

The ideal dental luting agent should have the mechanical, biological, and esthetic properties that are discussed below.

High Compressive, Tensile, and Bond Strength

A luting agent should have the ability to withstand compressive, tensile, and rotational forces transmitted to the restoration. During normal eating, the dental neuromuscular system develops forces below 30 N. One Newton (N) is the force of the Earth's gravity on an object with a mass of about 102 grams (such as a small apple). However, the maximum force developed in the molar region can be between 300 and 800 N. A weak interface between a tooth and restoration would result in eventual debonding or fracture. ADA/ANSI specification #96/1994 requires a compressive strength of 70 MPa; however, 31 MPa will give sufficient resistance to normal occlusal forces (Richter and Ueno 1975; Phillips 1996). Pascale (Pa) is a measure of force per unit area.

A restoration must also withstand forces immediately after cementation. Rapid development of high strength is especially important for cemented dowels and cores, because the dentist may be preparing the core for a final restoration with rotary instruments shortly after cementation.

Low Viscosity

Low initial viscosity or pseudoplastic behavior allows for the free flow of the luting material in all directions. This low viscosity is necessary for proper seating of the restoration. If the film thickness is high and the luting material also has a high solubility, the luting material at a wide margin will dissolve much faster than at a smaller margin. A film thickness of 25 μm is the ideal closed margin according to the ADA/ANSI specifications #8/1996.

Good Handling Properties

The luting agent needs to be easily mixed and manipulated. Those luting materials with simple mixing procedures that tolerate small variations in the ratios of the components are less likely to be mixed incorrectly. The storage and mixing of the materials is also critical to the successful outcome of the procedure.

Adequate Working and Setting Time

The initial phase of the setting time is used to insert the restoration while the second phase allows for the reaction of the molecules to form a strong bond. Auto-curing materials are formulated to follow ADA/ANSI specification #96/1994, which requires 2.5 to 8 minutes for the material to set. For dual-curing materials the chemical reaction needs to be completed using a light source. Light-curing materials use light activation only. This method allows the dentist to better control the setting reaction and cure on demand (O'Brian 2002).

Adhesion

Strong Adhesion to Mineralized Tissue

Good adhesion to mineralized tissue can reduce the risk of secondary decay and/or marginal leakage. It is important to differentiate between a chemical adhesion, as found in glass-ionomer cements, and micromechanical adhesion, as found in resin cements using an acid-etching technique. Bonded adhesion in contrast to frictional retention also permits more conservative cavity preparations, which preserves natural tooth structure. Classic preparation designs for indirect restorations have been based on concepts of cementation where retention of the restoration is obtained by the frictional fit between nonadhesive materials. These preparations often remove large amounts of healthy dental hard tissue. Conservative preparations are kinder to the pulp and are thus less likely to produce postoperative sensitivity (fig. 18-1).

Strong Adhesion to the Restoration (ceramic, alloy, etc.)

Successful adhesion between the cement and restoration is important to avoid leakage due to porosities that can allow cariogenic bacteria to colonize the interface and lead to failure. Usually there are no excellent adhesive properties inherent to the restoration itself. Metal restorations or high strength all-ceramic restorations can be sandblasted, and some ceramic restorations can be silanated to improve the bond to resin cements. The ideal luting agent should develop good adhesion to the tooth as well as to the restoration.

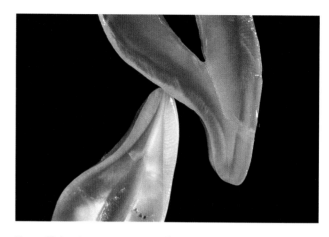

Figure 18-1. An upper Lava crown (3M ESPE) is opposing a lower natural central incisor, cross-sectional view. The Lava restoration appears very similar to the natural dentition (Courtesy of 3M ESPE).

Insolubility

The ideal luting material should be hydrophobic. This prevents structural changes to the restoration and does not jeopardize the occlusal function. Cemented restorations are surrounded at the margin by a cement line that may vary in thickness. If the luting material is exposed to the oral environment, it may dissolve, leaving a microgap that can be colonized by bacteria. Bacterial endotoxins may induce pulpitis by causing the receptors within the pulp to become hypersensitive (Curro 1990). Postcementation pain also occurs when there is fluid movement within the tooth caused by chemical reactions resulting from cementation; the degree to which it is felt by the patient often reflects the inflammatory state of the pulp.

Color Stability and Translucency

The aesthetic properties of luting materials are important for indirect restorations placed with translucent materials where no opaque substructure was used. Long-term color stability is crucial in maintaining the esthetic appearance of the restoration (Asmussen 1983; Imazato et al. 1995). A luting material with unfavorable color stability can dramatically reduce the aesthetic outcome of most feldspathic full-ceramic restorations such as IPS Empress or VITA PM.

Biocompatibility

Luting materials should not be toxic to pulpal tissue. Acids from some luting agents may be hydraulically extruded into the dentinal tubules when a casting is cemented. This can cause sensitivity during or shortly after cementation. The ideal luting material will not induce pulpitis directly or indirectly and will provide a long-lasting seal that inhibits fluid movement. The luting agent should have favorable thermal, chemical, and galvanic insulating properties (Casselli and Martins 2006).

Caries Resistance

The ability of luting materials to prevent caries is strongly correlated to their insolubility in oral fluids. The higher the molecular stability, the lower the risk of bacterial invasion. Some materials, for example, glass-ionomer cements, have intrinsic, fluoride-releasing properties that can reduce the susceptibility to caries (Lutz 1977; Wilson, Groffman, and Kuhn 1985).

Radiopacity

A luting material should be radiopaque for ease of identification; this is helpful in diagnosing excess cement in the periodontal tissue after cementation (Baratti, Dorigo, and Telesca 1985).

Permanent Cementation

Review of Properties of Water-Based Luting Materials

These luting agents have a relatively high solubility in the mouth and also set due to an acid-base reaction between the powder and the liquid. The rate of the reaction can be manipulated by variations to the liquid-powder ratio.

Zinc Phosphate Cement

Because of its long history, zinc phosphate cement is the standard by which cements have been measured for many years. It has had a wide range of applications from the cementation of fixed cast restorations, core-reinforced porcelain restorations, and orthodontic bands to its use as a cavity liner or base. The cement is available as a powder that is mixed with an acid liquid. The powder consists primarily of zinc oxide with up to 10% magnesium oxide, and the liquid contains 45%–64% phosphoric acid (fig. 18-2; Noort 2002).

Advantages of Zinc Phosphate Cement
- Easy to mix
- A well-defined setting time
- A working time that can be prolonged by adjusting the mixing technique
- Low cost

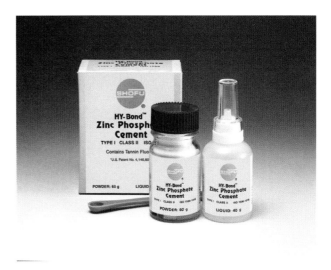

Figure 18-2. HY Bond zinc phosphate cement (Shofu Dental Corp).

Disadvantages of Zinc Phosphate Cement
- Potential for pulpal irritation due to its low pH (2)
- No antibacterial function
- Brittle
- No adhesive qualities
- More soluble than most other cements
- Opaque
- Exothermic reaction

A cool glass slab can be used to overcome the heat produced by the exothermic reaction and increase setting time. The right consistency is achieved during spatulation when a cement string 3 cm in length can be lifted from the slab. Mixing time is from 60 to 90 seconds, and the setting time is from 2 to 8 minutes.

Polycarboxylate Cement

These cements are generally used for cementation of castings, core-reinforced porcelain restorations, and orthodontic bands. They may be used as cavity liners or bases and as provisional restorative materials. These products come as a powder and a clear viscous liquid. The components of the powder are generally zinc oxide and magnesium oxide, and the liquid is mainly a 30% to 40% aqueous solution of polyacrylic acid (fig. 18-3).

Advantages of Polycarboxylate Cement
- They bond to enamel and dentin with a similar mechanism found in glass-ionomer cements, which may include the formation of a chemical bond.
- There is low irritation to the pulp tissue.
- Strength, solubility, and film thickness are comparable to that of zinc phosphate cement.
- They provide antibacterial action.

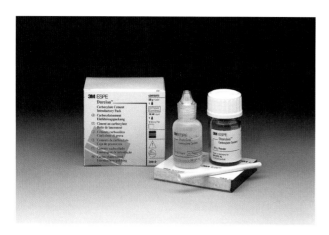

Figure 18-3. Durelon polycarboxulate cement (3M ESPE).

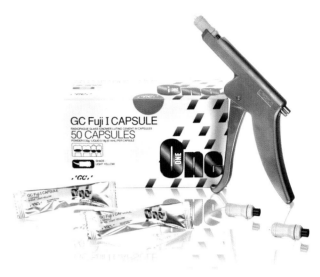

Figure 18-4. GC Fuji I glass ionomer luting cement (GC America).

Disadvantages of Carboxylate Cement
- Their properties are highly dependent upon the mixing procedure.
- They have a short working time and their viscosity rises quickly after mixing.
- They have a longer setting time than other cements and have a rubbery stage.
- Clean-up is difficult if the excess is allowed to harden; however, if the excess is removed too early it can result in a pitted margin.

Glass-Ionomer Luting Cements

Glass-ionomer luting cements have similar compositions to glass-ionomer filling materials that were discussed in chapter 10; however, luting cements contain smaller glass particles that allow for a thinner film thickness during cementation. Glass-ionomer cements were introduced in the early 1970s and have been modified many times since then. The setting mechanism is an acid-base reaction. They have lower solubility in the oral cavity than zinc phosphate and polycarboxylate cements (Hersek and Canay 1996). Their strength is the highest of the acid-base cements if they are not prematurely exposed to saliva, blood, or water (White and Yu 1993; Rosensteil, Land, and Crispin 1998). The setting reaction is slow and the material reaches its greatest strength several weeks after placement. They adhere to calcified hard tissue because they contain polyalkenoic acids that chelate with calcium in the enamel and dentin (Walls 1986). Glass-ionomer cements are used for the cementation of cast-alloy crowns, bridges, inlays, onlays, metal-ceramic crowns and bridges, and orthodontic bands and brackets. They are available in hand-mixed and predosed capsules (fig. 18-4).

Advantages of Glass-Ionomer Luting Cement
- Fluoride release due to ion exchange
- They have a "cariostatic" potential, especially on root surfaces (Erickson 1994; Featherstone 1994).
- They have a similar coefficient of thermal expansion when compared to calcified hard tissue.
- Chemical adhesion to dentin and enamel
- Compared to zinc phosphate, the glass-ionomer luting cement is available in predosed capsules that ensure a consistent powder-to-liquid ratio and low incorporation of air during mixing.
- Lower opacity compared to zinc-phosphate cements

Disadvantages of Glass-Ionomer Luting Cement
- They have less favorable mechanical properties when compared to resin cements in the categories of fracture toughness, brittleness, higher solubility and wear.
- They also absorb moisture during the initial setting phase.

When glass-ionomer luting cements were first introduced, there were reports that the use of these materials resulted in a higher incidence of postoperative sensitivity (Charbeneau, Klausner, and Brandau 1988). However, now it is generally agreed that there is no significant difference in postoperative sensitivity between glass-ionomer and zinc phosphate cements. Several theories have been proposed to explain the sensitivity (Leinfelder 1993; Rebitski and Donly 1993), but it is probably related more to tooth treatment procedures before cementation than the chemistry of the cement itself (Lacy 1994).

Review of Properties of a Combination of Water- and Resin-Based Luting Materials

Resin-Modified Glass-Ionomer Cement

These versatile cements are sometimes called hybrid ionomers, resin-reinforced ionomers, resin-modified ionomers, resinomers, ionomer-modified resins, and various other contrived names (Hammesfahr 1994; McLean, Nicholson, and Wilson 1994). They have many uses: cavity liners, bases, core buildups, and luting agents. The applications include the cementation of cast-alloy crowns and bridges to orthodontic appliances and core buildups. This group of materials covers the spectrum from primarily acid-base reaction glass-ionomer cements reinforced with polymerizable resins to nearly 100% composite resin containing reacted glass-ionomer particles as fillers. The chemistry, dentin-bonding capability, and clinical handling technique vary widely among these products. It is highly advised that the manufacturers' instructions are followed precisely. Most companies provide their materials as a hand-mixed as well as predosed capsule version. The latter has the advantage of fewer air bubbles during mixing and the right powder/liquid proportions. This ensures a better and homogeneous quality of the freshly mixed luting components. For luting, the cement is applied to an undesiccated tooth to avoid possible postoperative sensitivity (fig. 18-5).

Advantages of Resin-Modified Glass-Ionomer Cement
- Better tensile and compressive strength compared to water-based materials
- Less sensitivity to moisture during the initial setting phase
- Capable of bonding to composites
- Some fluoride release

Disadvantages of Resin-Modified Glass-Ionomer Cement
- Hydrophilic behavior
- Water absorption and hygroscopic expansion
- Leakage is less than water-based materials but more than resin-based materials

Resin-modified glass ionomers are twice as flexible as water-based glass ionomers. They have a lower modulus of elasticity. A high modulus of elasticity indicates increased stiffness and will therefore provide better resistance to deformation under occlusal force (ADA Professional Product Review 2008). This can have unfavorable consequences for long-term success if there is a thick layer of luting material remaining between the restoration and the tooth (Attin et al. 1995). Also, resin-modified glass ionomers have been found to expand on setting, possibly due to the absorption of water. This expansion is greater than for resin cements. Therefore, resin-modified glass ionomers are not recommended for luting all-ceramic crowns (silicate ceramics) or veneers, to avoid possible expansion stresses and ceramic fracture (Irie and Nakai 1995).

Polyacid-Modified Composites (Compomers) for Cementation

Polyacid-modified composites are indicated for cementation of cast alloy crowns, bridges, post and cores, inlays, and onlays. For cementation of all-ceramic materials this cement should not be used. Compomers often have three setting mechanisms: a self- and light-curing polymerization reaction as well as an acid-base reaction that might occur when it is in contact with oral fluids.

Advantages of Polyacid-Modified Composites for Cementation
- High values of retention, bond strength, compressive strength, flexural strength, and fracture toughness
- Low solubility (similar to resin-based cements)

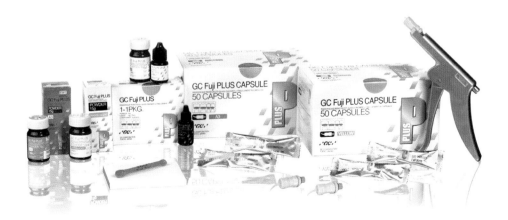

Figure 18-5.   Resin-modified glass-ionomer luting cement: GC Fuji Plus capsules (GC America).

Disadvantages of Polyacid-Modified Composites for Cementation

- Hygroscopic expansion can cause fracture of all-ceramic restorations, especially with veneers

Review of Properties of Resin-Based Luting Materials

Resin cements formulated with methyl methacrylate have been on the market since 1950 for use in inlay and crown cementation; however, the formulation of present-day resin composites was introduced in the early 1970s. Currently, the cementation of metal restorations is being accomplished more frequently than ever before with self- or dual-cured, self-adhesive resin cements due to their superior characteristics (fig. 18-6).

Rules to Follow When Selecting a Resin Cement

1. If there is enough translucency for a bright curing light (see chap. 10) to penetrate the restoration, use a light-curing resin cement (fig. 18-7). However, it has been shown that light transmission through porcelain with thicknesses ranging from 0.5 to 2 mm can be as little as 2% to 3% (Noort 2002). Therefore, increasing the light polymerization time may be prudent to ensure adequate polymerization. These materials have the advantage of a very nominal shade change during the lifetime of the restoration compared to dual- or self-cure cements. They are most useful for thin porcelain restorations such as veneers (fig. 18-8).

2. If there is some translucency to the restoration, use a dual-cure material. If both types of curing systems are combined in one material, this can assure the practitioner of the best result. These situations can include thicker and more opaque all-ceramic restorations, composites, and porcelain inlays and onlays (fig. 18-9). Remember that working time is shorter than with a light-cured cement. With chemically activated polymerization, the curing will continue after the light is removed.

3. If there is little or no light penetration through the restoration, a self-curing resin cement is the one to use (fig. 18-10a and 18-10b).

A dual cure product might also work in selected cases. Some of these applications could be metal crowns, high-strength all-ceramic restorations, or dowels.

There are dual-cured resin-based cements that can be purchased to serve as either one-paste or two-paste systems. Some of the available systems are Variolink II (Ivoclar Vivadent), Calibra (Dentsply Caulk), or NX3 (Kerr; fig. 18-11). No mixing is necessary if you use only the base paste without the catalyst. The base paste is usually a microfilled or hybrid composite formulated primarily from bis-GMA or urethane dimethacrylate resins and inorganic fillers such as fumed silica and/or glass fillers. The base paste/cement will set when

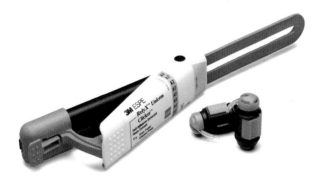

Figure 18-6. Self-adhesive resin cement RelyX Unicem (3M ESPE).

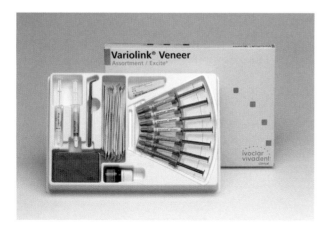

Figure 18-7. Purely light-curing adhesive resin cement: Variolink Veneer (Ivoclar Vivadent, Amherst, NY).

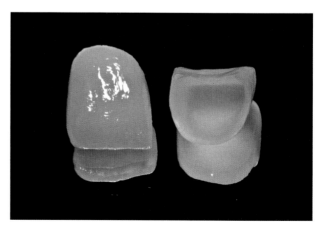

Figure 18-8. IPS Empress veneer (Courtesy of Philipp Striebe).

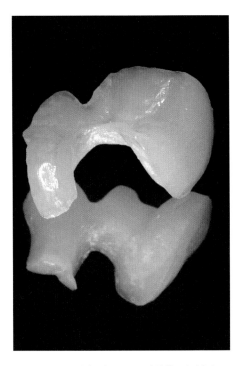

Figure 18-9.   IPS Empress inlay (Courtesy of Philipp Striebe).

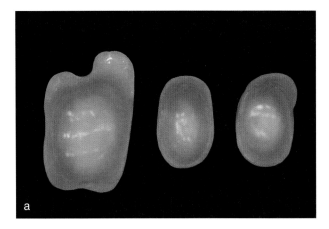

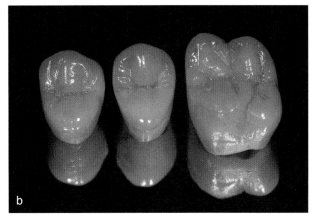

Figure 18-10.   a. Coping of high-strength all-ceramic crowns made of zirconia ceramic (Courtesy of Prof. Joachim Tinschert). b. Zirconia ceramic crowns prior to cementation (Courtesy of Prof. Joachim Tinschert).

exposed to light because of the presence of a photo-initiator such as camphorquinone. When you desire to initiate the autopolymerizing function, you would incorporate the catalyst into the base paste by mixing them together in a ratio advised by the manufacturer.

The dual-cured systems discussed above come in a base-catalyst form and must be mixed before use. They combine an initator-accelator system as well as a photo-initiator system in the base. The resin composition for both pastes mentioned above is primarily the same. With either the automixed or the dispensed dual-cure resin system, it is easier to obtain the correct proportions of each paste.

The totally self-cured resin-based cements are typically hand- or auto-mixed two-paste systems. One major component is a diacrylate oligomer diluted with lower-molecular-weight dimethacrylate monomers. The other major component is silanated silica or glass. The initiator-accelerator system is usually a peroxide-amine.

Resin-Based Cement in Combination with Bonding Procedures

The increased bond strength of resin-based cements is a result of the additional tooth treatment prior to the cementation process. The treatment could be an acid-etching system (e.g., Variolink II, Ivoclar Vivadent; Calibra, Dentsply Caulk), or it may require a separate self-etching bonding agent (e.g., Panavia F 2.0, Kuraray America; or Multilink Automix, Ivoclar Vivadent), or

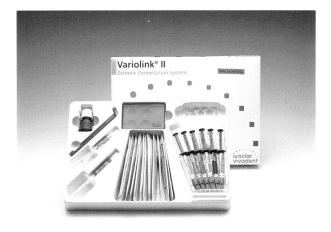

Figure 18-11.   Dual-curing resin cement: Variolink II (Ivoclar Vivadent, Amherst, NY).

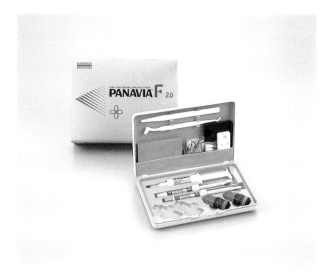

Figure 18-12. Dual-curing adesive resin cement: Panavia F2.0 (Kuraray America).

Table 18-1. Current self-adhesive resin cements.

Cement	Manufacturer
RelyX™ Unicem	3M ESPE, St. Paul, MN
Multilink® Sprint	Ivoclar Vivadent, Amherst, NY
BisCem™	BISCO, Inc., Schaumburg, IL
Breeze™	Pentron Clinical Technologies LLC, Wallingford, CT
EMBRACE™ WetBond™	Pulpdent Inc, Watertown, MA
G Cem™	Shofu Dental, Menlo Park, CA
Maxcem™	Kerr Corporation, Orange, CA
MonoCem™	Shofu Dental, Menlo Park, CA

it may contain an incorporated self-etching bonding agent (e.g., Rely X Unicem, 3M ESPE or MaxCem, Kerr; fig. 18-12).

Clinicians have reported more tooth sensitivity when using total-etch systems versus self-etching bonding agents prior to cementation (Clinical Research Associates 2003b). However, controlled studies have not shown sensitivity differences (Perdigão, Geraldeli, Hodges 2003; Perdiagao et al. 2004; Perry 2007). To avoid the likelihood of any postoperative sensitivity, use the total-etch technique when enamel is the primary retentive feature. These situations usually occur when veneers or inlays and onlays are bonded to enamel.

Custom-made post and cores or prefabricated posts can be cemented using self-adhesive resin cements (table 18-1) such as RelyX Unicem (3M ESPE). Figure 18-13 illustrates a case where high-strength ceramic (Lava, 3M ESPE) was the material of choice for the custom-made post and core on a central incisor. If there is enough remaining dentin after the cementation of the post and core, as shown in figures 18-13 a through e, the acid-etch technique in combination with a dual-curing cement (e.g., Variolink II, Ivoclar Vivadent) would be sufficient to cement the IPS Empress crown.

The self-etching resin cements are recommended when the strength of resin is needed and dentin is present for additional adhesion (Clinical Research Associates 2003a). This is basically true for all cast-alloy and high-strength all-ceramic restorations if a conventional cement could be used but additional adhesion would be helpful for long-term success. The goal of these materials is to include a dentin bonding agent, a ceramic bonding system, and a metal bonding system into the resin cement and have the entire assembly polymerized at once.

The resin cements containing a self-etching bonding agent (RelyX Unicem, 3M ESPE; and MaxCem, Kerr) are becoming more popular due to their clinical success, but long-term observations are still needed (Kramer, Lohbauer, and Frankenberger 2000; Browning et al. 2002).

Be aware that there is the potential for incompatibility between adhesives and resin cements based on their curing mode and other chemical incompatibilities. It is prudent to use similar curing modes for adhesives and resin cements and to always follow the recommendation of the manufacturer. It is risky to use a light-cured bonding agent with a self-curing cement and vice versa (fig. 18-14).

Advantages of Resin-Based Cements
- High compressive and tensile strength (White and Yu 1993; Rosensteil, Land, and Crispin 1998).
- Good biocompatibility
- Intraoral solubility is the least among the luting agents (Yoshida, Tanagawa, and Atsuta 1998).
- Superior adhesion compared with water-based cements
- They reach maximum strength in a short time and can resist forces of mastication much faster than water-based cements

Disadvantages of Resin-Based Cements
- Higher film thickness (15–40 μm) compared to resin-modified glass-ionomer cements or glass-ionomer cements
- Much more difficult to remove any excess once the material is cured.
- When used in conjunction with acid-etching techniques they can cause postoperative sensitivity

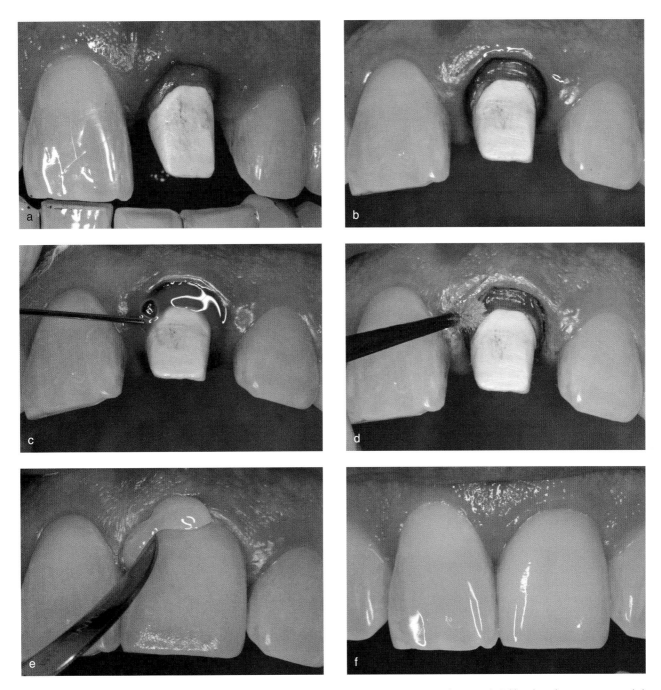

Figure 18-13.   a. Custom-made zirconia post and core on tooth #9 in place prior to IPS Empress crown placement. b. Rubber dam placement was too challenging; therefore, cord was placed to expose margins. c. Acid etching of the exposed dentin surface. d. Application of bonding agent to the dentin. e. IPS Empress crown has been placed with dual-curing resin cement. Excess is removed with scalpel. f. Crown on #9 after cementation.

Temporary Cementation

The use of a non-eugenol zinc oxide combination as a temporary luting agent for restorations that will use a resin cement for the final cementation is a time-honored concept, but there is recent evidence that it may no longer hold true with new materials (Woody and Davis 1992; Jung, Ganss, and Senger 1998; fig. 18-15). The base materials in the traditional and noneugenol products are similar: zinc oxide, mineral oil, and cornstarch (Kerr Corporation 2006). The accelerator component that can contain eugenol will have other ingredients such as oil

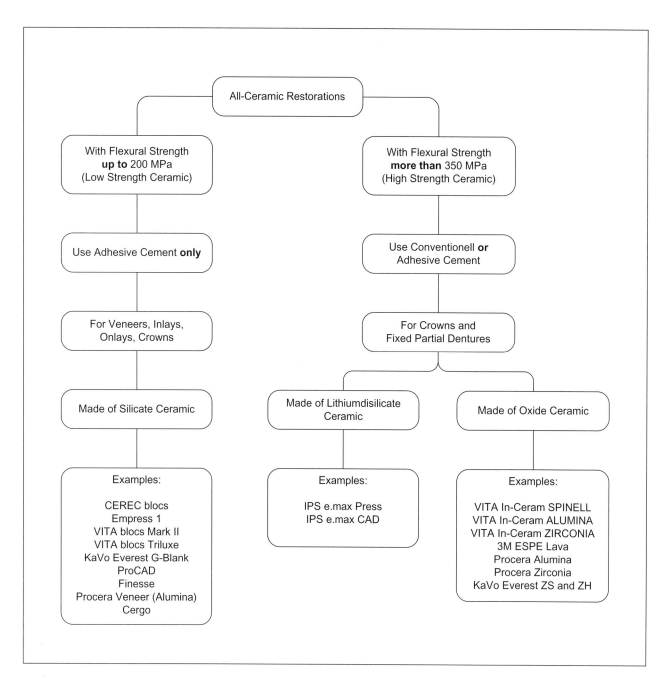

Figure 18-14.   All-ceramic restorations and their classifications; cement selection based on material used and physical properties.

of cloves (historical dental office smell), resin, and carnauba wax. An accelerator that does not have eugenol may possibly contain components such as uncured urethane diacrylate ester monomers, dibutyl phthalate, ortho-ethoxybenzoic acid, and 4-Allyl-2-Methoxyphenol. One manufacturer's product, TempoSil (Coltene/Whaledent), is silicone based and requires an acrylic liner if a polycarbonate or aluminum shell crown is used.

The components of each manufacturer's product will likely be specific for their product. Because of the wide variety of manufacturer's formulations, be careful to review the instructions that come with the product you are using. The same product from the same manufacturer may modify its composition with a subsequent change in the handling or mixing directions.

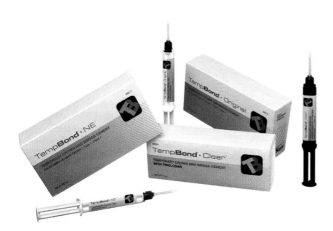

Figure 18-15. Temporary cements: Temp Bond NE, Temp Bond, and Temp Bond Clear (Kerr Corporation, Orange CA USA).

The Use of Luting Materials Classified by Type of Restoration

All-Ceramic Restorations

Use adhesive cement systems for ceramics with a flexural strength up to 200 MPa (low-strength ceramics) and use conventional cement (zinc-phosphate or GIC) or adhesive cement systems for the high-strength ceramic restorations with a flexural strength more than 350 MPa (Kunzelmann et al. 2006).

Low-Strength Ceramic Restorations

Applications: Veneers (IPS Empress).

Recommended Material: light- or dual-cure cement (Variolink II, Ivoclar Vivadent, Amherst NY; Calibra, Dentsply Caulk). For preparation of a ceramic restoration, etch the internal surface with hydrofluoric acid followed by a ceramic primer (silane). For better wetting purposes, a thin layer of bonding agent can be applied but should not be cured. It will be cured in combination with the resin cement.

For treatment of prepared tooth surface(s), follow the manufacturer's instructions for light- or dual-cure cements.

Applications: Inlay, Onlay, Full Crown (IPS Empress, VITA PM).

Recommended Material: dual- or self-cure cement (Variolink II, Ivoclar Vivadent; Panavia 21, Kuraray America). Make sure that the bonding agent is compatible with the specific brand of material that is selected. Hydrofluoric acid and silane must be used if the luting agent directs you to do so. Moisture and contamination control are essential.

High-Strength Ceramic Restorations (Lava, Procera Zirconia)

Applications: Core-Reinforced Full-Ceramic Crowns, Fixed Partial Dentures (FPDs), and Posts and Cores

Recommended Material: conventional cement (zinc-phosphate or glass-ionomer) or a dual- or self-cured resin cement for adhesive cementation (fig. 18-16).
A conventional cementation procedure can be used without the need for bonding materials, etching, or silanization (Kunzelmann et al. 2006; Tinschert et al. 2007). In one study, 155 crowns were cemented with composite resin or glass-ionomer cement. The crowns were placed in the molar, premolar, and anterior areas. Only one crown fractured. The others survived to the end of the study seven years later. The survival was not influenced by the core thickness, core design, or with a reduced or conventional margin (Galindo et al. 2006).

A self-adhesive resin cement containing acidic monomers (RelyX Unicem, 3M ESPE; MaxCem, Kerr; Multilink Sprint, Ivolar Vivadent) can be used without the need to prepare the tooth surface or the restoration surface. Long-term studies need to be conducted (see table 18-1; Christensen 2007).

Another way to lute core-reinforced ceramics, such as zirconia materials, is with the application of phosphate monomers that are contained in Panavia F 2.0 (Kuraray America). The cement acts as a self-adhesive on the oxide ceramic restoration while the tooth surface needs a primer. For all oxide ceramics, sandblasting with aluminum oxide (50–110 μm, 2.5 bar) on the inside of the restoration is beneficial for better retention and long-term success. Figures 18-17 a and b are photomicrographs of a sintered ceramic surface and a nonsintered surface of an oxide ceramic. No sandblasting has been performed (Zhang et al. 2004).

Indirect Resin Restorations

Applications: Inlay, Onlay, Full Crowns, Veneers (bellGlass)

Recommended Material: dual- or self-cure resin cement (RelyX Unicem, 3M ESPE; Panavia 21, Kuraray America). One method to cement composite/reinforced polymer crowns, inlays, and onlays would be to use a self-adhesive universal resin cement. Composite surface treatments are important for adhesion of indirect composite restorations (D'Arcangelo and Vanini 2007). The utilization of sandblasting or roughening the area of adhesion plus silanization can improve the resistance to tensile load. The above study suggested that sandblasting treatment was the main factor responsible for the improved retentive properties of indirect composite restorations (D'Arcangelo and Vanini 2007).

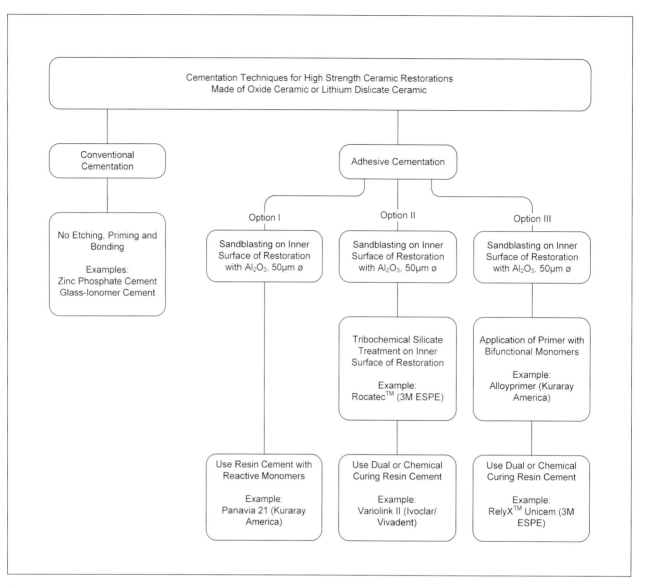

Figure 18-16. Cementation techniques for high-strength all-ceramic restorations.

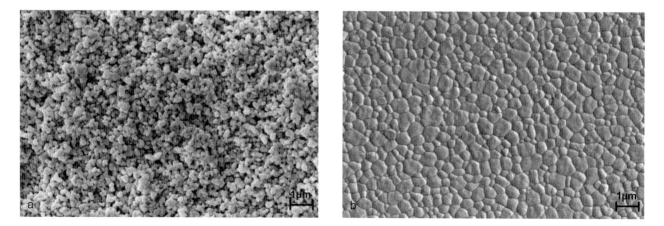

Figure 18-17. a. YZ Cube zirconia ceramic, not sintered (Courtesy of VITA Zahnfabrik, Bad Säckingen/Germany). b. Lava zirconia ceramic sintered; notice the highly condensed surface after the sintering process (Courtesy of 3M ESPE).

Alloy-Based Restorations

Applications: Inlay, Onlay, Full or Partial Crowns, FPDs, and Cast Post and Cores

Recommended Material: dual- or self-cure resin cement, glass-ionomer cement, resin-modified glass-ionomer cement, zinc-phosphate cement, and carboxylate cement (RelyX Unicem, 3M ESPE; Panavia 21, Kuraray America; RelyX Luting, 3M ESPE; GC Fuji Cem, GC America; Fleck's Cement, Mizzy).
The prime consideration in the seating of any precision restoration is that the film thickness is no greater than twenty-five microns. This is determined basically by the particle size of the powder. The type of restoration being cemented influences the ease of the cement escaping from around the margins of the restoration. A full-crown cast alloy presents the greatest problem in obtaining maximum displacement of the cement.

Implant Abutment Cement-Retained Restorations

Applications: Cast Crowns and FPDs

Recommended Material: temporary as well as permanent cements (Temp Bond, Kerr; UltraTemp, Ultradent; Premier Implant Cement, Premier; Improv Temporary Implant Cement, Salvin Dental; Fleck's Cement, Mizzy; Ketac Cem, 3M ESPE; Fuji Plus, GC America).
The amount of desired retention between castings and implant abutments determines the type of luting agent to use for cementation. Ultratemp regular (Ultradent) provides stronger retention, while if a lubricant like K-Y Jelly is placed on the abutment prior to placement of the mixed cement, a low (temporary) retention can be achieved (Sheets, Wilcox, and Wilwerding 2008).

Works Cited

ADA Professional Product Review. 2008. edited by David C. Sarrett. 3(1):9.

Asmussen E. 1983. Factors affecting the color stability of restorative resins. *Acta Odontol Scand* 41(1):11–18.

Attin T, Buchalla W, Kielbassa AM, Helwig E. 1995. Curing shrinkage and volumetric changes of resin-modified glass ionomer restorative materials. *Dent Mater* 11(6):359–62.

Baratti M, Dorigo E, Telesca G. 1985. Radio-opacity of lining cements. *G Stomatol Ortognatodonzia* 3(1):41–16.

Browning WD, Neson SK, Cibirka R, Myers ML. 2002. Comparison of luting cements for minimally retentive crown preparations. *Quintessence Int* 33(2):95–100.

Casselli DS, Martins LR. 2006. Postoperative sensitivity in class I composite restorations in vivo. *J Adhes Dent* 8(1):53–8.

Charbeneau GT, Klausner LH, Brandau HE. 1988. Glass-ionomer cements in dental practice: A national survey. *J Dent Res* 67(Special issue):283(Abstract#1365).

Clinical Research Associates. 2003a. Self-etch primer dual-cure resin cement. *CRA Newsletter* 27(9):1–2.

Clinical Research Associates. 2003b. Self-etch primer (SEP) adhesives update. *CRA Newsletter* 27(11/12):1–5.

Christensen GJ. 2007. Should resin cements be used for every cementation? *J Amer Dent Assoc* 138(6):817–19.

Curro FA. 1990. Tooth hypersensitivity in the spectrum of pain. *Dental Clinics of No. America* 34(3):429–37.

D'Arcangelo C, Vanini L. 2007. Effect of three surface treatments on the adhesive properties of indirect composite restorations. *J Adhesive Dent* 9(3):319–26.

Erikson RL. 1994. Root surface treatment with glass ionomers and resin composites. *Am J Dent* 7(5):279–85.

Featherstone JD. 1994. Fluoride, remineralization and root caries. *Am J Dent* 7(5):271–4.

Galindo ML, Hagmann E, Marinello CP, Zitzmann NU. 2006. Long-term clinical results with Procera AllCeram full ceramic crowns. *Schweiz Monatsschr Zahnmed* 116(8):804–9.

Hammesfahr PD. 1994. Glass ionomers: The next generation. In: *Proceedings of the 2nd International Symposium on Glass Ionomers*, 1st ed., edited by Hunt PR (44–47). Phiadelphia: Int. Symposia in Dentistry, PC, 44–7.

Hersek NE, Canay S. 1996. In vivo solubility of three types of luting cement. *Quintessence Int* 27(3):211–16.

Imazato S, Tarumi H, Kobayashi K, Hiraguri H, Oda K, Tsuchitani Y. 1995. Relationship between the degree of conversion and internal discoloration of light activated composite. *Dent Mater* 14(1):23–30.

Irie M, Nakai H. 1995. Effect of immersion in water on linear expansion and strength of three base/liner materials. *Dent Mater* 14(1):70–7.

Jung M, Ganss C, Senger S. 1998. Effect of eugenol-containing temporary cements on bond strength of composite to enamel. *Oper Dent* 23(2):63–8.

Kunzelmann KH, Kern M, Prospiech P, Mehl A, Frankenberger R, Reiss B, and Wiedhahn K. 2006. *Vollkeramik auf einen Blick*, 2nd ed. Ettlingen, Germany: Arbeitsgemeinschaft für Keramik in der Zahnheilkunde e.V.

Kerby RE, McGlumphy EA, Holloway JA. 1992. Some physical properties of implant abutment luting cements. *Int J Prosthodont* 5(4):321–5.

Kerr Corporation. 2006. Temp-Bond NE (No-eugenol) base. *Material Safety Data Sheet.*

Kramer N, Lohbauer U, Frankenberger R. 2000. Adhesive luting of indirect restorations. *Am J Dent* 13(Special number):60D–76D.

Lacy AM. 1994. Observations on glass ionomer [letter to the editor]. *J Am Dent* 125(2):126, 128.

Leinfelder KF. 1993. Glass ionomers: Current clinical developments. *J Am Dent Assoc* 124(9):62–4.

Lüthy H, Loeffel O, Hammerle CHF. 2006. Effect of thermocycling on bond strength of luting cements to zirconia ceramic. *Dent Mater* 22(2):195–200.

Lutz F. 1977. The effect of fluoride application following enamel etching on the adaptation and adhesiveness of adhesive fillings [in German]. *SSO Schweiz Monatsschr Zahnheilkd* 87:712–23.

McLean JW, Nicholson JW, Wilson AD. 1994. Suggested nomenclature for glass ionomer cements and related materials [editorial]. *Quintessence Int* 25(9):587–9.

Noort R van. 2002. *Introduction to Dental Materials*, 2nd ed. New York: Mosby.

O'Brian WJ. 2002. *Dental Materials and Their Selection*, 3rd ed. Chicago: Quintessence.

Perdigão J, Geraldeli S, Hodges JS. 2003. Total-etch versus self-etch adhesive: Effect on postoperative sensitivity. *J Amer Dent Assoc* 134(12):1621–9.

Perdigão J, Anauate-Netto C, Carmo AR, Hodges JS, Cordeiro HJ, Lewgoy HR, Dutra-Corrêa M, Castilhos N, Amore R. 2004. The effect of adhesive and flowable composite on post-operative sensitivity: 2-week results. *Quintessence Int* 35(10): 777–84.

Perry RD. 2007. Clinical evaluation of total-etch and self-etch bonding systems for preventing sensitivity in class 1 and class 2 restorations. *Compend Contin Educ Dent* 28(1):12–14.

Phillips RW. 1996. *Science of Dental Materials*, 10th ed. Phiadelphia: W.B. Saunders.

Rebitski G, Donly KJ. 1993. Dentin pretreatment and caries inhibition by a fluoride-releasing resin. *Am J Dent* 6(4): 204–6.

Richter WA, Ueno H. 1975. Clinical evaluation of dental cement durability. *J Prosthet Dent* 33(3):294–9.

Rosensteil SF, Land MF, Crispin BJ. 1998. Dental luting agents: A review of current literature. *J Prosthetic Dent* 80(3): 280–301.

Sheets JL, Wilcox C, Wilwerding T. 2008. Cement selection for cement-retained crown technique with dental implants. *J Prosthodont* 17(2):92–6.

Tinschert J, Natt G, Mohrbotter N, Spiekermann H, Schulze KA. 2007. Lifetime of alumina and zirconia ceramics used for crown and bridge restorations. *J Biomed Mater Res B Appl Biomater* 80(2):317–21.

Walls AW. 1986. Glass polyalkenoate (glass ionomer) cements: A review. *J Dent* 14:231–46.

White SN, Yu Z. 1993. Physical properties of fixed prosthodontic, resin composite luting agents. *Int J Prosthodont* 6(4): 384–89.

Wilson AD, Groffman DM, Kuhn AT. 1985. The release of fluoride and other chemical species from a glass-ionomer cement. *Biomaterials* 6(6):431–3.

Woody TL, Davis RD. 1992. The effect of eugenol-containing and eugenol-free temporary cements on microleakage in resin bonded restorations. *Oper Dent* 17(5):175–80.

Yoshida K, Tanagawa M, Atsuta M. 1998. In-vitro solubility of three types of resin and conventional luting cements. *J Oral Rehab* 25(4):285–91.

Zhang Y, Lawn BR, Rekow ED, Thompson VP. 2004. Effect of sandblasting on the long-term performance of dental ceramics. *J Biomed Mater Res B Appl Biomater* 71(2): 381–6.

Chapter 19
Restoration Delivery

Marc Geissberger DDS, MA, BS, CPT

After significant time has been invested in treatment planning, case design, preparation, impression fabrication, provisional fabrication, and laboratory communication, it would be tragic to encounter significant problems during the delivery phase of any aesthetic case. With the multiples steps required to successfully deliver an esthetic case, the clinician must allow an appropriate amount of time for the delivery appointment. Additionally, the clinician must ensure that attention to detail is observed during the bonding or cementation process. Proper bonding of esthetic restorations will decrease the potential for postoperative sensitivity, increase the potential longevity of the prosthesis, and ensure optimum esthetics is obtained. To ensure the proper success of each esthetic case the practitioner must pay close attention at each step of the delivery process.

The delivery of esthetic restorations can be broken down into several key phases.

1. Inspection and approval of the laboratory work
2. Anesthesia
3. Provisional removal and tooth surface preparation
4. Initial try-in and patient approval of esthetic restorations
5. Isolation
6. Restoration seating and cementation or bonding
7. Final adjustment, finishing, and polishing

Each of these steps will be outlined in detail in this chapter. Several cases will be presented to demonstrate slight variations on the cementation or bonding process. It is critical to recognize the importance of each of the steps outlined in this chapter. Several forms (checklists) will be provided as guides for clinicians to follow during the delivery process. Form 19-1 will enable practitioners to assess and provide feedback to their laboratory team regarding the quality of the esthetic restorations they have produced. Form 19-2 is a step-by-step checklist for the delivery and cementation of multiple full-coverage restorations utilizing a dual-cured cement. Form 19-3 is a step-by-step checklist for the delivery and cementation of porcelain veneers or other restorations that will be bonded with a light-cured cement system. These forms may be reproduced and used chairside. Additionally, this chapter contains a sample "esthetic restoration patient approval form" (form 19-4) that can be placed in the patient record once consent to definitively place the restoration(s) has been obtained.

Inspection and Approval of the Laboratory Work

Many practitioners prefer to appoint their patients for the delivery appointment at the time of the preparation appointment. While this has several advantages, adequate time between appointments must be provided for the laboratory to fabricate the prescribed restorations and for the practitioner to examine the finished product. Examining the laboratory work on the date of delivery should be avoided. If the laboratory did not produce the desired results, the patient will need to be rescheduled. This will inconvenience all parties involved and can lead to anxiety for both the patient and practitioner. Allowing adequate time for inspection of all esthetic restorations is essential and will lead to greater patient satisfaction.

The examination process of all laboratory work should follow a standard protocol that assesses each element of the laboratory prescription. This process will help establish a better working relationship between the practitioner and the laboratory. Additionally, it will help the laboratory understand the particular preferences of the practitioner and ultimately improve future products they deliver. Any deviations from the prescribed design should be noted and the case should be returned to the laboratory for correction. Several key elements must be examined during this process (see form 19-1).

1. Contours and proportions of the restoration(s)
2. Shade
3. Occlusion
4. Surface finish
5. Proximal contacts

Contours and Proportions of the Restoration(s)

Once the laboratory work has been returned, it is essential to assess the adherence to the prescribed esthetic design. A number of key elements should be checked in a logical and sequential order. First of all, did the laboratory create shapes in the proper proportions individually and with each other? When assessing this aspect of the laboratory work, it is critical to evaluate the position of the facial line angles and the incisal embrasures. These anatomic features will have the greatest impact on the general appearance of the final restorations (see Chapter 6). Careful management of these features is critical in achieving optimal esthetic results. If the facial line angles are positioned laterally on the restorations, teeth will generally appear wider. When the facial line angles are moved medially, the restorations will naturally appear narrower. When the incisal embrasures are kept small, teeth generally appear square. When the incisal embrasures are opened and rounded, the restorations will generally appear rounder and smaller.

Another critical area to assess in overall appearance is the contours on the facial aspect of the restorations. If the facial aspect of the restorations is relatively flat, the restorations may appear brighter than those that possess subtle undulations. Generally speaking, anterior teeth possess facial depressions that reflect light in different directions and create the natural color variation of anterior teeth. When restorations are created, careful reproduction of these anatomic features is essential if the restorations are to appear natural. Often, laboratory technicians fabricate restorations with appropriate axial shapes that lack the necessary facial depressions to appear natural. The tendency is to create flat surfaces that will make restorations appear higher in value, even when the appropriate shade has been selected.

Shade

Shade must be assessed prior to appointing the patient for delivery of the restoration(s). When assessing the laboratory efforts, it is essential that the requested shade be verified in several different light sources. Utilize a shade guide to check the laboratory efforts under natural, fluorescent, and incandescent light. If significant color variations were requested, confirm that the location of color transitions was placed as prescribed. Practitioners must understand that laboratory technicians often utilize surface stains to establish some requested color variations. When this technique is employed, contouring the restorations chairside becomes problematic. The practitioner runs the risk of removing surface color variation during the contouring process.

It is important to ascertain whether the color variations have been established with porcelain application or surface staining. If they have been established with surface staining, caution must be employed if any contouring is necessary. Oftentimes, modifying the shapes of restorations with surface staining and characterization will require reapplication of surface stain and reglazing of the restorations.

Occlusion

There are three critical areas to check when assessing the occlusal scheme established by the laboratory technician with any esthetic restoration. First of all, did the laboratory establish appropriate centric stops on the restorations? Second, did the laboratory establish the appropriate excursive guidance in both working and nonworking movements? Finally, were the prescribed protrusive contacts established properly? These occlusal contacts and excursions should be confirmed prior to the patient try-in and delivery appointment. Any modifications to the occlusal scheme should be documented and returned to the laboratory for modification.

Surface Finish

The overall surface finish plays a critical role in establishing appropriate esthetics. Even if contours and shade are completely accurate, the ultimate esthetic result can be hampered if the surface finish is not appropriate. Generally speaking, as the smoothness of the surface of a restoration increases, so does the value and reflective properties of that surface. When a laboratory errs on surface finish, they usually do so on the overglazed side of the glazing spectrum.

The surface finish of restorations can range from an eggshell finish to a highly glazed finish. Eggshell finishes will reflect the least amount of light and have the closest finish to natural teeth. As the glaze of a restoration increases to a smoother surface, so will the light reflection off that surface. The finish of the restoration should follow that prescribed by the practitioner. Careful attention to surface finish can ensure maximum esthetic results and must not be overlooked.

Proximal Contacts

The size and location of the proximal contacts can influence both function and esthetics. It is critical that the laboratory technician place the proximal contacts in the prescribed location. Moving proximal contacts on anterior teeth too gingival will open incisal embrasures and potentially impinge on the interdental papilla.

Moving the proximal contact areas too far lingual can create food impaction areas on the facial aspect of anterior teeth.

On posterior teeth, moving the proximal contacts too far to the lingual can create food impaction on the buccal surfaces. If the contacts are too wide either buccal-lingually or occlusal-cervically, the interdental papilla may become unnecessarily impinged. Careful attention to the appropriate size and location of the proximal contacts must be observed to establish and maintain appropriate gingival health and esthetic results.

Anesthesia

Because the soft tissues play such a critical role in the overall balance and appearance of esthetic restorations, careful management of anesthesia must be employed at the delivery appointment. Although profound anesthesia is critical for discomfort management during any dental procedure, its effects can alter the ways in which the soft tissues interact with the esthetic restorations. Profound anesthesia will affect the patient's ability to smile correctly and may ultimately interfere with his or her ability to make an appropriate decision concerning the appearance of their new smile.

Two strategies may be employed to allow the patient to make an accurate determination of the acceptability of the esthetic restorations. The first strategy is to remove the provisional restorations and try in the definitive restorations without the use of anesthesia. This strategy will not work well with individuals with low pain thresholds or extremely sensitive teeth. However, it can work quite well in individuals with receded pulp canals, high pain thresholds, or advanced age. After the patient has reflected on the esthetics of their new restorations and given approval for cementation or bonding, profound anesthesia can be obtained using traditional techniques.

The second strategy is to administer palatal anesthesia for the maxillary arch and/or lingual anesthesia for the mandibular arch. With this technique, small amounts of a 4% solution of Septocaine (or a similar anesthetic) delivered adjacent to the root apices can be utilized. This technique will provide adequate pupal anesthesia without affecting the muscles of facial expression. The patient will be able to provide appropriate feedback regarding the esthetics of the restorations without the negative effects of buccal anesthesia. After the approval for cementation or bonding is obtained, additional anesthesia may be obtained through buccal infiltrations for the maxillary arch or block anesthesia for the mandibular arch.

Provisional Removal and Tooth Surface Preparation

Care must be employed when removing provisional restorations to prevent damage to the remaining tooth structure. This is critically important with endodontically treated teeth due to their increased brittleness and greater potential for fracture. If multiple units are splinted together, it is advisable to section the provisionals between the incisal embrasures or through the straight facial aspect of each restoration. An instrument can be placed in the facial portion and the provisional can be spread apart mesiodistally. The use of a hemostat is contraindicated on full-coverage anterior provisional restorations because of an increased risk of tooth fracture.

Veneer provisionals can be safely removed by sectioning through the incisal embrasure of adjacent restorations (fig. 19-1). Care should be taken to avoid damaging the underlying preparation during this process. Once the incisal embrasures have been sectioned, a large spoon may be employed to remove the provisional restorations (fig. 19-2).

After the provisional restorations have been removed, excess cement should be cleaned from the prepared surface. This is best done with an anterior scaler or spoon. The preparations may be cleaned with flour of pumice and a prophy cup. Fluoride-containing polishing pastes should not be used to remove excess cement as the fluoride may decrease the bond strength between tooth structure and restoration. If any surface stain is present on the preparations, it can be easily removed with a small cotton pellet soaked in hydrogen peroxide.

Due to the nature of provisional restorations, hygiene issues associated with provisional restorations, and length of time between the preparation and delivery

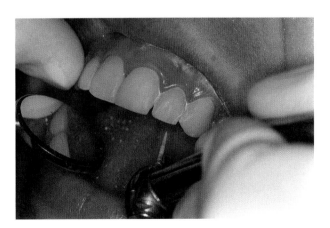

Figure 19-1. Use of a fine diamond bur to section between splinted provisional veneer restorations.

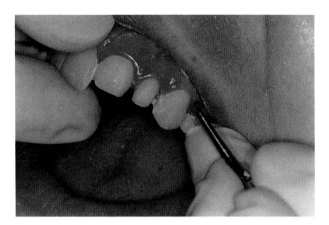

Figure 19-2.   Use of a spoon excavator to remove sectioned provisional restoration.

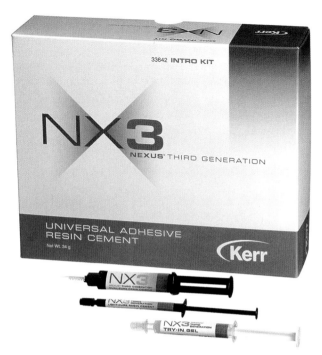

Figure 19-3.   Sample of a dual-cure and light-cure resin cement system ideal for the delivery of veneer restorations (Nexus 3, Kerr).

appointment, the surrounding tissue may be inflamed and prone to bleeding. Gingival tissues must be treated very carefully during the provisional removal and cleaning process. If bleeding does occur, a hemostatic agent may be applied to control the situation.

Initial Try-in and Patient Approval of Esthetic Restorations

The goal of this portion of the delivery appointment is to obtain consent from the patient to cement or bond the definitive restorations. Initial verification of fit, contacts, and occlusion is not necessary at this point. If the patient does not approve the esthetic component of the restorations, these factors are irrelevant.

For translucent restorations, the final cement shade should be obtained during this portion of the appointment. This is particularly important for thin facial veneers where the cement can have a significant effect on the final color of the restorations. The use of a resin bonding system that utilizes try-in pastes should be employed. Nexus 3 from Kerr (fig. 19-3), Variolink II from Ivoclar (fig. 19-4), and Calibra from Dentsply are examples of resin cement bonding systems that possess try-in pastes. These pastes allow the patient and practitioner to preview the final color the restorations will assume after they have been placed.

Isolation

There are several techniques that can be employed for isolating the teeth to receive bonded or cemented restorations. If the restorations will be cemented, traditional

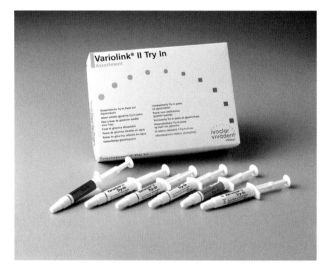

Figure 19-4.   Try-in paste from a resin bonding system that allows the practitioner to vary and choose the cement shade (Variolink II, Ivoclar).

isolation techniques using cotton may be employed. This holds true for porcelain-fused-to-metal or zirconium restorations that will be cemented with zinc phosphate, glass ionomer, resin-modified glass ionomer, or self-etching resin cements.

Restorations that will be cemented with resin cement such as porcelain veneers, ceramic or laboratory processed composite inlays or onlays, or crowns

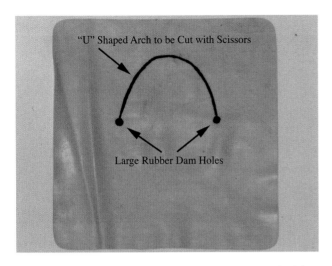

Figure 19-5. Picture of the punch position and arch shape utilized for a "slot dam" technique.

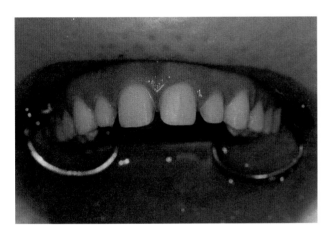

Figure 19-6. Rubber dam clamp position for a case where veneers will be bonded on eight maxillary teeth.

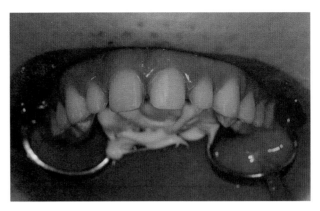

Figure 19-7. Slot dam with bite registration material placed to stabilize the rubber dam clamps and seal the palatal area. This will prevent accidental ingestion during the try-in and bonding process.

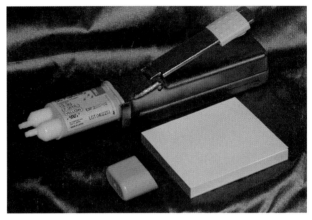

Figure 19-8. Fuji-cem, resin-modified glass-ionomer cement (GC Corporation).

should be isolated using rubber dam isolation. There are two versions of rubber dam isolation that may be employed. The first is a traditional rubber dam that isolates individual teeth. The second technique is a "slot dam" technique that isolates several teeth simultaneously. The dam is prepared by punching two holes midpoint from top to bottom and approximately two inches apart from each other. A U shape is cut from one punch to the other to within approximately one inch from the top of the rubber dam (fig. 19-5). Rubber dam clamps are placed two teeth distal to last tooth on each side of the arch to receive restorations (fig. 19-6). After the dam has been placed, the palatal area may be sealed with a fast-setting bite registration material (fig. 19-7).

Restoration Seating and Cementation or Bonding

All esthetic restorations may be bonded to tooth structure using light- or dual-cured resin bonding systems. Porcelain-fused-to-metal restorations, porcelain-fused-to-zirconium or -aluminum, and milled zirconium restorations do not require the use of resin bonding systems and may be more easily cemented with resin-modified glass ionomers (fig. 19-8) or self-etching resin cements (fig. 19-9). Porcelain veneers, pressed ceramic restorations, and laboratory processed composite restorations should be placed using composite resin bonding systems. There are a great number of techniques that can be utilized to cement or bond esthetic restorations. The remainder of this chapter will be dedicated to highlighting several techniques that are most predictable in the beginning practitioner's hands. When utilized, these techniques will yield superior clinical results.

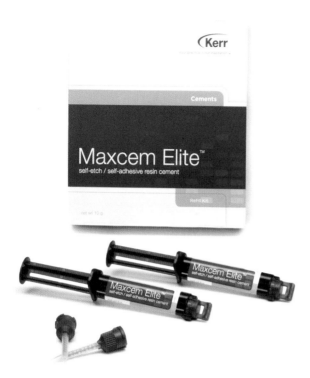

Figure 19-9. Maxcem Elite, self-etching resin cement (Kerr).

Placement of a Single Bonded Porcelain or Laboratory Processed Composite Inlay or Onlay

The placement of a single inlay or onlay with composite resin cement can be challenging. These restorations are small and often difficult to place and remove during the try-in process. Because of their relatively low strength, the occlusion should not be adjusted until the restoration has been completely bonded. Checking occlusion prior to bonding greatly increases the risk of fracturing the restoration or introducing cracks that may propagate later.

When the margins are above the tissue level, a traditional rubber dam technique may be utilized (fig. 19-10). A thin strip of Teflon tape may be laid across the occlusal aspect of the preparation (figs. 19-11 and 19-12). This will allow for easy removal after the restoration has been seated and the margins have been assessed. Teflon tape is so thin that it will not affect the seating of the restoration during the try-in. Any necessary adjustments to the proximal contacts should be made until complete seating has occurred.

Once the restoration has been successfully adjusted, it is prepared for bonding. The restoration's internal surface is etched with hydrofluoric acid (if the lab did not perform this procedure for you). Silane coupling agent is applied to the surface and the excess is removed with air. A light-cured bonding agent is applied to the surface and thinned with air. This material should not

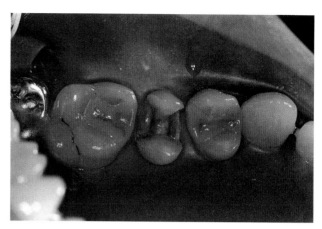

Figure 19-10. Placement of a traditional rubber dam for the bonding of ceramic restorations that are above the tissue level.

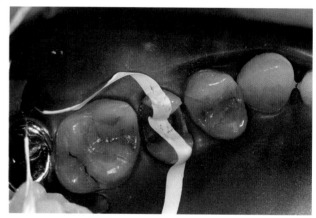

Figure 19-11. Teflon tape placed across the occlusal portion of a MOD (mesio-occlusodistal) inlay preparation to aid removal of restoration following try-in.

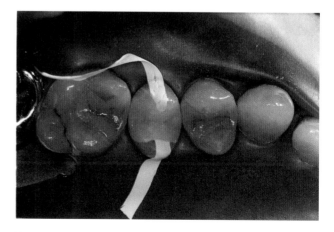

Figure 19-12. Ceramic restoration placed over the Teflon tape to assess initial fit of the restoration.

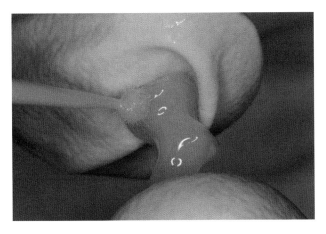

Figure 19-13. Light-cured resin cement being spread evenly over the internal surface of a ceramic inlay.

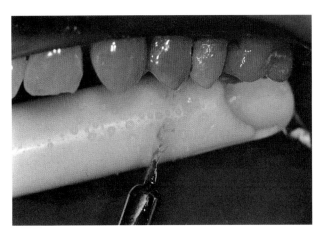

Figure 19-15. Copious amounts of water are used to remove acid from the surface to be bonded.

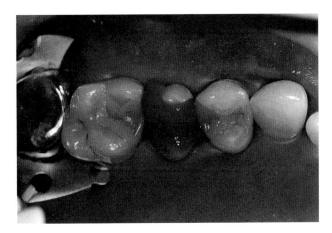

Figure 19-14. Twenty-second acid etching of the surface to be bonded with 37% phosphoric acid.

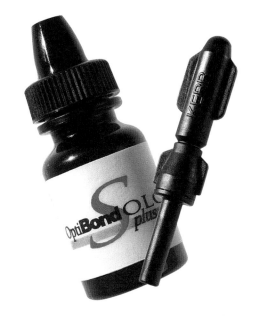

Figure 19-16. Optibond Solo Plus, fifth-generation resin bonding agent (Kerr).

be cured. Light-cured resin cement is applied to the surface and evenly coated with a microbrush (fig. 19-13). The prepared inlay is set aside under the protection of an orange storage container to prevent photo initiation of the resin cement from ambient light.

Attention may now be directed to preparing the tooth for bonding of the restoration. The surface is etched with 37% phosphoric acid for twenty seconds (fig. 19-14). The acid is removed with copious amounts of water. The preparation should be cleared of all excess water with air, then blotted dry with a cotton pellet (fig. 19-15). If a fifth-generation boning agent is utilized, care must be observed to prevent the surface from becoming unnecessarily desiccated. Teflon tape can be wrapped around the proximal surfaces of adjacent teeth to prevent resin cement from adhering to their surfaces. The preparation is coated with a light-cured, fifth-generation adhesive bonding agent and thinned with air (figs. 19-16

and 19-17). Resin cement is applied to the preparation surface, and the restoration is seated with apical pressure. While the restoration is being held in place, a curing light is activated to "spot" cure the restoration for ten seconds. Excess resin cement is removed at this stage, and then additional light is applied to the restoration to complete the cure.

Once the curing is completed, the rubber dam can be removed, occlusion adjusted, and a final polish obtained with intraoral porcelain polishing points and cups. The completed restoration should blend seamlessly with the surrounding tooth structure. In figure 19-18, note the contrast between the new restoration and the ceramic restoration on adjacent teeth placed thirty years earlier.

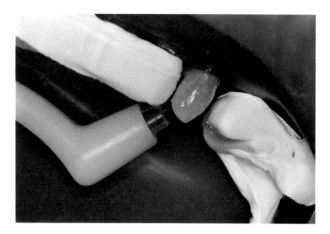

Figure 19-17.   Placement of fifth-generation bonding agent on the etched, moist bonding surface.

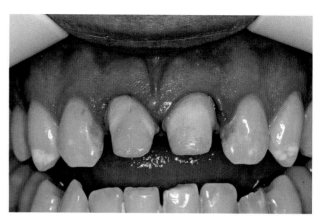

Figure 19-19.   The use of photographic cheek retractors to isolate the maxillary central incisors for bonding.

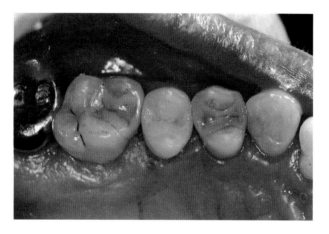

Figure 19-18.   Completed restoration of the maxillary right second premolar with a MOD Empress inlay (Ivoclar).

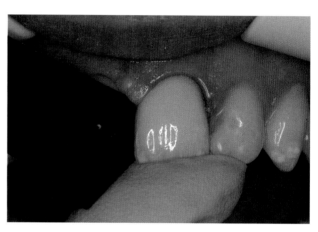

Figure 19-20.   The use of articulating paper to mark the proximal surface that is preventing the restoration from completely seating.

Placement of Multiple Bonded Ceramic Full-Coverage Crowns

The bonding process for full-coverage crowns is very similar to the one described in the previous section. The case shown here is the delivery of two restorations on endodontically treated maxillary central incisors. The location of the gingival margins on anterior crown preparations often necessitates the use of cheek retractors or a slot dam technique rather than a conventional rubber dam technique (fig. 19-19). Inflamed gingival tissue must be managed with hemostatic solutions to prevent bleeding during the bonding process. Each restoration should be tried in individually. The distal contacts may be adjusted until complete seating of each individual restoration is confirmed. Once each individual restoration is seated, both may be tried in simultaneously. If the restorations do not seat as a pair, the mesial proximal surfaces should be marked with articulating paper and adjusted with a porcelain adjustment kit (figs. 19-20 and 19-21).

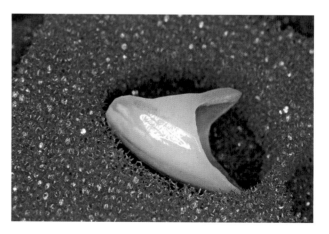

Figure 19-21.   The mark left by the articulating paper indicating the surface that needs adjustment.

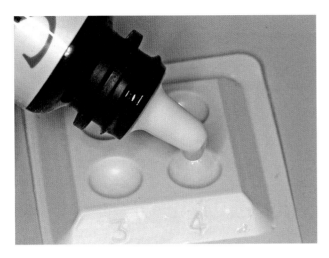

Figure 19-22. Dispensing of bonding agent immediately prior to the bonding process. The volatile nature of these products requires that they are dispensed only when needed.

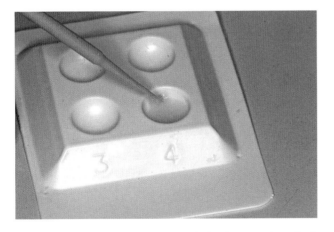

Figure 19-23. Dipping a microbrush into the bonding agent immediately after dispensing.

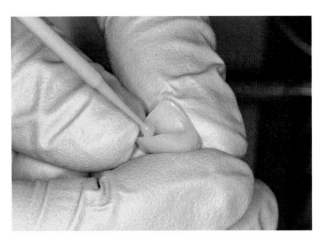

Figure 19-24. Application of bonding agent on the internal aspect of an Empress restoration (Ivoclar).

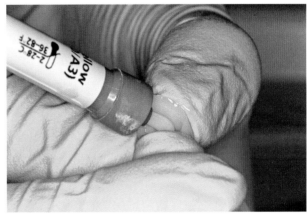

Figure 19-25. Light-cured resin cement being dispensed into the restoration.

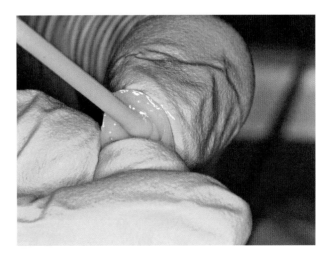

Figure 19-26. Light-cured resin cement being spread throughout the internal aspect of a crown restoration using the blunt end of a microbrush.

The restorations may now be prepared for the bonding process. If the internal aspect of the restorations has not been etched with hydrofluoric acid by the laboratory, that process should be completed at this stage. Silane coupling agent is applied to the etched surfaces. The surfaces are then coated with a fifth-generation bonding agent (figs. 19-22, 19-23, and 19-24). Light-cured resin cement is placed into the crown restorations and evenly distributed on all internal surfaces (figs. 19-25 and 19-26). The crowns are labeled, set aside, and covered in a light-protected carrier (figs. 19-27 and 19-28).

Now that the crowns have been prepared for bonding, attention is directed to the preparations. It is advisable to seat both restorations at one time to ensure proper alignment and positioning. Both preparations are etched using 37% phosphoric acid for twenty seconds (figs. 19-29 and fig. 19-30). Teflon tape is wrapped around the

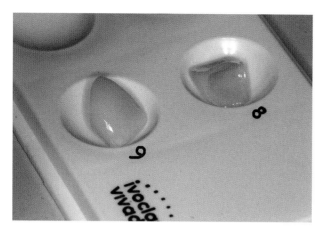

Figure 19-27. The restorations are placed in a protective well and labeled to prevent confusion during the placement process.

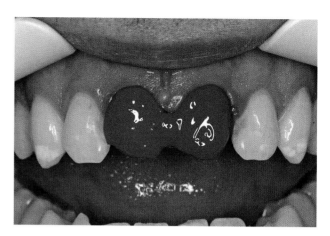

Figure 19-30. Completed placement of gel etchant.

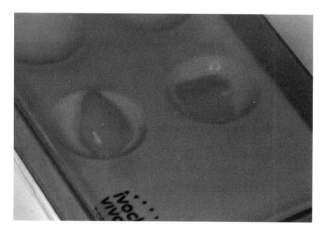

Figure 19-28. An orange cover is placed over the resin-filled restorations to prevent ambient light from initiating the polymerization of cement.

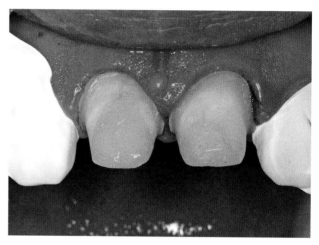

Figure 19-31. Teflon tape placed on the mesial aspect of the adjacent teeth to prevent resin cement from inadvertently bonding to their surface.

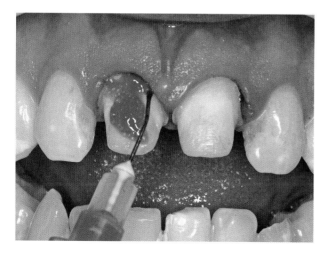

Figure 19-29. Dispensing of 37% phosphoric acid on the surface to be etched.

mesial aspect of both lateral incisors to prevent bonding agent and resin cement from adhering to their surfaces. This will dramatically improve the cleanup process (fig. 19-31). Fifth-generation bonding agent (Optibond Solo Plus, Kerr) is applied to all etch surfaces with a microbrush (fig. 19-32). The excess material is expelled using air. The crowns are seated over the uncured bonding agent with apical pressure and held in place during the light-curing process (fig. 19-33). Upon completion of the curing process, excess resin cement can be removed with either an anterior scaler or a curved #12 blade. Adjustments to the occlusion can be accomplished with an intraoral porcelain adjustment system. The completed restorations in figures 19-34 and 19-35 met the desires expressed by the patient esthetically.

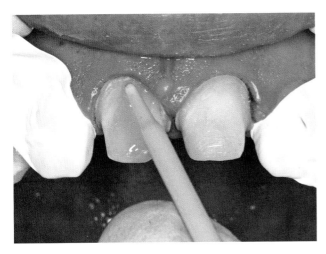

Figure 19-32. Application of a fifth-generation resin bonding agent (Optibond Solo Plus, Kerr).

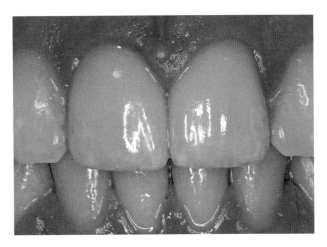

Figure 19-35. 1:1 ratio of the completed restorations of the maxillary central incisors.

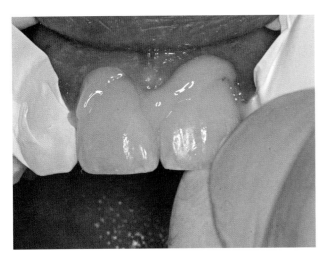

Figure 19-33. Simultaneous seating of both restorations on the maxillary central incisors.

Placement of Multiple Porcelain Veneers

There have been several techniques discussed in the dental literature for the seating and bonding of porcelain veneers. Many are touted as quick and easy. The process outlined in this section will lead to well-seated, predictable results and maximize the longevity of the final restorations. The process works extremely well for practitioners with limited experience bonding multiple porcelain veneers.

A rubber dam is placed using the slot dam technique. The preparations will be exposed for a long period of time and run the risk of being dehydrated, which could increase the likelihood of postoperative sensitivity. For this reason, it is imperative that the preparations are kept moist with a cotton "2 × 2" soaked in water. This will minimize the potential for dehydration (fig. 19-36).

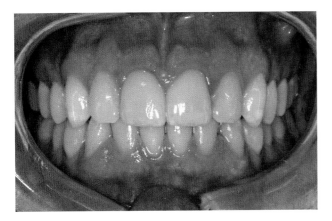

Figure 19-34. 1:2 ratio of the completed restorations of the maxillary central incisors.

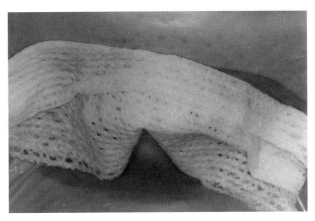

Figure 19-36. Placement of a wet 2 × 2 gauze to prevent dehydration of the tooth surfaces to be bonded to.

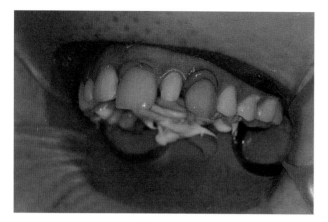

Figure 19-37. Try-in of two porcelain veneer restorations using a low-viscosity impression material to disclose potential internal discrepancies.

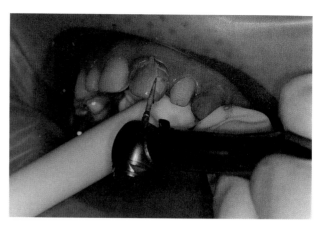

Figure 19-39. These small discrepancies can be adjusted with the use of a fine diamond bur.

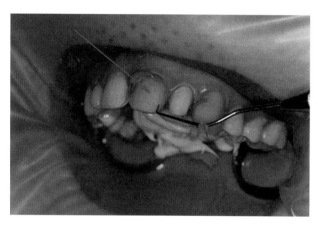

Figure 19-38. The area showing through the impression material demarcates a small discrepancy that is preventing the restoration from being completely seated.

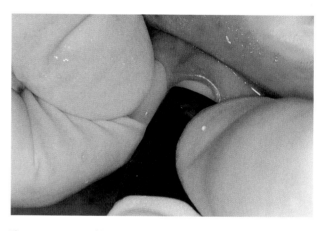

Figure 19-40. Acufilm (Parkell) articulating paper is used to mark the proximal surfaces of adjacent restorations for adjustment.

The first portion of the delivery process is to ensure the complete seating of each individual porcelain veneer. This can be accomplished using a low-viscosity vinyl polysiloxane impression material (Aquasil LV, Dentsply) dispensed into the internal aspect of two non-adjacent restorations at a time. The preparation should be dry and the internal aspect of the restoration should be damp. This will ensure that the set material remains on the tooth structure upon removal of the restoration. In the example shown in figure 19-37, the maxillary left central incisor and canine are being tried in together. This eliminates the possibility of proximal contacts affecting the seating of any one restoration. The restorations are removed using a #17 explorer, and any area of show-through may be identified and marked for adjustment (fig. 19-38). All adjustments are made on the preparation. Avoid making adjustments to the porcelain as this can increase the propensity for fracture propagation. The areas may be adjusted using a fine diamond bur (fig. 19-39).

Generally speaking, well-fabricated restorations made from an accurate impression require minimal adjustments. The process should be repeated with all remaining restorations until all margins are fully closed. At the completion of this process, each restoration should be completely seated individually. If multiple adjustments are required to seat porcelain veneers, a distorted impression could be the potential cause.

The process continues with the adjustment of the proximal surfaces of the two maxillary central incisors. When these restorations are placed over their corresponding preparations, they should seat completely. If they do not, one can attribute this to the proximal contacts. The proximal contacts may be marked with articulating paper and adjusted with porcelain polishing wheels (figs. 19-40 and 19-41). Once both restorations have been seated completely they are prepared for bonding.

The restorations should be etched with hydrofluoric acid, coated with silane coupling agent and bonding

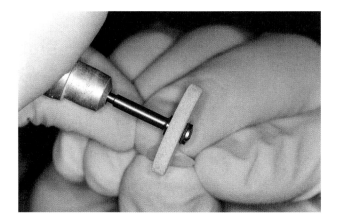

Figure 19-41. The proximal surface can be adjusted using a rubber porcelain adjustment wheel.

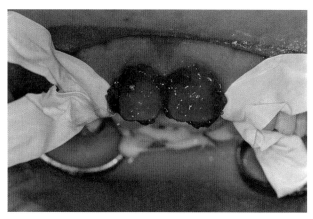

Figure 19-43. Placement of 37% phosphoric acid gel etchant on the maxillary central incisors.

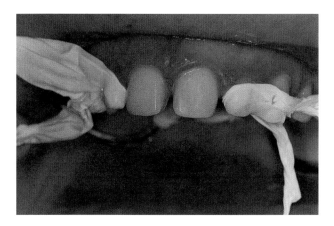

Figure 19-42. Isolation of the bonding surfaces and protection of adjacent tooth preparations with Teflon tape.

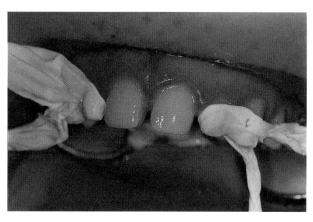

Figure 19-44. Veneer preparations coated with fifth-generation bonding agent after rinsing and air-thinning.

agent, and then loaded with light-cured resin cement and placed in a light-deprived container for bonding. Teflon tape is wrapped around the mesial surfaces of both maxillary lateral incisors (fig. 19-42). The maxillary central incisors are etched for twenty seconds with 35% phosphoric acid (fig. 19-43), rinsed, dried, and coated with fifth-generation bond agent (fig. 19-44). The restorations are placed and spot-cured for five seconds. The excess cement is removed with a curved #12 scalpel (fig. 19-45).

The next phase of the delivery is to check the seating of each lateral incisor. If they do not seat completely, the mesial contacting surfaces are the culprits and should be marked and adjusted accordingly. The bonding process continues in the same fashion as described for the central incisors. Based on experience and comfort level, the practitioner may choose to bond in subsequent restorations one at a time or in pairs. This protocol is

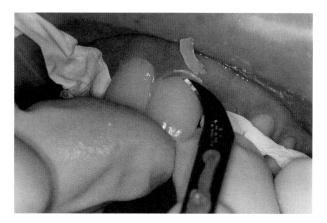

Figure 19-45. Curved scalpel blade is used to remove the excess, cured resin cement.

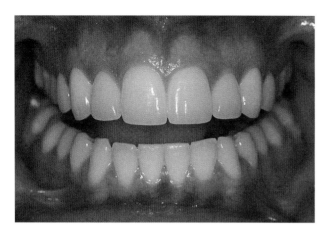

Figure 19-46. Completed veneer restoration on the maxillary anterior teeth and first premolars.

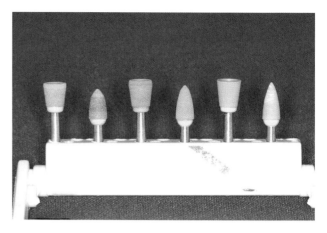

Figure 19-47. Intraoral porcelain polishing kit for the adjustment and polishing of bonded ceramic restorations.

repeated for each subsequent set of restorations until all have been successfully bonded into place.

The previously described technique minimizes chances for error, is kind to surrounding soft tissues, and ensures maximum longevity of the restorations. The final restorations should blend harmoniously with the surrounding tissues and achieve the desired esthetic results (fig. 19-46).

Final Adjustment, Finishing, and Polishing

Once the restorations have been bonded and excess cement has been removed, they are ready for final occlusal adjustment. Centric occlusal contacts and lateral guidance adjustment should be made to achieve the prescribed occlusal scheme. This is accomplished using a fine football-shaped diamond bur and an intraoral porcelain adjustment kit (fig. 19-47). The surfaces of the bonded restorations and adjacent teeth can be cleaned with rubber cup and prophy paste.

The patient should be appointed for a one-week check appointment. At this appointment, the clinician should address any irritated gingival tissue (generally indicating the presence of excess cement) and occlusal issues, as well as perform any final contouring that may be deemed appropriate. Final photographs should be taken at this appointment.

Suggested Reading

Chan DCN, Wilson AH Jr, Barbe P, Cronin RJ Jr, Chung C, Chung K. 2005. Effect of preparation convergence on retention and seating discrepancy of complete veneer crowns. *Journal of Oral Rehabilitation* 32:58–64.

Derbabian, Krikor, Marzola, Riccardo, Arcidiacono, Alessandro. 1998. The science of communicating the art of dentistry. *CDA Journal* 26(2):101–6.

Nohl FSA, Steele JG, Wassell RW. 2002. Crowns and other extra-coronal restorations: Aesthetic control. *British Dental Journal* 192:443–50.

Palacios, Rosario, Johnson, Glen, Phillips, Keith, Raigrodski, Ariel. 2006. Retention of zirconium oxide ceramic crowns with three types of cement. *Journal of Prosthetic Dentistry* 96(2):104–14.

Ruiz J-L. 2004. Simplifying the cementation of porcelain onlays. *Dentistry Today* March, 76–9.

Small, B. 1998. Laboratory communication for esthetic success. *General Dentistry* November/December, 566–74.

Small B. 2001. Avoiding failures during insertion of all-ceramic restorations. *General Dentistry* July/August, 352–4.

Small B. 2001. A review of devices used for photocuring resin-based composites. *General Dentistry* September/October, 457–60.

Wassell RW, Barker D, Steele JG. 2002. Crowns and other extra-coronal restorations: Try-in and cementation of crowns. *British Dental Journal* 193:17–28.

Warden D. 2002. The dentist-laboratory relationship: A system for success. *Journal of the American College of Dentistry* 69(1):12–14.

Doctor's Name: _____ Date __ / __ / __

Patient's Name: _____

Contours and proportions of the restoration(s)

❑ Appropriate contours and proportions established

❑ Modification to general contours required (see note)

❑ Modification to general proportions required (see note)

Note: _____

_____

Shade

❑ Appropriate shade established

❑ Modification to shade required (see note and/or diagram)

Note: _____

_____

Occlusion

❑ Appropriate occlusion established

❑ Modification to occlusion required (see note)

    ❑ Centric contact   ❑ Lateral excursions   ❑ Protrusive

Note: _____

_____

Surface finish

❑ Appropriate surface finish established

❑ Modification to surface finish required

    ❑ Overglazed   ❑ Underglazed

Note: _____

_____

Proximal contacts

❑ Appropriate proximal contacts established

❑ Modification to proximal contacts required (see note)

    ❑ Too light   ❑ Too heavy   ❑ Too buccal   ❑ Too lingual   ❑ Too cervical   ❑ Too occlusal/incisal

Note: _____

_____

Form 19-1. Laboratory Restoration Assessment and Feedback Form

1. Inspect internal of restorations.
2. Check marginal integrity on master model.
3. Try restorations on stump dies with water.
4. Remove provisionals, pumice all teeth.
5. Try in restorations one at a time.
6. Try in restorations collectively, dry.
7. Show patient restorations.
8. Obtain patient acceptance.
9. Remove restorations and clean, rinse, then dry.
10. Prepare slot-dam with heavy rubber dam.
11. Place rubber dam clamps, rubber dam napkin, and rubber dam with young frame.
12. Fill palatal area with bite registration.
13. Control any hemorrhaging.
14. Try in a single restoration with Aquasil LV and adjust areas showing through (prep).
15. Repeat with remaining restorations.
16. Try in #8 and #9 together, marking proximal with articulating paper.
17. Adjust contacts as needed.
18. Repeat proximal check/adjustment with remaining restorations.
19. Polish adjusted contact areas with porcelain polishing kit (Brasseler).
20. Try in all restorations with non-cure try-in paste.
21. Confirm desired shade of cement.
22. Clean restorations with alcohol, rinse, and dry.
23. Apply a layer of the silane coupling agent to #8 and #9 restorations, then lightly air-thin with moisture-free air.
24. Clean preps with antibacterial agent.
25. Place Teflon tape around #7 and #10.
26. Etch preps 8 and 9 for 20 seconds with 37% phosphoric acid, then rinse thoroughly and lightly air dry.
27. Dispense equal amount of catalyst and base cement onto mixing pad and cover.
28. Mix one drop each of dual-cure bonding agents.
29. Apply two coats of bonding agent to preps 8 and 9, and air-thin with moisture-free air.
30. Apply one coat of bonding agent to internal surface of crowns 8 and 9 and air thin.
31. Mix dispensed resin cement and quickly load crowns 8 and 9.
32. Seat crowns completely and confirm marginal adaptation.
33. "Tack" #8 and # 9 with 2-mm light guide.
34. Remove as much excess resin cement as possible using brush and rubber tip.
35. Gently floss through all contacts.
36. Place an oxygen-inhibiting medium on all margins.
37. Light-cure all restorations.
38. Remove excess resin cement.
39. Try in #7 and #10 and check mesial contacts.
40. If adjustments are needed, repeat steps 17, 19, and 22 through 36. If no adjustments are needed, proceed to step # 22.
42. Repeat process for remaining restorations, one at a time per side (i.e., #'s 6 and 12, #'s 5 and 13).
43. After all restorations have been cemented, remove rubber dam and check and adjust occlusion.
44. Polish all margins and adjusted porcelain.
45. Schedule patient for one-week follow-up.

Form 19-2. Porcelain Crown Cementation Utilizing Dual-Cure Cement

1. Inspect internal of restorations.
2. Check marginal integrity on master model.
3. Try restorations on stump dies with water.
4. Remove provisionals, pumice all teeth.
5. Try in restorations one at a time.
6. Try in restorations collectively, dry.
7. Show patient restorations.
8. Obtain patient acceptance.
9. Remove restorations and clean, rinse, then dry.
10. Prepare slot-dam with heavy rubber dam.
11. Place rubber dam clamps, rubber dam napkin, and rubber dam with young frame.
12. Fill palatal area with bite registration.
13. Control any hemorrhaging.
14. Try in a single restoration with Aquasil LV and adjust areas showing through (prep).
15. Repeat with remaining restorations.
16. Try in #8 and #9 together, marking proximal with articulating paper.
17. Adjust contacts as needed.
18. Repeat proximal check/adjustment with remaining restorations.
19. Polish adjusted contact areas with porcelain polishing kit (Brasseler).
20. Try in all restorations with non-cure try-in paste.
21. Confirm desired shade of cement.
22. Clean restorations with alcohol, rinse, and dry.
23. Apply a layer of the silane coupling agent to #8 and #9 restorations, then lightly air-thin with moisture-free air.
24. Apply a thin layer of light-cure-only bonding resin inside #8 and #9 restorations, then load with a light-cure-only lutin resin.
25. Place restorations in orange Vivadent box to protect cement from curing.
26. Clean preps with antibacterial agent.
27. Place Teflon tape around #7 and #10.
28. Etch preps 8 and 9 for 20 seconds with 37% phosphoric acid, then rinse thoroughly and lightly air dry.
29. Apply two coats of bonding agent to preps 8 and 9, and air-thin with moisture-free air.
30. Seat restorations on #8 and #9 completely.
31. "Tack" #8 and #9 with 2-mm light guide.
32. Remove as much excess resin cement as possible using brush and rubber tip.
33. Gently floss through all contacts.
34. Place an oxygen-inhibiting medium on all margins.
35. Light cure all restorations.
36. Remove excess resin cement.
37. Try in #7 and #10 and check mesial contacts.
38. If adjustments are needed, repeat steps 17, 19, and 22 through 36. If no adjustments are needed, proceed to step 22.
39. Repeat process for remaining restorations, one at a time per side (i.e., #'s 6 and 12, #'s 5 and 13).
40. After all restorations have been cemented, remove rubber dam and check and adjust occlusion.
41. Polish all margins and adjusted porcelain.
42. Schedule patient for one-week follow-up.

Form 19-3. Porcelain Veneer Cementation Using Light-Cured Resin Cement

My signature below indicates that I have looked at my dental work and that I approve its appearance. Consent to cement or bond the restorations is hereby given. (Please note that it may be impossible to make changes in the dental work after it has been approved.)

Patient Signature: _____

Date: _____

Form 19-4. Dental Esthetics—Patient Approval

Chapter 20
Protective Occlusal Splints

Laura Reid DDS, BS

Richard H. White DDS, BA

An occlusal appliance, often called a splint, is a removable device, usually made of hard acrylic that fits over the occlusal and incisal surfaces of the teeth in one arch, creating a precise occlusal contact with the teeth of the opposing arch. It is commonly referred to as a bite guard, a night guard, an interocclusal appliance, or even as an orthopedic device.

Occlusal appliances have several uses, one of which is to temporarily provide a more orthopedically stable joint position. They can also be used to introduce an optimum occlusal condition that reorganizes the neuromuscular reflex activity; this encourages a more normal muscle function. Occlusal appliances are also used to protect the teeth and supportive structures from abnormal forces that may create breakdown, tooth wear, or both (Okeson 2007).

General Considerations

After delivery of restorations, the last phase of treatment should be ensuring the long-term stability and protection of restorations. A well-trained assistant can discuss dietary habits and administer oral hygiene instruction. However, nocturnal bruxism or daily clenching habits deserve a different approach, such as protection with an occlusal splint.

When tooth morphology or tooth position is restored or changed, new ingrams for occlusion must be developed in the central nervous system. These new learned reflexes are not always immediate and may take longer for some people to develop (Rufenacht 1990). Newly placed restorations can fracture if a patient is adjusting to a changed occlusal scheme or has a bruxism habit. Delivery of a hard acrylic occlusal splint after the final restorations are cemented will serve to protect new restorations from fracture.

Parfunctional Activities

We will only address parafunctional activities as they relate to the long-term maintenance of the dentition. Most parafunctional activities occur at a subconscious level. In other words, individuals are often not even aware of clenching or bruxism habits. In many instances, once the clinician makes the patient aware of the possibility of clenching activities, they can be recognized and decreased. This is the best treatment strategy for destructive activities that occur during the day. Some practitioners have implemented biofeedback training as a simple neuromuscular learning model to extinguish damaging habits during waking hours. However, with this treatment strategy, patient motivation is important for a successful outcome (Dahlstrom 1984). Another approach is to instruct patients who clench to blow out through the mouth with the teeth apart. Then allow the lips to close and practice maintaining this open-tooth or relaxed muscular position regularly throughout the day (Tanaka 2007).

While some individuals demonstrate only diurnal muscle activity, it is more common to find people with nocturnal bruxism. A certain amount of nocturnal bruxism is present in most normal subjects, and for those where the activity results in damage to the dentition, an occlusal guard or night guard is prescribed as a means to protect the natural and restored dentition from damage. Night guards have been used to distribute occlusal forces across teeth (Kurita and Ikeda 2000) and are the final phase of many implant cases, as they protect the implants from an overload of occlusal forces during nighttime bruxism events (Lobbezoo and Brouwers 2006). Because appliance therapy is dependent on patient compliance, patient education and commitment are important components of treatment success.

Despite protection with night guards, research indicates bruxism continues (Tosun and Karabuda 2003).

Studies of healthy patients being prescribed a night guard show immediate decrease in nighttime muscular activity, but no prolonged decrease in activity. Harada and Ichiki (2006) studied the effect of oral splint devices on sleep bruxism and found that splints significantly reduced sleep bruxism immediately after insertion of the devices, but no reduction in bruxism was observed two, four, or six weeks after insertion. Other researchers have studied masseter muscle activity after insertion of a night guard only to conclude that any reduction in activ-

ity was transient (Dahlstrom 1984; Tosun and Karabuda 2003; Harada and Ichiki 2006).

Types of Occlusal Appliances

The various types of occlusal appliances are listed in table 20-1. The combination splint described by the Pacific School of Dentistry, the stabilization splint described by Tanaka (2007) and Okeson (2007), the

Table 20-1.   Types of occlusal appliances.

Name	Described by	Design	Purpose
1. Combination stabilization splint	Pacific School of Dentistry	Lab processed, dual-layered CR bite position Anterior disclusion ramps on canines for lateral excursions and all anterior teeth for protrusive	Protect restorations that have steepened angle of anterior guidance or protect the dentition from nocturnal bruxism. Sum of daily wear not to exceed 10 hours/day.
2. Stabilization splint or centric relation appliance	Okeson	CR bite position, lab processed Anterior disclusion ramps on canines through all excursions. Can include incisors in protrusive guidance.	Protect restorations that have steepened angle of anterior guidance or protect the dentition from nocturnal bruxism.
	Tanaka	CR bite position, lab processed Flat-planed posterior occlusion Anterior ramps for posterior disclusion	Protect teeth after restoring worn teeth or changing canine guidance. Protect teeth and restorations in any patient who has a history of bruxism.
3. Night guard	Rosentiel, Land, and Fujimoto	CR bite position, lab processed Anterior disclusion ramps on canines for lateral excursions and all anterior teeth for protrusive	Protect TMJ, teeth, and restorations from parafunctional activity in the maintenance phase after restoration—after attempts to resolve underlying etiology have been exhausted.
4. Michigan stabilization splint	Ash, Ramfjord, and others	Lab processed, hard acrylic CR bite position, with freedom in centric Anterior disclusion ramps on canines through all excursions. Mandibular incisors included in protrusive movement only when necessary.	Primary dental treatment for controlling the effects of parafunction, protection against lip and cheek biting, limiting periodontal trauma from occlusion, controlling forces on implants.
5. Nighttime occlusal appliance	Dawson	CR bite position, lab processed Contact on all posterior teeth with an anterior ramp	Indicated whenever the envelope of function must be restricted to achieve an improved esthetic result. Can be used on patients with perfected occlusion who continue to exhibit bruxism or are symptomatic bruxers.
6. Mandibular stabilization splint	Okeson and others	Similar to maxillary stabilization splint. For class III occlusions.	Used in patients with skeletal class III occlusion who have an anterior cross-bite.
7. Anterior positioning appliance	Okeson and others	For same-day treatment. Can be fabricated from vacuum-formed splint with orthodontic resin added for ramps.	For treatment of disc derangement disorders. Preferably used short-term at night only to facilitate healing of the TMJ. This treatment would usually be provided by a dentist specializing in TMD conditions.
8. Nighttime resin appliance with anterior contact only	Dawson	Contacts anterior teeth only. NTI-TSS is one version that is recognized by many labs.	For symptomatic bruxers. May prevent a pattern of bruxism by deprogramming muscles, but should only be used short-term. This may help a delta stage bruxer if it is made at an increased VDO of 8 mm with anterior contact only.

Note: CR = centric relation; TMJ = temporomandibular joint; TMD = temporomandibular disorder; VDO = vertical dimension of occlusion.
See Dawson 2007; Okeson 2007; Ramfjord and Ash 1994; Rosenstiel, Land, and Fujimoto 2006; and Tanaka 2007.

Michigan stabilization splint described by Ramfjord and Ash (1994), and the nighttime occlusal appliance described by Dawson (2007) are quite similar in their design and purpose. They are fit to the maxillary arch, are laboratory fabricated, designed in the centric relation (CR) position, and have anterior ramps that provide posterior disclusion of teeth through all excursive movements. They can all be used to protect teeth and restorations against nighttime bruxism, particularly if the angle of anterior guidance has been made steeper. The Michigan splint design varies slightly from the others in that the anterior guidance ramps are placed on canines only for all excursive movements. Incisors are included in protrusive movement only when necessary.

The mandibular stabilization splint is indicated for patients with a skeletal class III occlusal pattern and an anterior cross-bite. This splint is retained on the mandibular arch with a ramp design that discludes the posterior teeth through excursive movements. The anterior positioning appliance is more commonly fabricated at the dentist's office, using a vacuum-formed splint fitted to the teeth for retention and orthodontic resin to form the disclusion ramps. This design can be fabricated on the same day for patients who need an immediate splint.

The nighttime resin appliance with anterior contact only described by Dawson (2007) may help disrupt a pattern of bruxism, but it has several distinct disadvantages. Its small size allows possible accidental swallowing or inhalation. It cannot be worn for an extended period of time, as supereruption of the posterior teeth may occur. In addition, overloading of the TMJ can occur if the patient continues their pattern of bruxism with the appliance in place.

Diagnosis: Which Patients Are Candidates for an Occlusal Splint?

Patients who may be prone to nocturnal bruxism following esthetic restoration of the dentition are candidates for a protective occlusal splint. This is particularly true of a patient who may have requested esthetic improvement of his or her teeth after experiencing severe wear from bruxism. Even if the dental restorative process has eliminated occlusal interferences and provided appropriate guidance patterns in lateral and protrusive movements, clinical experience has shown that patients who have a history of bruxism habits will often continue to exhibit bruxism even with an optimized or perfected occlusal scheme in place (Tanaka 2007).

Before a decision is made to fabricate an occlusal splint for a patient, an assessment of mandibular structures and function as well as orofacial structures and

Mandibular Structures and Function
  Asymmetrical, deviated or guarded mandibular gait. L/R _____mm.
  Limited interincisal, lateral, or protrusive movement
  Pain response to mandibular movement
  Pain response to digital palpation
    Masseter muscle area
    Temporalis muscle area
    Temporomandibular joint area
  Joint sounds
    Click, pop, crepitis
  Excessive joint function (subluxation)

Orofacial Structures and Function
  Facial asymmetries
  Profile abnormalities: skeletal class I, II, III
  Anterior or posterior tongue thrust
  Compromised nasal or oral airway
  Abnormal dental function (bruxing, clenching)
  Excessive dental wear (facets)
  Lack of balanced dental support
  Dental abfraction sites
  Localized periodontal bone loss, without signs of infection
  If there are 2 or more findings in either category, consider referral or consultation.

Chart 20-1. Clinical observations and function of mandibular and orofacial structures.

function should be made (see chart 20-1). If two or more abnormalities are noted on either mandibular structures or orofacial structures, consider referral or consultation with a TMD specialist before proceeding with night guard fabrication.

In a patient who has significantly worn anterior teeth, restoration of protrusive guidance, producing a steepened anterior guidance, almost always promotes parafunction (Dawson 2007). An occlusal splint will position muscles at a length greater than their optimal force-generating length, thus reducing forces generated by bruxism. Dewitt Wilkerson (1993) studied muscular contraction using jaw-tracking instrumentation in combination with electromyography and joint vibration analysis. In accordance with Glassman's (2002) work, he demonstrated that occlusal splints reduce elevator muscle contraction force by 80% in severe clenchers. Additionally, the utilization of an occlusal appliance may decrease pressure on the temporomandibular joint. Nitzan (1994) found that when a simple occlusal appliance was utilized, intra-articular pressure decreased by more than 80%.

The occlusal splint has some advantages for severe bruxers. Coverage of all teeth in one arch has the effect of diminishing the mechanoreceptive response in individual teeth covered by the splint. The splint coverage may also prevent the minute rebound effect from occurring in teeth that have been intruded (Dawson 2007). In addition, the hard acrylic surface will be worn over time instead of healthy tooth structure or restoration. The acrylic splint is certainly easier to replace than tooth structure or restorations. Finally, the occlusal splint distributes the forces generated by bruxism over multiple teeth, thus reducing the chance of restoration fracture or trauma to the periodontal ligament. According to Spear (1997), the goal of treatment is to control the loading of the TMJ, teeth, and occlusal surfaces. This can be accomplished simply by the use of an occlusal device.

Patients should be properly educated about the occlusal splint and informed that it will require compliance on their part. It may need occasional adjustment and will likely need replacement after some normal wear. A recall three months after insertion is recommended to check wear on the splint. Korioth, Boliq, and Anderson (1998) found asymmetric wear between sides of the occlusal splint after this amount of time.

Finally, since the occlusal splint is a stabilizing appliance, it may be used an unlimited amount of time, particularly when definitive occlusal therapy is not practical or when damaging signs and symptoms persist despite attempted occlusal therapy (Ash and Ramfjord 1995).

Record Taking for a Protective Splint

Accurate records and good quality impressions will minimize the adjustments required at the delivery appointment and ensure a well-fitting functional splint (chart 20-2).

1. *Take an Accurate Impression of the Maxillary and Mandibular Arches* (fig. 20-1). The mandibular impression can be a good quality alginate impression, poured within one hour to prevent distortion. The maxillary impression should be a good quality polyvinyl or polyether impression of the full arch, showing all the occlusal anatomy, the facial and lingual embrasures, and a small band of palatal mucosa adjacent to the free gingival margin. Avoid touching the teeth to the tray. Teeth that touch the tray during impression fabrication can be intruded, creating a slight distortion in the impression. These teeth will have heavier contact internally in the splint, causing a pressure point needing internal adjustment for patient comfort. Attempting to mark and adjust these internal pressure points can be difficult and time consuming. Fortunately, the dual layered or "combina-

1. Review mandibular and orofacial structure and function
2. Take quality maxillary polyvinyl or polyether impression of full arch.
3. Take quality mandibular alginate impression and pour within one hour.
4. Using leaf gauge discluder, take open bite CR record.
5. Take facebow transfer record.
6. Evaluate CR/MI positions
   a. Initial tooth/teeth contacts _____
   b. Vertical slide _____mm
   c. Horizontal/forward slide _____mm
   d. Lateral slide _____mm to R or L

Prescription for laboratory should include fabrication of combination splint with the following specifications:

1. Uniform, bilateral, shallow centric stops across all teeth.
2. Shared protrusive disclusion across anterior teeth.
3. Lateral disclusion ramps for canine guidance.
4. Minimum 2.5- to 3.0-mm thickness in thinnest or posterior segment of splint.

Chart 20-2.   Clinical appointment I.

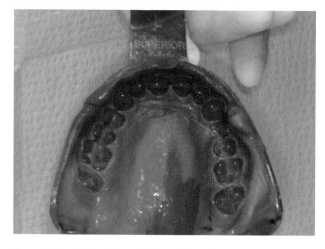

Figure 20-1.   High-quality PVS full maxillary arch impression.

tion" methylmethacralate/ethylmethacralate occlusal splint that we will be describing here can easily accommodate small discrepancies to maintain patient comfort and secure fit.

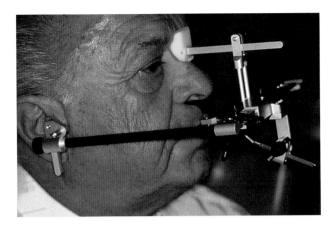

Figure 20-2. Facebow transfer record.

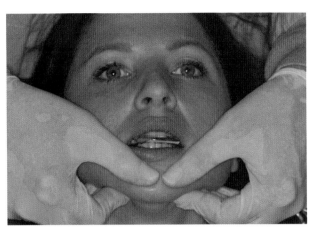

Figure 20-4. Two-handed technique to locate CR position.

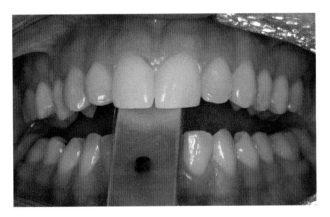

Figure 20-3. Leaf gauge deprogrammer.

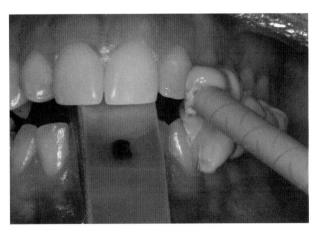

Figure 20-5. Bite registration material recording CR position.

2. *Take a Facebow Transfer Record* (fig. 20-2). This can be accomplished quite quickly using an earbow-type facebow. This quality record of the hinge axis can greatly reduce errors that occur if the lab needs to open or close the vertical bite position provided by the dentist. Once again, this can reduce the adjustments needed at delivery and speed the delivery process.

3. *Using a Leaf-Gauge Discluder, Take an Open-Bite CR Record.* A properly adjusted splint fabricated with this record will allow the patient's mandible and condyles to relax into the centric relation position while the occlusal guard is in place. This is the most restful position for the muscles.

Use an anterior deprogrammer such as a wax-lined metal ramp bent over the anterior teeth or a leaf gauge to relax the muscles of mastication (fig. 20-3). Using the leaf gauge is the easiest method for adjusting the CR bite to the desired height or separation of the posterior teeth. The bite should be open enough to be able to view a

2.5- to 3-mm vertical space between the cusp tips of the maxillary and mandibular second molars.

Use a one-handed or two-handed technique to gently guide the mandible to the hinge position. This should seat the condyles in the most superior and anterior position of the fossa (fig. 20-4). Once this CR position has been achieved, dry the posterior teeth and inject quick-setting bite registration material between the posterior teeth (fig. 20-5). Generally the best technique is to inject laterally across the upper and lower occlusal surfaces so that all the cusp tips and central grooves are included. Start expressing registration material in the molar region then move anteriorly to the canine region. When the material has set, gently remove the deprogrammer and then inject the quick-set bite registration material in the anterior region while the patient bites securely on the already polymerized posterior bites.

4. *Record CR and Maximum Intercuspation (MI) Positions.* Find the CR position using the anterior deprogrammer

and one- or two-handed technique. Record initial tooth contact at this position. The patient can assist you by pointing to the teeth they feel are touching in this position.

Mark the facial surfaces of the central mandibular incisor with a horizontal and vertical line to record its position with respect to the incisal edge of the maxillary incisor and midline. Note the position of the mesiobuccal cusp of the maxillary first molar with respect to the buccal groove of the mandibular first molar. Instruct the patient to gently close into the MI position. Note the shift of the mandible and record vertical, horizontal, and anterior slides in millimeters from the CR to MI positions. These records can be used to verify the CR mounting of your casts before laboratory fabrication of the splint.

5. *Instruct Laboratory to Fabricate a Combination Splint with Uniform, Bilateral Centric Stops for All Opposing Teeth, Shared Protrusive Disclusion Across All Anterior Teeth, and Canine-Guided Disclusion in Lateral Excursions.*

Laboratory Fabrication of the Protective Splint

The dental laboratory will mount your casts on a full-sized, semiadjustable articulator using the facebow transfer and CR bite records that you have provided. The lab will make small vertical adjustments of the pin position to establish room for 2.5 to 3.0 mm of splint material in the second molar region. A wax pattern of the maxillary splint is created with molars and premolars occluding on a flat plane and the canines and incisors occluding on a vertical stop, which transitions into a ramp. The ramp is designed to create posterior disclusion in lateral and protrusive excursions. The lingual surface and the occlusal half of the facial surfaces of teeth are included in the wax pattern for retention (fig. 20-6). The wax pattern is invested and boiled out. Methylmethacrylate is first pressed into the mold to form the biting surface of the splint. Then the internal soft material, ethylmethacrylate, is placed into the mold and heat cured (figs. 20-7 a through d).

Delivery of the Protective Splint

Despite best efforts to equilibrate a splint at the delivery appointment, studies show a patient with a history of bruxism will continue their habit even with an occlusal guard in place (Dahlstrom 1984; Tosun 2003; Harada and Ichiki 2006). Due to asymmetric patterns of wear on occlusal splints (Korioth, Bohliq, and Anderson 1998),

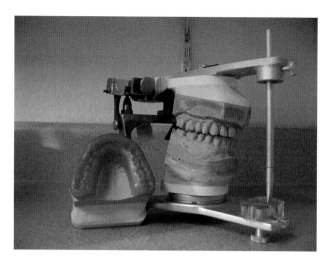

Figure 20-6. Wax pattern of occlusal guard ready to invest.

they require periodic adjustment. Wear of the occlusal splint will be different for each patient; thus, check fit and equilibration three months after delivery and then every six months at recall appointments (Ramfjord and Ash 1994).

As with many treatments, the patient is an active partner in the success of this treatment; therefore, an instruction sheet detailing specifics about care of the occlusal guard should be presented to him or her during the delivery appointment (chart 20-3).

Adjustment of the Occlusal Splint

Figure 20-8 shows occlusal marks on a splint approximately six months after delivery. For ease of marking, horseshoe-shaped articulating paper was used, with blue marks indicating a long centric anterior-posteriorly and red marks indicating right lateral, left lateral, and protrusive movements (figs. 20-9a and 20-9b).

The patient reported that the splint was fairly comfortable but felt slightly high on the right side. Note that on the right side of the splint, there are two functional contacts for each molar, buccal, and lingual cusp, while the left side has only one functional contact on the buccal cusp (fig. 20-8). The splint was adjusted so that only buccal cusps of the mandibular molars remain in function and all centric stops are roughly equal in force.

The long centric evidenced by the blue marks (fig. 20-10) indicates that the muscles of mastication have relaxed somewhat after approximately six months of night wear, allowing retrusion of the mandible toward CR position.

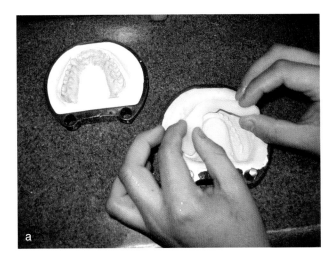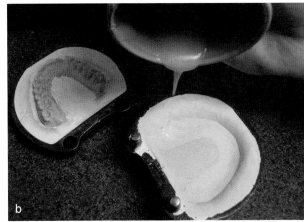
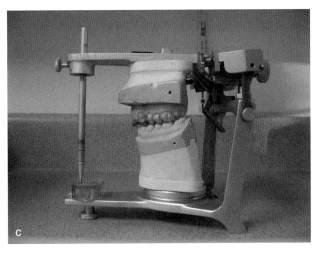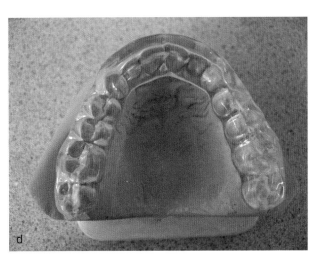

Figure 20-7   a, b, c, and d. Dual-layered splint being fabricated.

If posterior teeth touch the splint in lateral or protrusive excursions (fig. 20-11), adjust the splint so that contact is only in centric or long-centric positions. Figure 20-10 shows articulating paper marks on a completely adjusted splint. The anterior segment of the splint should be adjusted to distribute the protrusive guidance over anterior segment of the splint to disclude the posterior teeth (fig. 20-12). After adjustment of the splint is complete, the splint is polished to achieve a smooth surface, being careful not to remove occlusal contact areas.

Principles of the Full Occlusal Splint Design (adapted from Dawson 2007; Ash 2007; Ramfjord and Ash 1994)

The design of a full occlusal splint should incorporate four main principles:

1. The splint should allow uniform, equal-intensity contacts of all teeth against a smooth splint surface when the joints are completely seated in CR.
2. The splint should have flat contact in centric, providing a freedom in centric of 0.5 mm to 1.0 mm, and have an anterior guidance ramp angled as shallow as possible for horizontal freedom of mandibular movement.
3. The splint should provide immediate disclusion of all posterior teeth in all excursive jaw movements without restricting freedom in centric.
4. The splint should fit the arch comfortably and have stable retention.

Splint design is based on developing an appliance that is functional and comfortable for the patient long-term. CR is chosen as the position for splint fabrication because it is considered by most to be the most orthopedically stable position for the temporomandibular joint (Okeson 2007; Glossary of Prosthodontic Terms 1999). The

Your decision to purchase an occlusal splint indicates your desire to invest in the protection of your natural teeth and the dentistry that has been completed.

The following is a list of instructions that will help to protect your appliance over time.

1. The liner of the occlusal splint is a soft material that changes with heat. It should be comfortable, without any excess pressure on any teeth after being in your mouth for several minutes. Specific adjustments are made at the time of delivery to insure your comfort.

2. When not in your mouth, the appliance should be stored in a plastic carrying case, purchasable at any drug store. Do not soak or store the appliance in water. Please store it in the plastic container over a moist piece of paper towel.

3. Clean the appliance with a toothbrush, soap, and water or toothpaste. Do not soak it in denture cleaners.

4. Keep the appliance away from dogs. They have been known to chew and damage them.

5. The sum total of night and day wear should not exceed ten hours per day.

Once the initial adjustments have been made, it is important to have the splint adjusted when the biting force on both sides is no longer even or if new dental procedures have been completed.

Please consult your dentist if any symptoms develop with your teeth, gums, or facial muscles. Please bring your appliance to your cleaning appointment for evaluation and adjustment.

Chart 20-3. Occlusal splint care instructions.

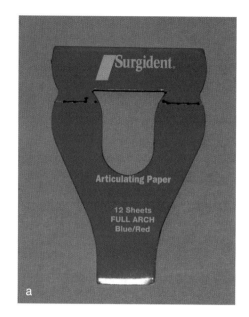

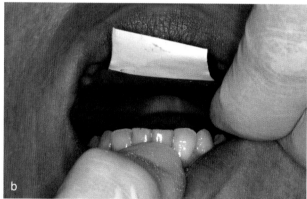

Figure 20-9. a and b. Horseshoe-shaped articulating paper useful for marking entire surface of occlusal splint.

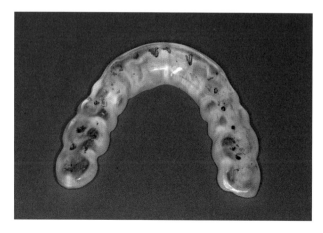

Figure 20-8. Photo of occlusal splint after six months of wear. Note uneven wear, with heavier and more numerous marks on the right side.

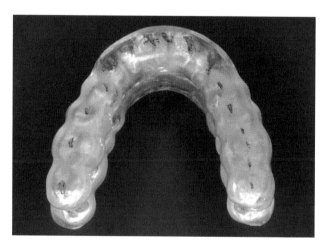

Figure 20-10. Long centric markings after adjustment.

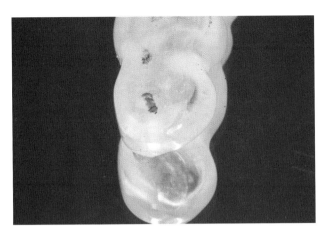

Figure 20-11. Posterior tooth interference in excursive movements.

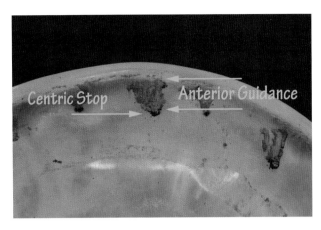

Figure 20-12. Anterior guidance with protrusive marks.

muscles controlling movements of the mandible are most relaxed and comfortable in CR, as long as there is even centric contact on all teeth and some freedom in centric without interferences (Dawson 2007).

Patients with a history of bruxism are often not able to tolerate a large change in the angle of the cuspid or path of protrusive guidance. Thus, change in protrusive guidance in anterior restorative cases and fabrication of the occlusal splint should be kept to a minimum. The splint design least likely to trigger bruxism is one with a gradual transition from freedom in centric to the guidance ramp (Dawson 2007; Tanaka 2007).

Protrusive guidance can be established with all anterior teeth participating, thus dividing forces among many teeth and accommodating deep bite situations. If the patient is exhibiting bruxism on the splint in protrusive movements, consider establishing protrusive guidance with the canines only. It is difficult to adjust a splint with even protrusive contact for all anterior teeth; therefore, adjusting the splint for canine-guided protrusion is simpler and has been shown to reduce muscle activity in some patients (Ramjford and Ash 1994).

It is not always possible to fabricate or deliver a splint with the condyles fully seated in centric relation. Accordingly, tooth contact with the splint occurs on flat areas that provide both freedom in centric and allow for slight retrusive movement of the mandible. As the muscles of mastication relax with wear of the occlusal splint, the patient will settle more completely into a CR position.

Protection with the occlusal appliance will extend the life of the natural dentition and restorations against the damaging effects of a bruxism habit. Delivery of an occlusal appliance at the finish of restorative cases is a necessary component of a complete dental treatment, particularly for patients who exhibit evidence of a bruxism habit.

Works Cited

Ash MM Jr. 2007. Occlusion, TMDs and dental education. *Head and Face Medicine* 3(3):1.

Ash MM, Ramfjord SP. 1995. *Occlusion*, 4th ed. Philadelphia: W.B. Saunders.

Dahlstrom L. 1984. Conservative treatment of mandibular dysfunction: Clinical, experimental and electromyographic studies of biofeedback and occlusal appliances. *Swedish Dental Journal Supplement* 24:1–45.

Dawson PE. 2007. Functional occlusion: From TMJ to smile design. St. Louis, MO: Mosby.

Glassman B. 2002. The aqualizer's role. *Dentistry Today* 21(11): 12.

Glossary of Prosthodontic Terms. 1999. *Journal of Prosthetic Dentistry* 81(1):39–110.

Harada T, Ichiki R. 2006. The effect of oral splint devices on sleep bruxism: A 6-week observation with an ambulatory electromyographic recording device. *Journal of Oral Rehabilitation* 33(7):482–8.

Korioth TW, Bohliq KG, Anderson GC. 1998. Digital assessment of occlusal wear patterns on occlusal stabilization splints: A pilot study. *Journal of Prosthetic Dentistry* 80(2):209–13.

Kurita H, Ikeda K. 2000. Evaluation of the effect of a stabilization splint on occlusal force in patients with masticatory muscle disorders. *Journal of Oral Rehabilitaion* 27(1): 79–82.

Lobbezoo F, Brouwers JE. 2006. Dental implants in patients with bruxing habits. *Journal of Oral Rehabilitation* 33(2): 152–9.

Nitzan DW. 1994. Intraarticular pressure in the functioning human temporomandibular joint and its alteration by uniform elevation of the occlusal plane. *Journal of Oral Maxillofacial Surgery* 52(7):671–9.

Okeson JP. 2007. *Management of Temporomandibular Disorders and Occlusion*, 6th ed. St. Louis, MO: Mosby.

Ramfjord SP, Ash MM. 1994. Reflections on the Michigan occlusal splint. *Journal of Oral Rehabilitation* 21(5):491–500.

Rosenstiel SF, Land MF, Fujimoto J. 2006. *Contemporary Fixed Prosthodontics*, 4th ed. St. Louis, MO: Mosby Elsevier.

Rufenacht CR. 1990. *Fundamentals of Esthetics*. Chicago: Quintessence.

Spear FM. 1997. Fundamental occlusal therapy considerations. In *Science and Practice of Occlusion* (chap. 31). Chicago: Quintessence.

Tanaka TT. 2007. Aesthetics and occlusion: How are they related and why are they important? American Dental Association Annual Session, 26–30 September, Moscone Center, San Francisco, CA.

Tosun T, Karabuda C. 2003. Evaluation of sleep bruxism by polysomnographic analysis in patients with dental implants. *International Journal of Oral Maxillofacial Implants* 18(2): 286–92.

Wilkerson DC. 1993. Monitoring the vital signs of the masticatory system health: A simplified screening to TM problems. *Dental Economics* 83(2):72–3.

Suggested Additional Reading

Van der Zaag J, Lobbezoo F. 2005. Controlled assessment of the efficacy of occlusal stabilization splints on sleep bruxism. *Journal of Orofacial Pain* 19(2):151–8.

Index